CONTENTS

HOW TO USE THIS BOOK

So you want to make a baby. Or at least you're thinking about it. You've come to the right place! In this book, you will find everything you need to know about fertility and queer conception that was left out of your high school biology curriculum—and all the things your primary care doctor didn't know to tell you, that your fertility doctor overlooked, and that would have taken you months to glean off the internet, wading through cis/het-centered information. Here, you'll find evidence-based information that *actually* applies to LGBTQ+ people building families via pregnancy. Whether you pick up this book when you are ready to build your family, or years before, you will find vital information here.

If you are doing some exploratory research in hopes of someday building a family, please be sure to take a look at Chapter 1: Making Decisions and Creating a Timeline. This chapter will guide you in thinking about your options as well as when to get started, including the ideal time to cryopreserve your gametes (sperm or eggs) if you know you want to make a baby someday but you're not ready now.

If you are ready to begin the process of seeking pregnancy, start with Chapters 1 to 3, which provide an overview of the options, help with initial decision-making, and assist in preparing for conception and pregnancy. This is foundational and will support you as you dive into the specifics covered in Chapters 4 to 6, including donor selection, surrogacy, and insemination. For those conceiving via insemination, special attention is given to helping you feel confident about when you are ovulating, so you can get the timing right, which is covered in Chapter 6. If you plan to start inseminating within the next three to six months, don't wait to review this chapter. If you are considering IVF (in vitro fertilization) or reciprocal IVF (conceiving via IVF with your partner's egg), Chapter 1 addresses success rates and costs, while Chapter 8 will walk you through what to expect during treatment.

If you are pursuing a surrogate pregnancy, you will find information that applies to you throughout this book. Chapters 1 to 4 cover the preparatory stages, Chapter 5 is dedicated to surrogacy, and Chapters 8 to 11 walk you through the clinical details related to conception and early pregnancy, including information about how to cope emotionally in Chapter 9.

If you are already in the process of inseminating when you pick up this book, be sure to take a look at the success rates and recommended timelines in the second half of Chapter 1. This will provide guidance for deciding how long to try and when to seek additional support if needed. It will also put your efforts to conceive into perspective with your age, assisting you in big-picture thinking to support you in moving to the next level of care at the appropriate time, before your fertile time runs out. You might then skip to the list of checkpoints at the beginning of Chapter 7: Troubleshooting and Complicated Conceptions. You can use this list to guide where in the book you turn to next. If you find there is information on the checklist you have not yet considered, back up to the recommended chapter provided on the checklist.

If you are about to dive into the IVF process yourself, as a partner, as a surrogate, or as a parent-to-be via surrogacy, start with Chapter 8: In Vitro Fertilization and Embryo Transfer. This chapter is designed to demystify the IVF process and provide anticipatory guidance to help you stay grounded as you go through it. Be sure to also flip back to Chapter 2: Fertile Health for Every Body to make sure you are doing what you can to support your reproductive system and/or prepare your body for pregnancy.

If you have been diagnosed with PCOS (polycystic ovary syndrome), fibroids, or endometriosis, Chapter 7: Troubleshooting and Complicated Conceptions is for you. A detailed exploration of the evidence for supporting these conditions is included here. This chapter, as well as the rest of the book, is written from a body-positive, anti-fat-shaming perspective. If you've simply been told you need to lose weight to conceive, you will find a more nuanced approach here.

If you are newly pregnant or your partner or surrogate is pregnant, turn directly to Chapter 11: Early Pregnancy and Lactation Induction. While this book is primarily focused on fertility and achieving pregnancy, this chapter is included for guidance in the early weeks after conception. Additionally, it contains information that is hard to find elsewhere, including protocols for inducing lactation, which ideally start three to six months before your babe arrives. Guidance is provided for choosing a care provider, caring for your mental health, getting the support you need, and queering pregnancy. Considerations for bonding and attachment, feeding after chest masculinization surgery, and ensuring that your baby gets a good latch are included as well.

If you are a midwife or other health care provider who cares for conceiving queer and trans families, you will glean a great deal of information by witnessing the transmission of information provided for families in this book. There are notes for you at the end of each chapter to guide you in your practice. Consider this the preceptorship you never had.

A NOTE FROM THE MIDWIFE

Dear reader,

By way of introduction, I am a white, queer, nonbinary transmasculine empty nester parent of four grown children, one of whom I gave birth to in a freestanding birth center in central Missouri in 1995. Not only did my own experience of pregnancy and birth under the care of midwives spark my desire to enter the midwifery profession, something my midwife said to me during pregnancy struck a chord that has influenced everything about the way I practice. She said to me, "We were never meant to do this alone." This sentiment motivated me to reach out and create community during a time that otherwise could have been extremely isolating for me as a new parent. It has also underscored the work I do with the families in my care.

Once I decided to heed the call of becoming a midwife, I knew that creating space for new parents to connect with one another would be a core aspect of my practice. When I realized my calling was to serve queer and trans parents, specifically, my drive to build community among the clients I serve became integral for providing affirmation and cultivating resiliency during a time when most of us experience rampant cis/heterosexism, if not outright transphobia and homophobia, in receiving health care and within the culture at large.

My practice is therefore unique. I don't catch babies much anymore. Instead, I focus my energy and attention on filling the gaps in care that exist for my community. This means providing queer- and trans-focused preconception care for local families as well as for those at a distance via telemedicine, local in-home IUI, and an online program of education and support for queer and trans families throughout conception, pregnancy, and the early weeks of parenthood.

Although my clinical practice may be focused on making babies, at its core, my midwifery practice is about making parents. In creating spaces and facilitating conversations where new parents feel safe enough to be vulnerable, people experience feeling deeply held by their community. The stories I have witnessed over the course of my role as an educator, protector, and guide for new families are not covered in textbooks and are never witnessed by providers in models of care that are purely focused on clinical concerns and end within days after birth. Although I can share a great deal of knowledge, what truly informs my practice is the past twenty-six years I have spent listening. My work as a midwife is to utilize clinical knowledge and procedural skills alongside psychosocial aspects of care, including counseling, education, and community building. From my perspective, it takes all of these to truly nurture and protect each individual's transition to parenthood.

That being said, my lens is limited by my experience of walking through the world as a white person. While I take seriously my personal, steadfast responsibility to be aware of and actively undo internalized white superiority, and I utilize my privilege to address the impacts of racism wherever I can, I still move through a white supremacist world under the protection of white privilege. Naming and acknowledging this is vital in claiming the limitations of my perspective. I would like to express sincere gratitude and appreciation for every Black, Indigenous, and POC client who has felt safe enough to share their experiences within the spaces of my practice, as well as the BIPOC colleagues, mentors, and students who have been gracious enough to inform me by sharing their own experiences and engaging in conversations with me about racism. I am listening, and I am endlessly grateful to each and every one of you for speaking your truths.

In addition to my work with families, I also fill gaps in education for midwives and other care providers by providing online modules and training programs for queer/trans-affirming preconception care, midwife-led IUI, and gender inclusivity, as well as speaking at conferences and educational institutions and providing consulting services from time to time. Although I experience marginalization within my profession because of my gender and outspokenness about the needs of my community, I keep working for change, and I continue to create space for and provide guidance to queer and trans midwives entering the profession.

For you, dear reader, I offer this book as an ever-present guide to support you through the creation or expansion of your family. Queer conception is any conception that occurs outside of cis/heterocentric norms. Being queer means we forge our own way when culturally prescribed norms don't suit us. This book is about conceiving differently, in ways that suit our personal needs, affirm our identity, and reflect the level of intention with which we conceive. It's a book about how we go about creating our families and crafting our lives. As you step into the major life transition of becoming a parent, my hope is that this book will midwife you in ways you didn't even know you needed, and hold you in ways you didn't know you could be held.

With big queer love,
Kristin

MAKING DECISIONS
AND CREATING A TIMELINE

The decision to become a parent is monumental for anyone. While some in our community can make babies by having sex, the vast majority of us must utilize outside resources, and the decision-making on the way to conception can be overwhelming. Even the more obvious choices to be made, such as finding donor gametes or deciding who will carry the pregnancy, can be paralyzing for many families, whether you are single, coupled, or in a poly relationship. The complexity of each of these decisions intersects with every aspect of our identities, from racial background to gender identity to career and socioeconomic status, from religion and spiritual identity to where we live and who we call family. For every individual choice, there are implications for that decision that lead to further decision-making, like a never-ending series of Russian dolls that are opened, one after another, all based on the simple desire to hold a baby in our arms.

Deciding When to Have a Baby

While many people struggle with this question, those of us who must conceive with donor gametes and/or a surrogate have a lot more to consider than families who can conceive on their own. For any family, adding a child may depend on financial readiness; however, the additional costs associated with donor conception, IVF, or surrogacy are substantial. And for people who are considering future desires for parenthood in the context of pursuing gender-affirming hormone treatment and/or surgeries, the timing of seeking pregnancy can be even more complex. As you navigate life plans that include having a baby, consider the following age considerations.

WHEN TO CONCEIVE WITH YOUR OWN SPERM

Sperm production begins during adolescence, and while many people think there is no upper age limit on the fertile capacity of bodies that make sperm, sperm quality starts to decline over age forty. Chromosomal abnormalities are more common over age forty-five, so while you may be able to conceive at a later age, the chance of miscarriage is higher because of chromosomal issues.

If you started a gender transition during childhood and only took blockers to delay puberty, your reproductive capacity can be expected to return after blockers are stopped and puberty resumes—however, if you added gender-affirming estrogen, it is unlikely that your body will ever be able to make sperm. The same is true if you started your transition after going through endogenous puberty. Blockers alone simply put the reproductive system on pause, but adding estrogen causes changes in the testes that are often irreversible. While fertility medicine may be able to help you conceive even with a very low sperm count, the safest plan of action is to bank your sperm before hormonal transition.

Even if you are undecided about becoming a parent, gamete cryopreservation prior to hormonal gender transition is the best way to ensure the possibility should you someday decide to pursue genetic parenthood. Until health insurance companies provide coverage and/or sperm banks provide financing and payment plans (as they often do for other health indications such as cancer treatment), the costs must come out of pocket. Although you may need to ask your family or community for help raising funds (expect around $2,000) and it may take some time to build your count and provide the samples, you may be really glad you did. Get an analysis and test thaw to see what your sperm count is like. If you have been tucking or there are other fertility inhibitors in your daily life, you may need to take about three months to build your count before banking (see Chapter 2 for more information about how to do this). Once you start banking, you will go to the clinic every couple of days for about two weeks. Aim for eight to ten vials for every child you think you may want to have.

WHEN TO CONCEIVE WITH YOUR OWN EGGS

The golden years for conceiving easily with the lowest rate of miscarriage are between ages twenty-five to thirty-five. Conception rates are great under age twenty-five, but miscarriage rates are higher in the general population, so if you are in your younger reproductive years, rise above the statistics by taking excellent care of your body. If you are approaching age thirty-five but you are not yet ready to carry a pregnancy, think seriously about freezing your eggs. There are many reasons to delay pregnancy, but your eggs will continue to age whether you're ready to use them or not. Egg freezing, or oocyte cryopreservation, may seem cost prohibitive, but there may be options to offset the cost. Some companies offer fertility benefits that will cover this, so it's worthwhile to seek out one of these employers. Your parents may be willing to invest in having grandchildren someday, if that is something that feels right in your relationship with them, and if they are financially able. Some egg donor programs offer oocyte cryopreservation for personal use as part of their compensation package for egg donors, which is something to look into if you are willing to donate your gametes to another family. Whether or not oocyte cryopreservation is on the table for you, take a look at Chapter 2 to get a sense of the kinds of things you can do now to take care of your fertile health so that once you are ready to try, you will be in good shape to do so. But don't wait too long . . . age is still the single most predictive factor for conceiving successfully and avoiding miscarriage, and the stats start to change over age thirty-five.

Once you turn thirty-five, make sure you are putting plans in place to start trying to conceive by the time you turn thirty-seven. This gives you time to utilize the available options while success rates are highest. If you desire children but you are partnered with someone who does not, it is much better to reevaluate the relationship at age thirty-five than to wait until you are forty—especially given that many solo parents need to process some grief before taking steps to conceive on their own. If you are considering a career change or an intensive education program that is likely to bring about stress or take a toll on your body, you might be deciding between that and a pregnancy if you do so after age thirty-five. Factor in the costs of oocyte or embryo cryopreservation now and IVF later, or opt to have a baby first.

If you are over age thirty-five, how long you can safely wait depends on your sperm source. If you will be conceiving with a partner, coparent, or donor who will be providing fresh sperm, your chances of conception are limited by that person's age as well as your own. In other words, if you are combining the effects of age on both types of gametes needed for conception, your options become limited as each of you ages. As noted, sperm quality starts to decline over age forty. If self-insemination or intercourse is not successful and you end up needing to do IUI, and your sperm source is a similar age or older than you, your chances of success decline once you turn forty. If you aren't ready to conceive now but your sperm source is aging, consider having them freeze their sperm so that it will be as viable as it is today when you are ready to use it.

If you are over age thirty-five and conceiving with frozen sperm from a young, well-screened sperm bank donor, this might buy you some time. Donor IUI is still a viable option up to age forty-two; however, your options for assisted reproductive technologies become limited once you pass age thirty-nine. For instance, if you don't conceive within a reasonable number of cycles of IUI, the first-line medical approach is to stimulate the ovaries with oral medications such as letrozole or Clomid. If that doesn't work, injectable gonadotropins can be used for IUI cycles, which is still considerably less expensive than in vitro fertilization (IVF). However, over age thirty-nine, the success rate for IUI with gonadotropins is low enough that IVF becomes a more cost-effective option. Essentially, this means that once you are over age thirty-nine, you are looking at spending well over $10,000 to conceive via IVF if IUI doesn't work. By the time you are forty-three, IVF success rates are so low that they don't outweigh the likelihood of success with IUI, and regardless of how you conceive, the miscarriage rate is over 50 percent by the time you reach age forty-five. This is why so many people are encouraged to conceive with a donor egg once they pass age forty-three. You will find these options mapped out over time in the table on page 26.

If you are considering the implications of gender-affirming testosterone therapy on your fertility, you can be reassured that as long as you went through endogenous puberty before starting testosterone—even if that puberty was delayed by taking blockers during adolescence—current evidence indicates that your fertile potential is likely to return after stopping testosterone. (In contrast, circumventing endogenous puberty during adolescence with blockers and testosterone prevents development of the natal reproductive system, which is irreversible.) You will still be limited by the effects of age, so the previous paragraphs apply to you as well. If you have zero desire to ever carry a pregnancy but want a genetic connection to a child, think seriously about cryopreserving your eggs before you start testosterone, so that you don't have to stop taking hormones later on in order to have eggs retrieved. The other option is to start testosterone and then discontinue for about three to six months to harvest eggs at a later time. As mentioned before, this is best done under age thirty-five.

WHEN TO CONCEIVE WITH A PARTNER'S EGG

If you are planning to conceive via IVF so that you can carry a pregnancy created with your partner's egg, your chances of success are primarily based on your partner's age. Live birth rates with IVF are based on the age of the egg: around 55 percent per cycle under age thirty-five, 40 percent per cycle at age thirty-five to thirty-seven, 25 percent at age thirty-eight to forty, 13 percent at age forty-one to forty-two, and only 4.5 percent above age forty-three. If there is an age difference in your relationship, the passage of time might have a large bearing on whose eggs are used to conceive. Although there are stories of pregnancies being carried successfully over age forty-five, this option comes with greatly increased risks, including triple the chance of severe morbidity and increased rates of cesarean delivery, preeclampsia, postpartum hemorrhage, gestational diabetes, thrombosis, and hysterectomy.

Guiding Principles to Keep in Mind When Planning a Pregnancy

Once you are ready to pursue pregnancy, there are many decisions to be made. As you navigate the decision-making process, hold fast to the reasons you are doing this in the first place. For instance, most of us choose to become parents because there is love in our hearts that we have to give to a child. Let that love guide you. Keep it in the forefront of your mind, and let it keep you heart-centered when the thinking part of this process starts to bog you down.

Meanwhile, realize that you are going through a major life transition. You are not just bringing a new human into the world, you are stepping into the role of a parent, which will change everything about how you live your life. If you are already parenting, adding another child will change who you are as a parent. A lot of people make the mistake of thinking that having a baby will just be something that is added to your life, which any parent will tell you could not be further from the truth. Becoming a parent changes you. Who you are now will be integrated into your identity as a parent, not the other way around.

What this means, ultimately, is that the ways you come to know yourself, and the personal growth that happens along the way, are all part of investing in yourself as a parent. Recognize that you are embarking on a path of lifelong learning. The decisions you make as a parent will not end once conception has occurred, or even once the baby is born. The process of knowing your truth and acting on that truth is exactly what it takes to parent wholeheartedly.

Stepping into your truth, nurturing your capacity for resilience, and intentionally choosing life, love, and joy are what queerness is all about. We have so many tools as queer and trans people that serve us as parents. The very act of conceiving with intention means that our children are deeply wanted. The resiliency we have accumulated over a lifetime of existing outside cultural norms will help us navigate the ups and downs of fertility, pregnancy, and new parenthood.

Know that so many others have come before you, and that you are not alone in grappling with these decisions. Tackle them one at a time, stop and breathe deeply as needed, and take the time you need to integrate your thoughts and feelings each step of the way. If you have one or more partners, or if you are choosing to coparent with someone who is not your romantic partner, make sure each of you are doing your own soul-searching, then come together and compare notes. See where you match up, and where there are more conversations to be had. I promise, this will not be the last time you do this big work together. If you are becoming a solo parent, process your thoughts and feelings with the loved ones in your life, and then revel in the freedom of being the sole decision-maker of what is right for you. No matter the structure of your family, you are about to take the steps that will lead you into a life that will never be the same. Love yourself completely. Keep showing up. Together with your baby-to-be, you are creating a family.

Carrying a Pregnancy as a Solo Parent

No matter the number of parents, a family is a family. Know that throughout this book, the word "family" is used to refer to all families, including those with one parent, even if that parent is in the planning stages or currently trying to conceive.

While some people have always intended to become solo parents, many do so because there is no partner and time is running out. This means letting go of the dream of having a child within a romantic relationship while at the same time harnessing the strength to go it alone. Eventually, grief and loss give way to feelings of empowerment and relief at not having to navigate parenthood with another person. There is great freedom in making your own decisions without the need for processing them with a partner!

However, while the ultimate responsibility and decision-making power may be solely up to you, none of us parent in a vacuum. We are human, which means we are social creatures, and we need each other. It truly does take a village to raise a child, in part because it takes a village to raise a parent. Some people in your life will raise concerns about your decision to be a solo parent, which may feel like they are questioning your abilities or undermining your resolve. However, these comments often come from other parents who know just how much work it is to care for a baby, and the idea of solo parenthood may bring up feelings of isolation they experienced, even while partnered, in the early months and years of parenting. Rather than silently resolving to prove these naysayers wrong by never admitting to a need for support, gently acknowledge their privilege in having a partner when they became a parent, affirm your desire to have a child, and ask them if they are someone you can call on when you need a hand. Keep the door open to tangible displays of caring, support, and community. Raising a child is hard. You can totally do it. And there will be times when you call on your community, family, and friends to support you—just like any parent would do.

When More Than One Partner Has the Capability and Desire to Carry

If there is more than one partner in a relationship who wants to carry, deciding who should be pregnant first is not an easy choice to make. The person who carries first may harbor some guilt, and the one who doesn't can feel a range of emotions, from jealousy or loss to relief or even some guilt of their own during the parts of pregnancy that are difficult to bear. If the person carrying conceives with their own eggs, this may bring about additional concerns regarding who has a genetic connection to the child, but keep in mind that your child will pick up traits and mannerisms from each of you, and over time, your lived experience of parenting your child will far outweigh the cis/heteronormative concept that parenthood is defined by genetics alone.

The decision about who will carry a pregnancy first can also take into consideration how each of you are likely to be recognized as parents by the outside world. A butch, nonbinary, or transmasculine parent may go first when partnered with a femme, in attempts to circumvent the likelihood that their role will be overlooked in a society that conflates femininity with giving birth. A mixed-race family with a white partner may opt for a parent of color to go first because of the tendency of a racist society to assume that a person of color is a nanny instead of a parent. When one partner is estranged from their family of origin, they may opt to go first in order to affirm a sense of belonging and to offset the sense of marginalization that can happen when in-laws focus on genetic expression in your child. If one of you has a family member who can be a sperm donor, that may decide things for you—or you may ultimately decide that genetic relationship is not as vital as other factors.

Take the time to sort through the issues at hand and make the choice that is going to be most grounded given the circumstances. Take into consideration:

- How is your gender likely to inform your experience of pregnancy, and how is pregnancy likely to inform your gender? In some ways, it may be impossible to know the answers to these questions ahead of time, but the self-investigation is useful for planning the support you will need.

- What are the implications of your racial or ethnic background on biological parenthood? How do those intersect with your choice of a sperm donor, and how does the availability of donors affect that decision? (See Chapter 4 for more on this.)

- How are your families of origin likely to relate to a child you carry, versus a child your partner carries, and how do you see yourself setting boundaries to maintain one another's emotional safety as well as your sense of family integrity?

- What are the financial implications of one partner being out of work or on leave for an extended period of time? Is childcare affordable in your area, or does it make more sense for one parent to stay home? Does that need to be the parent who carries (or lactates)?

- Who loves their job? How can each of you be happiest in the long term? If lactation is in the plan, know that pumping at work is equivalent to working double time, not just for pumping but also because your baby will likely have extra night waking to get time feeding from you. If you truly love your job and your workplace is supportive of the needs of lactating parents, this can work out fine, but if not, you are likely to prefer an extended leave or a pause on your career if this is financially feasible for you.

- Who is the caretaker in your relationship? Who finds it easier to receive care, and will the physical demands of pregnancy fall easily into that role, or will there be a role reversal? A partner who is fiercely independent and prides themselves on not needing support may find pregnancy to be an isolating experience, while a partner who is comfortable asking for and receiving support may find pregnancy and postpartum recovery easier to navigate without feeling a loss of this aspect of identity.

- What other thoughts do you have about the lived experience of pregnancy and biological parenthood, and how do those inform your desire for or against carrying? What are the considerations your partner(s) has, and who has the greatest need for a biological connection? What are the ways you are each confident that you can support the central role of a nonbiological parent in your family?

Note that none of these questions have to do with who is younger or older or who has better fertile health. Although these are important factors, the lived experience of pregnancy and parenthood are too important to overlook, even if you mix it up by doing IVF with a partner's egg. I suggest you start with these questions, because even if you ultimately end up with health considerations that inform your decision, you will have already put a lot of aspects of the process on the table. That way, when feelings and experiences come up, as they surely will, you won't be surprised by them. Conception, pregnancy, and parenthood bring plenty of unknowns. The more you enter the experience with full awareness and solid connections within your relationship, the stronger the foundation of your family will be.

Considering Simultaneous Pregnancy

If two partners each have the ability and the desire to carry a pregnancy, at some point, you may consider carrying pregnancies simultaneously. It usually doesn't take much asking around to discover that the idea is not actually as dreamy as it may sound. If there are people in your life who have had simultaneous pregnancies, and they are still together (many aren't), ask them what made it work for them, and to be honest with you in sharing the parts that were hard.

The best-case scenario might include the financial means to pay for a night nurse, overnight doula, or nanny; emotional and logistical support from affirming and available extended family; and excellent physical and mental health. Without such privilege, there is a whole lot to lose for the sake of little gain. Based on the struggles I have witnessed new parents grapple with during my quarter-century-long career, simultaneous pregnancy is something I wholeheartedly discourage. There is no way to truly understand what it is like to be pregnant, let alone what it is like to be a parent of a newborn. The experience is so all-encompassing, with such intense highs and lows, that it can't be accurately described in words. It has to be lived to be truly understood.

Simultaneous pregnancy might be fun (when you're not fighting over the toilet bowl to puke every morning); however, watching your partner give birth shortly before giving birth yourself has the potential to be encouraging, intimidating, or distressing, depending on how it goes. It also means you will be a parent of a newborn when you go into labor, which means you will be utterly exhausted from the start. For a parent who is newly postpartum, attending a partner in labor means feeling torn about being there for them versus being there for the baby you already have. It also means reliving your own birth before you have had time to fully process it, and doing all of this while in the midst of your own healing and physical recovery, which may be recovery from major abdominal surgery if you have a cesarean birth. The lack of sleep faced by new parents, along with the major hormonal shifts of recovering from pregnancy, leave us vulnerable to imbalanced brain chemistry that can bring on postpartum anxiety or depression or exacerbate other mental health issues such as bipolar disorder or obsessive-compulsive disorder. If you choose to establish lactation and learn to feed your baby with your body, this process will be central to the experience of postpartum recovery, so much so that if it does not go well, the entire postpartum adjustment will be impacted for each of you. It often takes two parents to get the latch right in the beginning, one to do the nursing and the other to help with pillows, footrests, and holding the little one's hands out of the way when latching the baby on.

Ultimately, if both of you are pregnant at the same time, the intensity of the experience will not only be double, it will prevent each of you from really being there for the other in the midst of it. Once there are two babies, everything will be multiplied not just by two, but exponentially, because everyone in the family will need support, but there will be no one available to give it. Parents will get the experience of simultaneous pregnancy, but no one will get the experience of becoming a parent and *not* being pregnant, which is a true gift! Being a nongestational parent is beautiful, vital, and necessary. Caring for your partner and your baby simultaneously is a wholly valid way to be a parent. If you also each want the experience of carrying a pregnancy, I strongly advise doing it separately so that you and your partner each get to fully experience the role of being the pregnant parent, as well as the opportunity to parent separate from the physical experience of pregnancy.

Carrying a Pregnancy by Default

If you have no desire to be pregnant but your partner is unable to carry, you and your uterus might be called to the task. This brings up some pretty complex feelings. If your partner wanted to carry but was unable to conceive, or if your partner would love nothing more than to carry a pregnancy but they do not have the anatomy required, there can be a certain level of guilt as well as feelings of obligation. Just because you have a uterus doesn't mean you have to or should want to use it to carry a pregnancy. For some, making use of the tools you've got can bring a sense of empowerment, but for others, it could prove to be a deeply dysphoric experience. However, it may seem that this is the only option for your family to have a child. Take some time to dig deep into this question if you find yourself in such a predicament. Is there work you need to do to get to a yes, or is there work you need to do both on your own and as a couple to be able to be affirmed in saying no? There are many ways to become a parent. If pregnancy is going to be harmful to your psyche, that is not an ideal way to bring a child into your life. On the other hand, if you feel up to the task but you know you are going to need extra support, be as up front about that as you can be, and also ask for the space to continue stating your needs as they become known to you. We often don't know what we will need until we aren't getting it, so be as gentle with yourself and with your partner(s) as you can while it all unfolds. As hard as it may be to come to this level of honesty with yourself—and to articulate your feelings to your partner(s)—this will only be the first of many such frank and deeply honest conversations that you will have as parents.

When More Than One Partner Can Provide Sperm

If there is more than one person in the family who has the ability to provide sperm for conception, you may be sorting out whose sperm will be used, especially if your clinic does not allow mixing of sperm samples. Before running out to get a semen analysis and awarding a gold star to the one whose sperm count is highest, consider the implications of biological parentage in your family system. Has one parent banked gametes prior to gender transition? Are there considerations around racial identity or a cultural history that make genetic connection especially important? Is there a history of adoption or estrangement from family of origin that has bearing on the decision to be genetically linked to this child? How might your extended family honor each parent's relationship to the child—and will a genetic relationship secure recognition for a parent who is vulnerable to being overlooked as a full parent? Is there a potential surrogate in your extended family, making traditional surrogacy an option that limits one of you from providing gametes for the pregnancy? Ultimately, you will each participate in affirming the validity of your family, correcting those who make thoughtless comments, fielding intrusive questions about your child's genetic origins, and setting boundaries around the language others use to refer to you and your parental relationships. Keep in mind that once you are parenting, genetics may fade into the background and become overshadowed by your child's unique personality and needs as well as your contributions as parents.

Pursuing Transmasculine or Nonbinary Pregnancy

Gestating new life can be an amazing and affirming way to experience living in your body. A lot of transmasculine and nonbinary people find many aspects of pregnancy to be empowering and awe-inspiring. As long as your reproductive organs completed pubertal development prior to taking testosterone, the growing body of research demonstrates that your fertile function can be expected to return quite seamlessly once you stop, with the same fertile potential as anyone your age. This means that all the information in this book on supporting egg health, preparing for pregnancy, timing inseminations, and the superior success rates of unmedicated donor IUI apply to you as well. Most people want to limit their time off of gender-affirming hormones and get pregnant as quickly as possible. The more you are willing and able to work with your body, the more quickly and easily you will be able to conceive. Pregnancy has the potential to be a deeply embodied experience, which means that the months leading into pregnancy are a time to navigate being at home in your body as it changes.

For most transmasculine and nonbinary pregnant people, the most difficult thing about being pregnant has to do with interacting with the outside world. It's important to find a care provider who is affirming of your gender identity, and to advocate and keep advocating for appropriate pronouns and terminology your providers use when they speak to you. If you go to a fertility clinic for assistance getting pregnant, be prepared for an environment that is heavily oriented toward the gender binary. The preconception period can be the most stressful part of pregnancy for transmasculine people due to the lack of control over how long it will take to achieve pregnancy while simultaneously finding little support and validation for your experience. Seek out support groups of all kinds so that you don't feel so isolated in this process, whether it's a Facebook group, a group that meets virtually, or a group that gathers in your local community. Recognize that trying to conceive is super stressful for everyone, and as a nonbinary or transmasculine person seeking pregnancy, there is even more at stake, so the stress for you is extra. Be sure to get extra support, extra validation, and extra love from all your people. You deserve it!

Once you stop testosterone, you can expect anywhere from one to six months for your cycles to return. Once you are ovulating again, your best chances of pregnancy are in the first three months of trying; however, most people will conceive within eight months. Adding in the nine months of pregnancy, and a month or so for hormonal recovery, you are looking at about two years off of testosterone. Any changes you had in your voice or hair patterns on testosterone will remain the same, so you may find that you still pass quite easily into the second trimester of pregnancy, and even longer if you have a large body size.

The most obvious and immediate changes of pregnancy are in the chest, which is why a lot of transmasculine people opt for top surgery prior to pregnancy. This brings up the question of infant feeding, which is a whole lot to think about before you have even conceived. Some people have zero desire to lactate and chestfeed, but others feel torn about not being able to feed their baby with their own milk after top surgery. (See Chapter 11 for more details about options for lactation and chestfeeding.) If you are on the fence about this decision, seek out others who have chestfed, with and without top surgery, to hear about their lived experience and see what comes up for you as you listen to their stories. While feeding is a huge aspect of caring for an infant, bottle feeding is pretty sweet too. Get as much information as you can, do some soul-searching, and settle on the decision that feels best to you. Parenting is a wholehearted journey, and the path that keeps you true to yourself and allows you to be as fully present as you can possibly be is the right choice for both you and your baby.

Once pregnant, those who have not had top surgery usually find binding to be prohibitively painful quite early in pregnancy, as the chest typically becomes swollen and sore right away. Those who have had top surgery prior to pregnancy often find that any lactiferous (milk-making) cells that still remain in the chest tissue respond to the pregnancy hormones, and the chest can take on a lumpy appearance. For this reason, it is recommended to delay any secondary surgeries for fine-tuning the appearance of your chest until after pregnancy. If you wait until after pregnancy to have top surgery, you will want to have weaned your baby and completely stopped making milk prior to the procedure so that there is not a painful buildup of milk in any ducts that may be severed or left behind.

Aside from these logistical questions, what most nonbinary and transmasculine parents-to-be grapple with on a daily basis are complex questions about identity, personal safety, and the unsettling feeling of not knowing what this whole experience is going to be like. Embarking on pregnancy brings up a range of conflicting emotions about wanting this yet hating this, using your body's tools yet feeling at the mercy of your body, and having no other way to become a parent yet at times wishing there was some other way. Masculine pregnancy is a complex experience, and while there are common themes, each person's experience is different. Take time for self-care every single day. Surround yourself with people who love and support you, and let go of any relationships that don't. Everything you do to keep yourself intact through this process makes you a better parent and ensures that there is more of you available to love and care for your child.

Approaching Pregnancy as a Trans Woman or Nonbinary Parent-to-Be

While pregnancy after uterine transplant has been accomplished successfully, this option has so far only been provided for cisgender women. Until reproductive science catches up with the needs of nonbinary and trans people who don't have a uterus, the best option for genetic procreation is to use your gametes to conceive a child that someone else carries through pregnancy. This may be easier said than done, and not just for the logistical reasons of needing a partner or surrogate to carry your baby. For many, there is some amount of grief to process regarding not being able to be pregnant and give birth to your child. However, many trans mothers and nonbinary parents are thrilled to find out that they can breastfeed their babies, either by inducing lactation or by using a supplemental nursing system to feed the baby at the breast. Any breast growth you may have had while on estrogen will help. (See Chapter 11 for more information about lactation induction.)

If you decide to conceive with your own gametes and you have already started hormone treatment, you will need to stop taking hormones in order to find out if you can regain fertile function. How long you have been on hormones, and what hormones and blockers you are taking, will determine your likelihood of success. Of course, stopping hormones as a trans woman is no simple thing. Any changes in fat distribution, muscle mass, and skin and hair texture will go back again, and your genitals will begin to function as they did before. Physical safety is a very real concern, and careful consideration must be given to maintaining your mental health through this process. Having a solid support system in place is of utmost importance. Take time for self-care every day, and be clear about your social and emotional boundaries. You get to take the space you need to keep yourself safe and sane during this process, and everything you do to build yourself up is only going to make you a better parent to your child, so go for it!

Carefully balance the choice to delay or go off of gender-affirming hormones with what you might gain from having a biological connection to your child. Due to the barriers presented by societal transphobia, biological parentage can be protective when your validity as a parent is questioned, whether it's an obnoxious query about who the child's "real" parent is or needing to defend your rights to your child in front of a judge. However, if not being on hormones is going to present a high degree of risk for you, consider if there is another way for you to become a parent besides genetic procreation, such as using a sperm donor, adopting, or coparenting (parenting together in a non-romantic relationship) with chosen family. Do some soul-searching and consider each option wholeheartedly before moving forward. Ultimately, what your future child needs most is you.

Decisions about Conception in a Poly Family

The dynamics in polyamorous families are complex, but you are likely accustomed to navigating them. As you make decisions about who will carry and who will provide gametes for conception, be sure to take stock of existing relationship dynamics and actively incorporate those into your decision-making. If there are already dynamics that take work in order to keep everyone feeling connected, this is likely to be exacerbated during the sleeplessness and emotional vulnerability of early parenthood. Is there someone who struggles with a sense of belonging because they are not legally recognized as a partner, they are not on the deed to the house, or for any other reason? If such a dynamic exists, be especially mindful of everyone's role in conception and pregnancy, ensuring that no one is in a position to feel they are the odd one out. Taking the time to set things up well in the beginning can be the gateway to enjoying the benefits of having multiple parents and ensuring a strong foundation for shared parenthood.

Intentional Coparenting Arrangements

Coparenting, which in this context refers to building your family with one or more people you are not romantically involved with, is about as queer as it gets. (In this book, I will use the term "coparenting" to refer to such familial relationships, and the hyphenated term "co-parenting" to refer to the act of parenting together.) Pursuing parenthood completely outside nuclear family norms takes creativity, open-mindedness, and a great deal of intentionality. And like all nontraditional relationships, it takes a lot of work, dedication to personal accountability, self-reflection, honesty, vulnerability, clear communication, and a commitment to putting the child's needs first while also taking into consideration the needs of all the parents. It means engaging in the work of a long-term relationship without the buffer of a sexual connection. On the flip side, it can be a relief to navigate coparenting and a chosen-family relationship without the responsibilities that go along with romantic partnership.

Just as with any committed, long-term relationship, choosing coparents means sorting through many aspects of how you fit together as individuals. It takes time to really get to know someone, not just the shiny first impressions we all put forth and allow ourselves to see in a new relationship but also how each person responds during times of anger, stress, and sadness, and how each of you is able to maintain respect when you disagree. Many people find that their ideas about parenting, and preformed expectations of appropriate parenting style, change once they actually become parents. The more parents are involved, the more variation there is likely to be. Who calls the shots? How will you come to agreements so that the child experiences continuity among households and/or with different parents? If there are power dynamics that emerge among you, don't overlook them. Nothing creates conflict more than a parent who loves and is invested in a child yet has no say in how they are raised.

While so many of these considerations are about the lives of each of the parents, it all must be examined through the eyes of a child. As long as everyone is aware of and committed to nurturing secure attachment for all the parent-child relationships, coparenting can be a wonderful way to create family without the stressors inherent in a two-parent nuclear family. However, the level of intention that it takes to create a family outside of culturally prescribed norms is something that requires a great deal of forethought, and an ongoing commitment to continuous co-creation, not only as your child grows but as each of you grows and changes.

If you decide that a coparent relationship is what you are looking for, then take the time to fully explore everything that this means before moving ahead with conception. Years of heartache, custody battles, and legal expenses can be avoided by having a solid foundation for this type of arrangement. Coparenting is the epitome of intentional family building, and the intention starts long before the child is conceived. Having all the important conversations now, and paying close attention to how the conversations feel and the ways in which you each deal with the hard topics, will inform how these types of conversations might unfold as circumstances in each of your lives (and your child's life) change in the future. Make sure you receive guidance from a family therapist or other family-building specialist who can help you think through common parenting scenarios that you may not be fully aware of before having a child. In fact, it is highly recommended that you maintain care with a family therapist and plan to see this person regularly throughout your coparenting journey. Once you articulate your understandings, create a written coparenting agreement under the guidance of legal counsel. Your family's needs may shift over time, so consider it a "living document" and be sure to have a process in place to make changes as needed.

TOPICS TO DISCUSS WITH POTENTIAL COPARENTS

- What is the history of your relationship with each other, and how does it inform your decision to parent together?

- What sort of history do each of you have with raising children?

- What values do you want to hold fast to in your coparenting relationship?

- What values do you each hold in raising a child? Think about spiritual or religious beliefs, education and discipline style, as well as approaches to nutrition and health.

- Who will decide on the baby's name, and who will be on the birth certificate?

- Will rights to make decisions for the child be shared equally, or will one parent have primary decision-making authority?

- Will you share financial responsibilities equally, or will this be determined by percentage of income or other determinants of financial ability? Think about clothing, food, housing, medical expenses, childcare, schooling, camps, rites-of-passage celebrations, college expenses, etc. Do you want to agree to maintain a certain level of income or financial contribution to the child's needs? Will you open a joint bank account, or will there be certain expenses that each of you pay for? Who will claim the child as a dependent on their taxes, or will it alternate in some way?

- Will you share time with the child equally, or will the child live primarily in one household?

- How might the child's living situation change over time? (For instance, most newborns need to be in close physical proximity with a lactating parent, and there is an adjustment period for a parent who gestates a child to feel secure in being away from the child, which can take a few months.)

- What level of geographic proximity do you want to maintain and for how long? Are there exceptions such as moving for a new job, to care for aging parents, or for a romantic relationship?

- How will you divide your time with the child, such as vacations, holidays, days off school, and time with your families of origin?

- How will you work together to provide consistency for the child if you live in different households, such as agreed-upon discipline style, screen time, bedtime, chores, etc.?

- What agreements do you want to have in place around your dating lives and when/how new partners will be introduced to and/or spend time with the child?

- What if some of the coparents are partnered, and they break up? How many different homes would you expect a child to live in, and how would you maintain parental relationships if the number of households exceeds what is healthy for the child?

- What happens if one of you dies or becomes unable to care for the child? Will you take out life or disability insurance to cover the child's needs in this scenario?

- What happens if one of you has another child on their own or with a partner or other coparent? How could this be done in a way that affirms the child's sense of family and continues to support each of your roles as this child's parents?

- How do you intend to nurture and support your relationship as coparents? To whom will you turn for guidance in your relationship?

- How often will you communicate with one another about parenting, and how often will you meet with your family therapist or other professional or spiritual guide?

- How often will you review and revise your coparenting agreement?

- What will you do when conflict or disagreements arise? Will you agree to seek mediation or collaborative law prior to legal arbitration? How will this be paid for?

Dealing with Overwhelm in the Decision-Making Process

In addition to all of the decisions mentioned so far in this chapter, you may also need to make decisions about gamete donors (Chapter 4), surrogacy (Chapter 5), and/or route to pregnancy (Chapters 6 and 8). There are so many decisions to be made on the path to parenthood, it is reasonable to sometimes feel mired down in overwhelm. Some decisions will come easy to you, while they bring up confusion and uncertainty for your partner(s) or coparent(s). Some options will be limited by biology, and others will be limited by finances, both of which may bring up resentment or regret that needs to be addressed. Get the support you need to examine not only the decisions you are making but also the feelings that come up in the process of decision-making. A therapist who is experienced in supporting new or prospective parents will be a helpful resource to have as you wade through the options. Reach out to others in your community who have gone through a similar experience, and listen carefully not just to the decisions they made but to the feelings they had about it at the time and how those feelings did or did not come into play over time.

Start with the decisions that seem most straightforward, so that you can build momentum and begin the process with a few of the easier choices already tucked away. For the more difficult decisions, allow time for self-reflection in therapy, by journaling, talking to friends, during workouts, or while making art—whatever you know is the best way for you to sort through your thoughts and feelings. Do this separately from others who are making the decision alongside you, and then come together so that you can compare notes on each person's priorities and start to put those together in a way that works best for the family as a whole. Set a timeline for when to regroup at each step, whether that is a week, two weeks, or a month.

If you are feeling stuck, or if you and your partner(s) or coparent(s) are at odds about a particular decision, get help. A relationship or family therapist is the best tool a family can have, so if you don't have one, this is a great time to start. Your midwife or family-building specialist may be able to assist you in asking the important questions and providing insight as you sort out what is going to be best for you and your family. If you need to take a break, do that, but make a plan about how long the break will be and when you will come back to the table again.

If you're a single parent, you are embarking on a lifetime of solo decision-making, so what you learn about yourself now will help you feel more grounded in this aspect of parenthood going forward. If you are parenting with a partner, partners, and/or coparents, you are learning and practicing what it is to make decisions with one another. In either case, the conclusions you come to are only part of what is actually taking place. You are discovering qualities in yourself and your loved ones as decision makers, and exploring ways to honor and respect your own truth as well as the truths of those you love. You are learning to navigate making decisions for your child, which is weighty and intense. This is only the beginning of a lifetime of making your own best choices—wholehearted, vulnerable, and authentic—and allowing one decision to unfold into the next, affirming and upholding that, at each step of the way, you are making the best possible decisions with the information you have. Love yourself, and trust yourself to move forward knowing that once you make a choice, you can let go and rest in it completely.

Creating a Timeline for Conception

While your timeline for having a baby may initially be determined by baseline financial concerns such as housing, covering parental leave, and paying for childcare, this must be weighed against the immutable reality of a ticking biological clock. As you age, conception itself can become more costly due to waning fertility and the increased likelihood of needing high-tech fertility medicine to help you. No one can ultimately predict how much it will cost for you to conceive, but be sure to keep the potential costs of achieving pregnancy in mind as you determine where the balance is for you.

If you are conceiving with a surrogate, expect up to a year of lead time once you start the process. If you know you are going to conceive via IVF, whether with your own egg, a partner's egg, donor egg, or donor embryo, the timing will depend on your clinic's schedule, which could be at least six months including wait time for an appointment, initial testing, and preliminary procedures. In these situations, the timeline of the conception process is primarily determined by logistical steps and clinic protocols, both of which are somewhat outside your control.

If you plan to conceive via insemination, the timeline will mostly be determined by you. There are considerations to keep in mind regarding your overall fertile life span, when to start prepping your body, how long it will reasonably take to conceive, and when to seek medical support if it's not working. Once you are in the process of trying, the ups and downs of conception attempts can start to take over your life, making the process feel like an endless roller-coaster ride. Having a timeline in place provides some containment, so that even though there are unknowns, you can at least locate yourself in time and know what the next steps will be.

It takes about three months for egg cells to come out of dormancy and prepare to ovulate, although it is ideal to start to prepare for pregnancy up to a year ahead of time. This means following the recommendations in Chapter 2 for supporting your fertile health, and getting lab work done to guide you in your efforts as outlined in Chapter 3. Don't make the mistake of putting off your preconception care when you could be taking advantage of lead time in making sure your body is ready to go. This is why preconception lab work is recommended at the beginning of your prep time (see Chapter 3). If medications, supplements, or lifestyle adjustments are needed, this allows you time to get those underway and retest to make sure you are in range before conceiving. It can take three to six months to arrive at the appropriate medication dose for thyroid conditions, and it can take the same length of time to normalize glucose levels if your A1c is high. On the other hand, low vitamin D and anemia can be adequately treated within about a month's time, as long as you utilize supplements that are highly absorbable at the proper dose (see Chapter 2).

You will also want to start identifying your ovulation using the information in Chapter 6, so that once your sperm is available, you will know the right time to inseminate. You can be choosing a sperm donor, creating a legal agreement with a sperm donor who is someone you know (a "known donor"), or waiting for a directed donor quarantine (as described in Chapter 4) simultaneously as you prepare to conceive. If you are using a known donor who needs to boost their fertility, this takes at least three months as well, which is why a semen analysis is the recommended first step when selecting a known sperm donor.

If you have very short or very long cycles (fewer than twenty-three days or more than thirty-five days from the start of one period to the start of the next period), or you sometimes skip periods, or you have a lot of pain or bleeding between periods, do not wait to get this checked out. Similarly, if you know that you have PCOS, endometriosis, or fibroids (see Chapter 7), you may need an extra six months to work on nutrition, exercise, and complementary treatments to support your reproductive health.

Comparing Costs and Success Rates of Assisted Conception

As you map out your timeline, there are a few things to be aware of that can inform your plan. For instance, a lot of people opt to self-inseminate with frozen sperm, but success rates double with IUI. Some people wonder if going to a clinic and doing medicated cycles will help them get pregnant more quickly, but the data does not support this unless you are over age forty or have diminished ovarian reserve. IVF success rates are much higher than IUI up to age forty-one, but that comes with a price tag that far exceeds the cost of IUI. The baseline cost for an IVF cycle is $12,000 on average, with additional costs ranging up to $8,000 for medications, genetic testing, and other aspects of assisted reproduction. In comparison, an unmedicated cycle of IUI without ultrasound monitoring is around $200 to $600 depending on location and provider.

What this means is that if you are under forty and conceiving with frozen donor sperm, you do not need infertility medicine—you just need IUI. Additional services available in a fertility clinic, such as ovarian reserve testing, ultrasound monitoring, and medications such as Clomid, letrozole, and hCG "trigger" are not needed at the outset of your conception process, and they may inflate your costs significantly. Even if you are over forty, you can still consider a few cycle attempts before seeking medical support, especially if you have never tried to conceive before.

Any way you look at it, trying to conceive is a game of odds. The factor that has the greatest impact is your age. If an egg is not genetically normal, the pregnancy will most likely miscarry, and the older you are, the more likely this will be the case. IVF can't correct for this, but it can help you get to the point of transferring a genetically normal embryo, if there is one to be had. The older you get, the less likely it is that IVF can improve your chances of success beyond what you would expect through insemination or intercourse. As your age goes up, the live birth rate goes down.

Pregnancy and Miscarriage Rates by Age with Frozen Donor Sperm

Age	Pregnancy Rate per Unmedicated Donor Self-Insemination Cycle	Pregnancy Rate per Unmedicated Donor IUI Cycle	Miscarriage Rate
‹ 35		17–22%	10%
35–40	6%	8–14%	19%
40+		3–6%	27%

Ferrara 2002, Cohlen 2011, Ripley 2015

Below the age of thirty-seven, you can reasonably expect to conceive with the lowest cumulative cost, no matter the method. The overall cost of conception may be lower with IUI, given that you are most likely to conceive within three to six cycles of IUI, which is still less than the cost of one cycle of IVF. If you do IVF, you will most likely have enough healthy eggs that the cost of genetic testing will not be warranted, and a single embryo can be transferred with a reasonable likelihood of success—this means your costs will be more like $12,000 to $15,000, and you may end up with extra embryos for future pregnancies as well.

IVF Live Birth Rate by Age per Cycle of Egg Retrieval

Age	Live Birth Rate per Cycle of Egg Retrieval in IVF
‹ 35	54.7%
35–37	40.6%
38–40	25.6%
41–42	12.8%
43+	4.4%

SART national summary report, 2017

Between ages thirty-eight to forty-two, genetic testing of embryos in the IVF process increases your chances of live birth while reducing the rate of miscarriage, but that adds another $2,000 to $3,000. Because egg health starts declining around this time, testing embryos and only transferring those that are genetically normal offsets rates of pregnancy loss from chromosomal abnormalities. You may need multiple cycles of stimulation and retrieval to end up with the number of frozen embryos needed for a successful transfer and healthy live birth, typically two healthy embryos for each anticipated child. This adds another $20,000 per retrieval and an additional $4,000 per frozen embryo transfer. Some added benefits of this method are that transferring frozen embryos allows you to focus on building your uterine lining in a separate cycle, which increases the likelihood of a successful transfer. This method also allows you to capitalize on getting more embryos cryopreserved with your own eggs before you get any older, which helps preserve your opportunity for future pregnancies during your forties.

Once you reach age forty-three, there is such a low number of healthy eggs that IVF cannot improve your odds over IUI. Both options have a low rate of success, and IUI is much less expensive for the same odds. This is why a donor egg or donor embryo is recommended by fertility clinics at this point. IVF with eggs this age just doesn't have anything more to offer if you've already tried with viable sperm and a clear pathway to the egg, and it would be unethical to take your money without any likelihood of it increasing your chances of success.

If IVF is on the table for you, you may want to go to a fertility clinic up front to get an assessment of your ovarian reserve (see Chapter 3) and likelihood for success with IVF, along with an estimate of costs (see Chapter 8). Even if you don't start there, it can give you a sense of the expenses that may lie ahead if you are unable to conceive via IUI. This can inform how many IUI cycles you decide to try before moving on to IVF.

Putting It All Together

The chart on pages 26–27 provides guidelines for pregnancy preparation time plus options for methods of insemination and fertility treatments based on age. It is derived from the available data on success rates for donor insemination with and without fertility medications at various ages, as well as cost-effectiveness of IUI versus IVF in light of the limitations of age.

The timeline represents the simplest-case scenarios. It doesn't take into account waiting to get in for an appointment at a fertility clinic, or the time it may take to change care providers if you find yourself in a clinic that doesn't honor your gender, your family structure, or your donor choice. For instance, in many states, clinics won't work with families who are using a known donor, so you may actually be more limited in your options than the chart implies—or you may need to add six months for directed donor sperm cryopreservation and quarantine (see Chapter 4).

Choosing a Care Provider

Depending on where you live, you may or may not have options to choose the clinic or provider you work with for conception. Ask around in your community to find out what others have experienced. Did your friends feel listened to and respected? Were partners welcomed? Did staff and providers get the pronouns right? Were there any blatant homophobic or transphobic experiences? What were the assumptions about gender and family structure? What was the clinic's approach to donor conception—did they have to go through additional tests or counseling sessions? Were there physicians or staff of color, or was the clinic predominantly white? Did your BIPOC friends experience racism at the clinic? How were your large-bodied friends treated? Were there differences in the clinical recommendations or alternate locations required for treatments based on body size, and was this discussed in a way that was respectful? Did the providers go slowly during exams, checking in and ensuring consent at each step? Did they take steps to ensure as much comfort as possible and provide support for unavoidable pain or discomfort during procedures? Did friends feel that they were treated as people rather than numbers?

While you may simply need some medical intervention, there is no such thing as a purely medical experience. You are a person who is receiving medical care, and you deserve to be treated as such. Take the time to select a clinic where you will be treated with consideration and respect. If you've got the capacity to cope and maintain resiliency, you may be able to navigate care in a clinic that doesn't always get the gender and orientation aspects right; however, it takes emotional energy and intentional reframing in order for this to not chip away at your sense of validity as a prospective queer or trans parent. For some, this will mean silently correcting the language you see and hear so that you

Timeline for Pregnancy Preparation Based on Age and Method of Conception

Age	Prep Time for Pregnancy	Identify Your Body's Ovulation Pattern	Get Preconception Health Tests	Booster Shots If Needed for MMR/Varicella/COVID-19	Complete Genetic Carrier Screening
‹ 35	Up to twelve months	Final three to six months of prep time	At beginning of prep time	At least one month before conceiving	At least one month before donor selection
35–37	Six to twelve months	Final three to six months of prep time	At beginning of prep time	At least one month before conceiving	At least one month before donor selection
38–39	Three to six months	Track ovulation simultaneously with prep time	At beginning of prep time	At least one month before conceiving	At least one month before donor selection
40–42	Do not delay— start trying simultaneously	Start trying while re-evaluating your timing plan after each cycle attempt	ASAP	At least one month before conceiving	At least one month before donor selection
43+	Do not delay— start trying simultaneously	Start trying while re-evaluating your timing plan after each cycle attempt	ASAP	At least one month before conceiving	At least one month before donor selection

and your family are validated, even if only inside yourself. For others, it will mean addressing the issue head-on by pointing out instances where the clinic's printed materials, forms, and language used is not appropriate to you or your family. Many providers are amenable to such feedback, and some will go the extra mile to make sure you are seen and heard and cared for appropriately.

Many families who are conceiving via insemination opt for preconception care from a provider who specifically focuses on the needs of queer and trans

Self-Insemination with Fresh Sperm	Self-Insemination with Frozen Sperm	Unmedicated IUI with Fresh or Frozen Donor Sperm	IUI and Letrozole/ Clomid	IUI and Gonadotropins
Up to twelve months, then do IUI	Up to three months, then do IUI	Three to twelve months	Up to six months	Up to six months, then IVF
Up to six months, then do IUI	Not recommended unless IUI is unavailable	Three to twelve months	Up to six months	Up to six months, then IVF
Up to six months, then do IUI	Not recommended unless IUI is unavailable	Three to six months	Up to six months	Up to six months at age 38, not recommended at age 39
Up to three months, then do IUI	Not recommended unless IUI is unavailable	Up to three months	Up to three months, then IVF (with donor egg or donor embryo by age 42)	Not recommended
If not opting for IVF with donor egg, twelve months or more as desired	Not recommended unless IUI is unavailable	If not opting for IVF with donor egg, 12 months or more as desired	Up to three months, then IVF with donor egg or donor embryo	Not recommended

families, even if that care is accessed at a distance by conducting visits online. This allows you to get the guidance, support, and preconception care you need in a model that is uniquely suited to you. You can combine this care with IUI services from a local provider, creating the best of both worlds. You can access preconception care and find a referral list of queer/trans-competent IUI providers on the MAIA website.

GUIDANCE FOR CARE PROVIDERS

Supporting families as they go through the initial decision-making process takes a great deal of "soft skills." If part of your training included counseling skills, they will be put to good use here. You can assist families by helping them organize their thoughts and feelings about various aspects of the process while providing clinical information and anticipatory guidance.

One of the central aspects of supporting families through this time is helping them manage decision-making fatigue. As one overwhelmed client expressed to me, "Where is the joy in this?" Keep bringing prospective parents back to the reason they are doing this in the first place: the love in one's heart that has space for a child. Holding people through this time requires being attuned to how decision-making fatigue may be overshadowing the ability to maintain heart-centeredness and embodiment. Clinical guidelines are not always cut and dry, which can lead to a sense of confusion when the stakes are high. Keep bringing people back to their hearts, and encourage the use of intuition and going with gut instincts. Remind parents-to-be that this is how many parenting decisions are made, mainly because when there is no "right answer," you must go with the answer that feels right to you.

When a family presents for preconception care, creating a timeline is an important part of the service you provide. A thorough preconception care plan will always include next steps and a timeline for follow-up. You can support the families in your care by listening carefully to their thoughts about when they want to start inseminating; however, you may also need to reframe some expectations to account for all the steps involved. Make clinical recommendations as appropriate. Some families will be accepting or even eager for medical intervention, while others will want to avoid this at all costs. Provide information about why you are recommending each step, and participate in shared decision-making as each family decides what is right for them.

Resources

Family-Building Consultations, Preconception Care, and Queer/Trans-Competent IUI Providers

MAIA Midwifery & Fertility Services: MAIAMidwifery.com

TWO

FERTILE HEALTH FOR EVERY BODY

Congratulations! Making the decision to bring new life into the world is one of the most incredible experiences a person can have in a lifetime. No doubt, this will change you. Creating a child with intention means you have the opportunity to nourish and prepare your body. Daily care and tending of your body can keep you connected to yourself, cultivating feelings of groundedness and embodiment as you navigate all the steps necessary to conceive. The first part of this chapter is for all bodies, while later in this chapter you will find sections with information that is specific to the type of reproductive system your body has. Given that fertile health is dependent on the underlying health of the human body, we are going to start with information that applies to everyone.

Boosting Your Fertility Means Boosting Your Capacity for Life

The magic of caring for your body well is that you will feel better, both physically and emotionally. Good nutrition, ample sleep, regular exercise, and well-tended mental health all work together cohesively to lower stress and increase feelings of well-being. It may take some time for the changes to become routine, but once you get going, you will start to notice that you have more energy, your moods are more balanced, and you sleep better at night. This means that the same things that help support your fertility also help you weather the stress of trying to conceive—so this applies to prospective parents who are not using their body to conceive as well!

It also means that societal barriers to health and well-being, such as direct and systemic racism, homophobia and transphobia, ableism, and the oppression of poor people are forces to be reckoned with in order to make space for what our bodies need. It means that every act of self-care becomes an act of resistance, and every step toward overcoming these barriers builds the resiliency that you will rely on for a lifetime of parenthood.

The guidelines in this chapter are provided as a best-case scenario, which may be more or less attainable on any given day, and in any given context, depending on the extenuating factors at play in your life. The goal is to create balance in ways that are accessible to you. For instance, when factors beyond your control affect the level of emotional stress you are experiencing, this can be offset by feeding yourself well and stepping up the strategies that bring your body into a state of calm. When racist violence and police brutality puts you at risk for simply exercising outdoors, seek ways to move your body that feel safe and secure, such as BIPOC-led yoga classes that simultaneously nourish and connect you with the power of community. When your budget relies on shift work that keeps you up at night, make sure to feed yourself well and get the sleep you need during the day. No matter what your circumstances, refrain from taking on guilt for not doing everything perfectly, and acknowledge instead that the goal is not perfection, rather, it's striking the best possible balance for yourself as an individual.

DO YOUR BEST TO GIVE YOUR BODY WHAT IT NEEDS

From a Western perspective, there are many body systems—the respiratory system, the cardiovascular system, the digestive system, etc. The body needs every system in order to remain alive—except one: the reproductive system. The reproductive system is connected in some way to every other body system; however, if the body is struggling, it will let go of reproductive function in order to save itself. But at this point in your life, you are not just looking to survive—you want your body to be healthy enough to support two. Think about it this way: if a body isn't getting everything it needs, why would it be open to the demands of an additional human life and/or all that a developing baby needs from the body carrying it? A young body can compensate more effectively, but as we get older, the body becomes less and less able to function without getting what it needs. In fact, as you enter your late thirties and early forties, caring for your body well is required in order to maintain your fertile capacity. As you read this chapter, take note of any area of self-care that you have been neglecting or avoiding—this is likely the missing piece that can make a huge difference not only in your fertile health but also in your capacity to emotionally navigate the process of conceiving and becoming a parent.

CONSIDER THE PAYOFF

Of course, how you take care of your body is ultimately up to you, and no one gets it right all of the time. But it is worth considering what you are willing to do to offset the potential costs of conception. The data is compelling—getting the nutrition, exercise, and sleep you need while avoiding fertility inhibitors such as smoking, alcohol, and environmental endocrine disruptors all support the health of your gametes as well as the hormones that develop them and guide their release.

Don't just invest in donor gametes—invest your time, money, and energy into supporting your body's ability to conceive and/or carry a healthy pregnancy.

Eating for Fertility

It's no wonder that what we put into our bodies will have an effect on our overall health. But what sort of diet is truly healthy? Low fat? Vegetarian? Vegan? Paleo? Keto? Mediterranean? The simple answer is that plant-based, whole-food nutrition is best for fertility. While keto or Paleo diets may work well for building muscle, you aren't looking to build muscle, you are looking to build a baby. Vegetarian and vegan diets are no better if they consist mostly of processed foods and large amounts of soy. Foods that are advertised as low fat are often high in sugar, not to mention that your body needs healthy fats for many functions, including manufacturing hormones.

UNDERSTANDING THE SCIENCE OF HOW EATING PATTERNS AFFECT THE ENDOCRINE SYSTEM

It's not just about what you eat—*when* you eat is also vitally important for the reproductive system. You could be eating the healthiest of foods, but going too long between meals or practicing intermittent fasting means that your body needs to focus on keeping your blood sugar stable instead of reproductive function. Every cell in the human body needs energy (in the form of glucose) to function, which means that if you aren't eating frequently enough, the body will shut down everything else for the sake of survival. In extreme circumstances, such as athletes in training or those struggling with eating disorders, reproductive function can literally be turned off in response to too few calories for the body's energy demands. On the other hand, if your intake of refined sugar and simple carbohydrates (potatoes, pasta, white rice) is too high, the cells of the reproductive system will be damaged by high glucose levels, and hormone production will be disrupted as the body works to store the excess sugar.

The most common scenario I see in my practice is one in which meals are skipped or delayed, resulting in ravenous hunger at mealtimes and/or sugar or carb cravings between meals, which results in the body having to cope with a roller coaster of blood sugar highs and lows throughout the day. Here's a typical example: You wake up, have a cup of coffee, and don't really feel hungry until midmorning, when you grab a scone or a bowl of cereal. You eat lunch on the go around noon, and around three in the afternoon you feel peckish so you grab some chips or crackers—or if you are feeling health conscious, maybe a piece of fruit. Some days, you feel low energy by this time, so you grab a second cup of coffee or tea. At dinnertime, you have a full meal, but during the evening hours, you can't help but have a bit of ice cream or a bowl of popcorn. This is a typical day for many of us, whether our meals are home-cooked or from a restaurant, composed of organic, whole foods or from the freezer section at Trader Joe's. But regardless of what you are eating, this pattern of eating is keeping your body very busy managing your blood sugar.

Here is what is happening to your endocrine system in this scenario: caffeine in your morning coffee, unmediated by intake of food, stimulates an adrenaline response. While this may be desired in terms of the short-term energy boost it provides, an adrenaline, or fight-or-flight, response mobilizes stored glucose and shunts blood flow away from the digestive system, suppressing appetite and raising blood sugar. This gets you through the first hour or two of the day, but by that time, your blood sugar drops again, bringing on an urge for simple carbs. The midmorning carb snack shoots your blood sugar up again, and although a balanced meal at lunch can level things out, you may feel sleepy as your body attempts to recuperate from the ups and downs of the morning. As the afternoon goes on, your blood sugar goes down, and a carb snack and/ or a caffeine pick-me-up raises your blood sugar again, only to crash by the time your day is done, making dinner prep a bit stressful, which may result in ordering out or opting for something processed to pop in the microwave at home. We often experience a day of blood sugar ups and downs as emotional ups and downs, so a late-evening snack may feel like an emotional reward, but meanwhile, the body is stowing away the excess glucose as it braces for another day in the struggle for glucose regulation.

If you are reading this and recognizing yourself, know that you are not alone. If this routine sounds familiar, except that you are often too busy to grab a midmorning or midafternoon snack, you are in good company as well. If you tend to go more than three hours at a time without any protein, whether or not you rely on carbs or caffeine to get through the day, I'm going to take a wild guess that you tend to wake up in the wee hours of the morning and have trouble falling back asleep. This happens because blood sugar fluctuations, and the accompanying stress response, are wreaking havoc on the adrenals. Normal adrenal function consists of a twenty-four-hour circadian rhythm that causes you to wake as the sun comes up. But if your adrenals have to work all day to keep your glucose levels steady, your body clock will be offset, causing you to wake up around two or three in the morning as cortisol levels rise prematurely.

This is a common example of how eating, sleep, and stress are interconnected. Adding in exercise can help blow off some steam, reducing stress and using up some of the carbohydrate intake, but without protein to maintain glucose levels, even exercise can contribute to the problem as the adrenals have to kick in for energy to get through workouts. The good news is that you can bring your body into balance by getting the nutrition, exercise, and sleep you need to maintain steady blood sugar, resulting in fewer emotional ups and downs, mediating stress and enhancing libido, and allowing the reproductive system to function at peak capacity.

There is a simple plan to accomplish blood sugar regulation: Eat protein every three hours throughout the day, and accompany each protein-based meal or snack with a fruit or vegetable from a variety of colors. Add in some whole grains and healthy fats at mealtimes. Listen to your body. If you actually get a little hungry, shaky, or moody closer to two hours than three, you may have a faster metabolism that needs protein every couple of hours. If you are nowhere near hungry at three hours, but at four hours you could eat something, do that. Watch out for sugar or carb cravings—this is your body telling you that your glucose levels are low. Note the time interval since you last had some protein, and step it up so that you don't go so long next time.

If you will be carrying a pregnancy, your body will go through massive changes while growing a small human inside. The need for frequent protein intake goes up even more in the early weeks of pregnancy. If you already have a habit of eating smaller, more frequent meals throughout the day, you are more likely to avoid first-trimester nausea, although you may find that you need to eat even more frequently (every two hours, or as much as every hour) to keep the nausea at bay.

FOCUS ON ANTI-INFLAMMATORY PROTEINS

All proteins are not created equal. Plant-based proteins (lentils, legumes, whole grains, nuts) and fish provide protein without increasing inflammation. Get most of your protein from these sources, adding in moderate amounts of dairy and poultry, and keeping intake of red meat to a minimum. Soy is also a good source of protein, but too much soy can be a problem for fertility because of high levels of soy isoflavones, which are phytoestrogens. Limit your soy intake to no more than twice a week.

The average person needs about sixty grams of protein daily. If you are smaller than average, or larger than average, you may need less or more. If you want to get technical about it, you can calculate 0.8 grams per kilogram (divide your body weight in pounds by 2.2 to get kilograms). A pregnant body needs even more protein daily—up to a hundred grams. While it may be useful to track your intake until you get a sense of how much protein you actually need to eat, the general idea is to eat more plant-based proteins and fish than animal proteins. If you are eating every three hours, your blood sugar will be stable, reducing sugar cravings as well as the propensity to eat larger meals. You will be able to listen to your body, and portion sizes will adjust based on your appetite.

Sources of Protein

Plant Proteins	Grams of Protein per ½ Cup	Animal Proteins	Grams of Protein per Serving
Peanuts	18	Salmon, 4 ounces	24
Edamame	16	Tuna, 4 ounces	20
Peanut butter	14.5	Pork, ½ cup	18
Sunflower seeds	14	Chicken/turkey, ½ cup	17
Pistachios	13.5	Beef, ½ cup	16
Almonds	12	Cottage cheese, ½ cup	14
Hummus	12	Cheddar, 2 ounces	14
Cashews	10	Mozzarella, 2 ounces	13
Tofu	10	Egg, 1	12
Lentils	9	Chèvre, 2 ounces	10
Split peas	8	Greek yogurt, ½ cup	9
Pinto, kidney, navy, and black beans	7.5	Cow milk, 1 cup	8
Whole grains	3-4	Yogurt, ½ cup	7.5

BE CAREFUL ABOUT THE FISH YOU EAT

While the FDA recommends eating eight to twelve ounces of fish every week, it is important to avoid fish sources that are high in mercury. Never eat king mackerel, marlin, orange roughy, shark, swordfish, tilefish (Gulf of Mexico), or bigeye tuna. The highest omega-3 and lowest mercury fish are salmon, sardines, mussels, rainbow trout, Atlantic mackerel, oysters, pollock, and herring. There are many options in between. You can reference information from the FDA or the Environmental Working Group for guidance about avoiding mercury and other contaminants in fish. The EWG recommends wild-caught salmon, in particular, due to high levels of PCBs, dioxins, and insecticides in farmed salmon.

EAT A RAINBOW OF FRUITS AND VEGETABLES

Fruits and vegetables provide the body with carbohydrates, while the antioxidants they contain support reproductive function by regulating oxidative stress. The vitamins and minerals contained in fruits and vegetables are necessary for all bodily functions. Along with whole grains, fruits and vegetables provide the fiber needed for digestive function and balanced microflora, enhancing gut health. While supplements can make up the difference when your food lacks ample vitamins and minerals, supplements do not provide fiber and carbohydrates. Eating fruits and vegetables is the best way to get what your body needs to function well, and to conceive and grow a baby. If you eat a fruit or vegetable every time you have a dose of protein, and the fruits and veggies you eat represent a rainbow of colors, you will get a broad range of vitamins and minerals from your food. Another good practice is to eat leafy greens every day, which helps ensure enough iron to adequately oxygenate your tissues.

BE INTENTIONAL ABOUT PESTICIDE-FREE FRUITS AND VEGETABLES

The reproductive years are an important time to focus on pesticide-free sources of fruits and vegetables. Not only are locally grown, organic fruits and vegetables higher in nutrients, conventional farming practices are one of the primary ways we are affected by endocrine-disrupting environmental pollutants. A 2019 study on dietary patterns and outcomes of assisted reproduction showed higher live birth rates with intake of low-pesticide fruits and vegetables and avoidance of those with high pesticide levels. Babies in utero are affected in a variety of ways by foodborne pesticides ingested during gestation, and pesticides in human milk disrupt the infant microbiome (the beneficial bacteria that keeps our bodies healthy) and central nervous system (the brain and the messages it sends to the body). Children are uniquely susceptible to pesticide toxicity, including links to pediatric cancers, decreased cognitive function, and behavioral issues. An excellent source of information on which foods to always buy organic versus those you can purchase from conventional sources without high levels of pesticides is the Environmental Working Group's annual list of the "Clean Fifteen" and the "Dirty Dozen" based on data on pesticide residue from the USDA.

Clean Produce Buying Guide

Always Buy Pesticide Free	OK to Buy Conventional
Apples, apple sauce, blueberries, celery, cherries, grapes, green beans, leafy greens, nectarines, peaches, pears, plums, potatoes, raisins, spinach, strawberries, sweet peppers, tomatoes, winter squash	Apple juice, asparagus, avocados, bananas, beans, broccoli, cabbage, cantaloupe, carrots, cauliflower, corn, eggplant, grapefruit, honeydew, kiwi, lentils, lettuce, mushrooms, onions, oranges, orange juice, papaya, peas, pineapple, prunes, summer squash, sweet corn, sweet peas, sweet potatoes, tofu, tomato sauce, zucchini

EAT WHOLE GRAINS

There is a big difference between processed grain products and whole grains. Whole grains contain the outer covering of the grain as well as the germ, which contain B vitamins, iron, copper, zinc, magnesium, vitamin E, and antioxidants. Whole grains also contain slow-burn carbohydrates, which are digested more slowly due to the high fiber content. Refined grains such as white rice, pasta, and white flour have the nutritive portion of the grain removed, leaving only starch, which causes rapid elevation of blood sugar as well as inflammation. One of the simplest changes you can make to your eating in support of your fertility is switching to whole-grain bread and pasta, and opting for whole-grain rice as well as other accompaniments to your meals such as barley, brown rice, buckwheat, bulgur, corn, kamut, millet, quinoa, rye, oats, spelt, teff, farro, and wild rice. Whole grains also increase the protein content of your meals by about 3 to 4 grams per serving. If white rice is a staple of your food culture, limit your portion size and offset the carbohydrate load with anti-inflammatory proteins and healthy fats.

EAT HEALTHY FATS

The fats we eat not only make our food taste good, they also help absorb vitamins A, E, D, and K, and they make up the cellular membrane that surrounds every single cell in our bodies (including the egg cell). Fats that are solid at room temperature, such as butter, coconut oil, and dairy products, are called saturated fats, and they contain mostly omega-6 fatty acids, which are pro-inflammatory. Unsaturated fats are found in nuts, seeds, avocados, and fish, and they contain omega-3 fatty acids, which are anti-inflammatory. To support your reproductive system, get most of your fat from unsaturated plant and fish sources, keeping intake of inflammatory fats to a minimum. In practice, this looks like cooking with olive or canola oil; eating nuts, seeds, and avocados every day; and eating fish twice a week. This is the time in life to opt for full-fat yogurt and whole milk and cheese, but maintain a ratio of these foods that is less than your intake of plant-based fats. And above all, avoid trans fats in the form of hydrogenated oils. These are chemically altered oils that appear in processed foods, and they contribute to insulin resistance (a state in which the body is no longer able to cope with high blood sugar levels), inflammation, and ovulatory infertility.

Fertility Foods Cheat Sheet

Eat Lots of These Foods	Limit These Foods
Seafood	Red meat
Poultry	Processed meats
Nuts/Seeds	Dairy
Whole grains	Pasta/White rice
Beans/Legumes	Soy products
Vegetables	Potatoes
Fruits	Sugar and soda
Olive oil	Trans fats

Fertile Living

What you put into your body, and when, is only one aspect of supporting your fertility. In addition to nutrition, there are a number of other important lifestyle factors to consider.

EXERCISE IS SUPER IMPORTANT!

When you exercise, you are putting your good nutrition to work. Exercise pumps blood all the way to the capillary beds that infuse the liver, kidneys, uterus, and ovaries and delivers nutrients to the organs that need them. On a cellular level, oxygen and nutrients are taken in, and carbon dioxide and waste products are released. The cellular respiration process is happening all the time, but when we move our blood via exercise, this process happens much more efficiently. Exercise is the most evidence-based thing you can do to support your fertility.

Regular low- to moderate-intensity exercise is ideal for fertility, while high-intensity exercise, extreme training regimens, and even heavy-exertion occupations can decrease sperm parameters and cause anovulatory cycles (when an egg does not release). This is not a time to train for a triathlon, but it is a great time to get some exercise every day, combining aerobic activities with strength building on alternate days. Exercise enough to get your heart rate up and break a sweat for about half an hour most days—at minimum three to four days per week. This could be done with a brisk walk, a swim at the YMCA, a yoga class, a run, or any other way you love to move your body—however, sperm producers need to be careful about cycling and other forms of exercise that increase heat in the reproductive organs (see page 51).

EXERCISE FOR STRESS REDUCTION AND MENTAL HEALTH

Exercise has the added benefit of lowering stress. The endorphin release that happens with exercise makes you feel good during exercise and immediately after. Exercise helps you sleep better and decreases symptoms of depression and anxiety. It can even have a positive effect on your relationships. It is no wonder that exercise is so important to human life. Be sure to gravitate toward activities you love. If you hate the gym, don't go to the gym—pick something else. If you love to be in nature, get there. If exercise classes provide you with the accountability and camaraderie you need to stick with it, find one that feels good to you.

EXERCISE IN A WAY THAT IS RIGHT FOR YOUR BODY

Make sure that the level of exercise you are doing is enough, but not too much. Making eggs requires enough calories to support the level of physical activity you do. If you regularly engage in high-intensity exercise, especially if your body is on the smaller side, this can cause you to stop ovulating. If your periods are irregular and you exercise a lot, cut back on the intensity of your workouts and add in more calories so that your body doesn't have to choose between the demands you are putting on it and what it has left for reproductive function. If you just don't feel the same without a strenuous workout, do this in the first half of your cycle, when the body is primed for physical exertion. After ovulation, cut way back—especially when you are actively attempting conception. Don't forget to find other ways to mediate your stress during this time, such as making art, meditation, or therapy.

On the other hand, if regular exercise has not been a part of your life for a while, you can jump-start your fertility by adding exercise into your routine. Along with the aforementioned dietary guidelines and ample sleep, increased physical activity can shift the endocrine system in support of conception. Building muscle results in greater insulin sensitivity, which reduces inflammation and oxidative stress on reproductive cells. For those who produce eggs and/or carry pregnancies, especially for those with a larger-than-average body size, you can increase your chances of conceiving by doing an intense workout once or twice a week in addition to moderate exercise on most days. This also supports the production of hormones that cause egg follicles to develop, release mature eggs with strong ovulation, and support the early weeks of pregnancy.

For those who produce sperm and have a body composition with greater-than-average fat tissue, that tissue can function as an endocrine organ, converting the body's testosterone into estrogen and affecting the production of sperm cells in multiple ways. The end result is lowered sperm parameters and reduced fertility. However, restrictive diets can also decrease fertility, and even bariatric surgery can decrease fertility for a time. This is why exercise is so important for reproductive health.

GET ENOUGH SLEEP

Along with physical activity, the body also needs rest. While we sleep each night, the body has a chance to regenerate in a way that it simply cannot when it is supporting mental and physical activity during the day. Although our fast-paced world does not value it, sleep is a vital aspect of physical and mental health. Without it, we start to suffer. The adrenal glands are often left to make up the difference, as we push ourselves in high-stress situations, fully caffeinated, on insufficient sleep. Pregnancy rates go down, sperm count decreases, and menstrual cycles become more irregular with fewer than seven or more than nine hours of sleep each night, especially for those with high levels of stress and those with depression. Too little sleep can contribute to hypothyroidism (low thyroid hormones), which interferes with ovulation and increases the chance of miscarriage; it lowers FSH (follicle-stimulating hormone) levels, which diminishes the development of sperm and egg cells; and it can increase prolactin levels, which is associated with anovulation, PCOS (polycystic ovary syndrome), and endometriosis.

If you work the night shift, it is highly recommended that you get on the day shift or find a different job while trying to conceive and during pregnancy if at all possible. Those who work at night have a higher risk of infertility, miscarriage, preterm birth, and impaired fetal development. Insulin resistance goes up, which contributes to PCOS and gestational diabetes. Inflammation is increased, which exacerbates endometriosis and impacts sperm health. Consider that shift work has been shown to increase the time to conception, so if you are making more money by working at night, but you are also spending more money buying donor gametes or paying for fertility treatments, you may not be coming out ahead.

If you are watching TV or working on your computer right up until bedtime, this may be delaying your sleep. Consider a screen curfew, and implement a bedtime routine such as a warm bath, light yoga and meditation, or even masturbation or sex prior to sleep. Try to go to bed at the same time every night. Keep your bedroom completely dark, cool, and quiet, and only utilize your bedroom for sleep or sex. Make sure you have a supportive mattress and pillow. Limit caffeine intake to one cup at breakfast, and never have caffeine after noon. Limit fluid intake after dinner. Exercise regularly, and keep your blood sugar stable throughout the day. If you have put all of these techniques to use and you still have trouble sleeping, try taking magnesium before bed. Pay attention to what you need to do in order to get ample sleep at night, and do that. Once your baby is born, you will no longer have this luxury—you will get your sleep when you can, because there will always be needs for nighttime parenting in one way or another until your kids grow up and leave home.

MEDIATE YOUR STRESS

It is no wonder that psychological stress can have an effect on fertility. When stress goes up, the body responds by going into a fight-or-flight adrenal response. Over time, chronic stress causes higher and higher levels of cortisol (one of the hormones that is activated by the adrenal response), which can inhibit the release of hormones necessary for ovulation to occur. This is how the body shuts down the reproductive system in times of extreme stress. Stress can even make target tissues, such as the uterine lining and the glands that produce cervical mucus, resistant to estradiol (the primary form of estrogen). In bodies that make sperm, times of psychological stress have been shown to increase oxidative processes in seminal plasma and reduce protective antioxidant activity, which ultimately damage sperm cells.

It is worthwhile to take note of the stress in your life and investigate ways to reduce or mitigate it. After all, trying to conceive is inherently stressful, so your stress level is about to go up simply by virtue of the task at hand, and becoming a parent will change everything. While it may be infused with joy, this major life transition will also bring about an extended period of increased stress. What might you need to rearrange in your life to make space for a baby, and for yourself as a parent? You may find that in making those structural changes now, you gain the time and space you need to slow down, breathe, and create calm in your body.

There are also forms of stress we cannot control. Systemic oppressions, racism, transphobia, and homophobia affect daily life, which means that every moment you take to care for your physical, mental, emotional, and social well-being supports your efforts toward pregnancy. If you suffer from post-traumatic stress, techniques such as EMDR (eye movement desensitization and reprocessing) or CPT (cognitive processing therapy) may ultimately support your efforts to conceive. If there is conflict in your relationship, taking some time for couples work will not only prepare you for co-parenting, it can ultimately support your efforts toward achieving pregnancy as your stress levels go down. Treatment of mood disorders such as depression or anxiety, whether through therapy or pharmacological treatment, can support your efforts to conceive.

Techniques and practices that can help balance the unavoidable stressors in your life include good nutrition, regular exercise, ample sleep, mindfulness meditation, psychotherapy, gratitude practice, yoga, massage and bodywork therapies, making art, connecting with friends and loved ones, and whatever else brings you peace. Every effort you make in support of your mental health and emotional well-being is well worth undertaking not only for your fertility but also for the health of the baby during pregnancy, the transition to parenthood, and the overall well-being of your family as you raise your little one.

FOCUS ON HEALTHY HABITS RATHER THAN WEIGHT LOSS

While many researchers and physicians point to high BMI as a culprit in decreased fertility, the issue is more complex than that. Trying to lose weight is psychologically complex, and additional psychological stress is also not good for fertility. Rather than honing in on BMI or pounds on the scale, which can carry so much negative messaging from our fat-shaming society, I encourage you to pursue healthy habits and let your body adjust without scrutiny. The approach presented here is to eat healthy foods, do moderate physical exercise, and get ample sleep, rather than focusing on trying to lose weight. Meeting these basic needs gives your body the building blocks it needs for optimal health. If the habits you had before were not in line with the recommendations in this chapter, expect your body to reconfigure its structure in some way in response to better nutrition, ample movement, and adequate sleep. In this case, your body size is likely to change; however, this is not the goal. The goal is to give your body what it needs to conceive.

Avoiding Fertility Inhibitors

Supporting your body for optimal fertile function is only part of the picture, especially when there are so many things in our modern world that negatively impact fertility. While it may not be feasible to completely eliminate these things from your life, it is helpful to do what you can to protect your health in a chemical-laden, industrialized culture that is often more concerned with profits than people. Even those living in communities affected by environmental racism can offset the effects by reducing toxins inside the home. For those in recovery from drug or alcohol abuse, know that you are not alone, and you are absolutely worthy of becoming a parent. The personal growth you have done to achieve and maintain your sobriety has made you a better parent already. Own your work, and let it continue to be your foundation and your guide as you enter this new phase of life.

CAFFEINE

Functionally speaking, caffeine diminishes appetite, so if you are having difficulty eating breakfast or you often skip your midafternoon snack, and you tend to drink caffeinated beverages at these times instead, it's time to reconsider caffeine's role in your life. Cutting back on caffeine is an excellent way to help ensure you are supporting your body's nutritional needs while also supporting your fertility. An eight-ounce cup of coffee contains 100 milligrams of caffeine, while an eight-ounce cup of green or black tea contains 30 or 50 milligrams respectively. For bodies that make sperm, consuming 300 milligrams of caffeine daily has been shown to cause DNA damage in sperm cells, and consuming no more than 200 milligrams daily renders the highest birth rates. Caffeinated sodas and energy drinks cause the most sperm damage because of the added effects of sugar and resulting oxidative stress. For bodies that make eggs and carry pregnancies, miscarriage rates double when caffeine consumption exceeds 200 milligrams daily. Consuming more than 100 milligrams daily during pregnancy has also been associated with fetal growth restriction and low birth weight. Although it is impossible to rule out all the factors at play, the safest approach for all bodies is to limit caffeine intake to one cup in the morning, with breakfast (not before).

ALCOHOL

The effects of alcohol on fertile health are clear. Studies on alcohol intake and fertility show that as the number of drinks per week goes up, pregnancy rates and sperm parameters go down. This makes sense when you consider that the body prioritizes the metabolization of alcohol because it is a toxin. Alcohol is processed in the liver, which also plays a central role in glucose regulation and the proper balance of testosterone and estrogen. This means that when alcohol is ingested, the liver's primary function is to process alcohol instead of supporting the reproductive system. In bodies that carry pregnancies, one study showed that consuming one to five drinks per week reduced the likelihood of pregnancy by 39 percent, and at more than ten drinks per week, the odds for pregnancy dropped by 66 percent. In bodies that make sperm, alcohol damages the "nurse" cells that produce sperm in the testes, resulting in lower counts of living, moving, normally shaped sperm cells. Alcohol consumption is so damaging to fertility that even low doses in the month or week prior to in vitro fertilization reduces live birth rates. In light of the data, the safest way to go is to stop drinking alcohol altogether; however, an occasional drink is fine. Red wine from moist regions (Washington; Oregon; and Mendocino County, California) is the best option due to the high resveratrol content, which has antioxidant benefits. Be sure to avoid drinking alcohol on an empty stomach, and as a general rule, don't drink enough to feel buzzed—that's the feeling of your liver working to process the alcohol toxin.

SMOKING AND VAPING

Inhaling toxic substances in the form of smoking and e-cigarettes causes birth defects and cancer, regardless of the type of reproductive system your body has. It takes smokers up to a year longer to conceive than nonsmokers, and this effect is even seen in those who are exposed to secondhand smoke. In addition to the increased likelihood of an earlier death due to lung cancer, prospective parents who smoke have more difficulty getting pregnant. Miscarriage rates are significantly increased when sperm-producing partners smoke, as well as when egg-producing partners smoke.

During pregnancy, nicotine concentrates in the fetus and placenta. It has been associated with sudden infant death syndrome, attention deficit hyperactivity disorder, substance abuse disorders, and aggressive behaviors in offspring. In addition to the increased risk of miscarriage, smokers who produce eggs have a shortened fertile life span due to earlier onset of menopause and reduced markers of ovarian reserve. Smoking even affects the reproductive systems of offspring.

In bodies that make sperm, those who smoke have a high concentration of lead and cadmium in their reproductive fluid, indicating heavy metal damage that decreases the number, physical structure, and motility of sperm cells. Additionally, smoking increases inflammation and oxidative stress, which affects sperm production at every level, from hormonal glands to the function of sperm cells to the DNA contained inside the cells. The DNA damage in smokers' sperm cells is so pervasive that it can even be observed in the cells of offspring. Nicotine has been shown to decrease sperm motility, so if you need to use the patch in order to quit smoking, consider this an intermediary step. The goal is to remove nicotine altogether.

While e-cigarettes are marketed to have lower levels of the toxins contained in cigarette smoke, they contain other chemicals that are just as harmful. Diacetyl used in flavoring causes major, chronic lung damage. In animal studies, e-cigarettes show reduced fertility, delayed implantation, and effects on the growing fetus.

CANNABIS

Regular, heavy cannabis use lowers sperm count, motility, and morphology. At high levels, cannabis blocks the production of reproductive hormones, and cannabis metabolites can even be found in seminal fluid. Because of these effects, it is thought that cannabis can exacerbate other problems with the creation of sperm cells, so quitting or greatly reducing your cannabis use is highly recommended when semen parameters are abnormal.

As for egg health, pregnancy, and lactation, research shows that cannabinoids (THC being the most psychoactive component) cross the placenta and are secreted in human milk. There is concern that research conducted over the past few decades may underestimate effects for offspring because modern strains of cannabis have much higher levels of THC than strains previously studied. Large-scale studies have found a higher likelihood of preterm birth (twice that of nonusers), placental abruption, small-for-gestational-age infants, NICU admission, low Apgar scores, and higher rates of neonatal morbidity and death (three times the risk), as well as neurobehavioral issues in children with cannabis use during pregnancy. One study of daily cannabis users during pregnancy showed resistance to blood flow in the placenta, which is believed to be the reason for impaired fetal growth. Outcomes are dose dependent, meaning the more you use, the greater the likelihood your baby will be affected. THC is stored in fat cells, which accumulate during pregnancy and then are utilized in the production of milk. For this reason, cannabis use during pregnancy contributes to what is passed to the baby during subsequent lactation. To date, there are no studies looking at the effects of the CBD cannabinoid in pregnancy, which many people use to address mental health concerns. While CBD is not psychoactive, it is unclear whether or not it has similar effects on placental blood flow and neonatal outcomes.

ENDOCRINE DISRUPTORS

Unfortunately, there are many substances found in the environment, from soil and water to food production to household products, that disrupt the endocrine system and have a negative effect on fertility. Being aware of the sources and taking steps to reduce your exposure will not only support your efforts to conceive, it will also support the health of your child, ultimately protecting their fertility for generations to come. The most important actions you can take are: use a water purifier, eat plant-based foods, seek low-PCB sources of fish and other seafoods, choose organic fruits and vegetables, get plastic out of your life, store food in glass containers, store water in glass or stainless steel, replace nonstick pans with cast iron or stainless steel, use fragrance-free products, avoid industrial chemicals and heavy metal exposures, and use nontoxic cosmetics.

Avoiding Endocrine Disruptors

Endocrine Disruptors	What You Can Do to Avoid Them
Bisphenol A (BPA) is an industrial chemical that has been used to make plastics since the 1960s. It imitates estrogen and is linked to breast and reproductive cancers. BPA has been detected in the human placenta, amniotic fluid, follicular fluid, and umbilical cord tissue.	Avoid plastics and BPA-lined cans, especially those marked "PC" or recycling label #7. Choose fresh produce and use water bottles made of glass or stainless steel.
Dioxin is pervasive in the environment, and it builds up in the body over time, disrupting sex hormones. This includes the bodies of animals we eat for food.	Cut down on meat proteins, and increase sources of plant-based proteins.
Atrazine is an herbicide used widely on US corn crops, and due to runoff, it is a common drinking water contaminant. It has been linked to prostate cancer in humans and has a range of effects on the reproductive systems of animals.	Choose organic produce and corn products, and drink filtered water (make sure your filter removes this substance).
Phthalates are chemicals found in plastics that cause hormonal changes, lower sperm count and motility, and cause defects in the reproductive systems of male offspring. They are also linked to diabetes and thyroid problems. Phthalates are also found in commercial fragrances.	Store food in glass rather than plastic containers. Do not use PVC plastic wrap, and avoid plastics with recycling label #3. Be careful to choose children's toys that are phthalate free. Choose fragrance-free personal care products.
Perchlorate is found in produce, milk, and drinking water. It blocks iodine absorption, which can lead to thyroid problems.	Use iodized salt and make sure your prenatal vitamin contains iodine.

Flame retardants (PBDEs) are found in upholstery and carpets, causing thyroid problems and impairing brain development. Over time, they concentrate in the bodies of humans and animals, and as a result, PBDEs are excreted in milk.	When doing home or furniture repairs, use PBDE-free materials, and use an N95 mask to protect yourself. If your home has carpet, be sure to use a HEPA-filter vacuum to keep these substances from being dispersed in the air.
Lead affects nearly every body system, and it is especially toxic to babies and young children, causing brain damage, hearing loss, and preterm birth. In adults, it disrupts sex hormone production and the hypothalamic-pituitary-adrenal axis.	Make sure your home does not contain lead paint, and ensure that your drinking water is lead free by using a purifier that removes lead. If the water in your community or home is contaminated by lead, use a filter on your shower and/or bathtub as well.
Arsenic is found in food and drinking water. It disrupts glucocorticoids, which can depress the immune system and cause insulin resistance, osteoporosis, protein wasting, and hypertension.	Use a water filter that removes arsenic from your drinking water.
Mercury enters our air and water as a result of burning coal for fuel. It can disrupt hormonal pathways, causing menstrual problems and ovulatory disorders, and during pregnancy, it can concentrate in the fetal brain.	Choose fish and seafood with low mercury content. Never eat king mackerel, marlin, orange roughy, shark, swordfish, tilefish (Gulf of Mexico), or bigeye tuna. Choose wild-caught instead of farmed salmon.
Perfluorinated chemicals (PFCs) are commonly found in nonstick cookware, and they are extremely pervasive in the environment. They are linked to low birth weight, decreased sperm quality, kidney and thyroid disease, and high cholesterol.	Use stainless-steel or cast-iron pans for cooking. Avoid water-resistant coatings that contain PFCs on clothing, furniture, and carpets.
Organophosphate pesticides are neurotoxins that kill insects in commercial farming; however, they also interfere with fertility and brain development and cause behavior issues, low testosterone, and thyroid dysfunction.	Choose organic, pesticide-free foods.
Glycol ethers are found in paint solvents, cleaning products, brake fluid, deicers, and cosmetics. They have been found to shrink testicles in rats, lower sperm counts in painters, and cause higher rates of asthma and allergies in exposed children.	Avoid all paint solvents, cleaning products, and cosmetics that contain 2-butoxyethanol (EGBE) and methoxydiglycol (DEGME). Wear an N95 mask when you must work with cars or deicing chemicals.

Start Supporting Your Fertility up to a Year Ahead of Time

It may sound obvious once you really think about it, but the real goal isn't just conceiving or getting pregnant—it's about creating a healthy pregnancy and having a healthy baby. Laying down healthy patterns of eating, exercising, and sleeping—and arranging your life to keep stress in check—can take time. Working through barriers to mental health, or investing in the health of your relationship, requires effort, but frankly, it is so much harder to do big emotional work once you have a baby to care for. If you know you have work to do, do it now, because investing in yourself means investing in the person who will parent your child. Fill your cup, put your own mask on first—the more you give to yourself, the more of you there will be for your child.

FOCUS ON THE THREE MONTHS BEFORE YOU CONCEIVE

The most impactful time period for preconception health is the three months before conception occurs. For those who produce eggs, this is the length of time it takes for dormant egg follicles to reach maturity in preparation for ovulation. For those who produce sperm, this is the length of time it takes for new sperm cells to develop. This means that the things you do to support your fertility now will take three months to come into full effect. If you are discontinuing gender-affirming hormones in order to conceive, allow at least three months for new sperm cells to form, or be prepared to allow three months for optimal egg health once your cycles resume.

Egg Health and Pregnancy Preparation

SUPPLEMENTS

PRENATAL VITAMIN WITH METHYLFOLATE

Prenatal vitamins are basically a multivitamin with extra folic acid or folate for the prevention of neural tube defects. All prenatal vitamins are not created equal, especially when it comes to folate. Folic acid is the synthetic form of the folate that occurs naturally in foods. Folic acid is cheaper to produce, so lower-quality prenatal vitamins contain folic acid, which must be converted by the body into the active form, L-methylfolate. Not all bodies do this effectively, so your best bet is to choose a prenatal vitamin that contains methylated folate, especially given that conditions that inhibit the conversion of folic acid are also associated with infertility. Research indicates that a daily dose of 800 to 1,000 micrograms (0.8 to 1.0 milligrams) is ample for most people.

OMEGA-3

Because dietary intake of essential fatty acids is so important for reproductive function, it is worthwhile to consider taking an omega-3 supplement, especially if you eat meat and dairy products. The primitive human diet consisted of a one-to-one ratio of omega-6 to omega-3 fatty acids; however, over the past hundred years, the typical American diet has devolved to a ratio of ten-to-one to twenty-five-to-one. The ratio of these essential fats can affect the entire reproductive process, from the creation and synthesis of reproductive hormones, to egg quality, uterine function, and prevention of preterm labor. If you are conceiving over age thirty-five, omega-3 supplementation is even more important for sustaining egg quality as you age.

The type and source of omega-3 supplement you take is important. Pollutants such as mercury and PCBs in water find their way into fish, which can become especially concentrated in fish oil supplements. Choose a brand that is well regulated and guarantees the absence of these toxins, such as Nordic Naturals. Opt for a concentrated DHA formula during pregnancy and lactation to support baby's brain and eye development. If you are a vegan or vegetarian, choose an algae formula rather than flax oil, because the type of omega-3 in flax often cannot be absorbed.

VITAMIN D

Ample levels of vitamin D are vital for healthy pregnancy and fetal development, as well as the vitamin D content of human milk. Even the minimal amount of supplemental vitamin D in most prenatal vitamins decreases the risk of preeclampsia, gestational diabetes, and low birth weight. Current research investigating the effects of increased dosages of supplemental vitamin D, up to 4,000 IU daily, are showing reduced risk for gestational diabetes and preeclampsia. Because there is no harm in taking this amount of vitamin D, and the benefits are so compelling, I recommend supplementing with 4,000 IU daily before and during pregnancy. During lactation, increasing the dose to 6,000 IU daily provides ample vitamin D content in human milk.

PROBIOTICS

The reproductive tract is colonized with beneficial microflora that are imperative for the health and function of these organs. Flora imbalance is implicated in a range of conditions, from yeast infections and bacterial vaginosis to infertility and preterm birth. The most important species is *Lactobacillus*, specifically *L. rhamnosus*, which helps maintain normal vaginal pH and inhibit the growth of pathogens, including HPV. Various studies have shown that a lack of ample *Lactobacillus* species is common in miscarriage and preterm birth. In fact, *Lactobacilli* are even found in the uterine lining, and research on IVF has shown increased endometrial receptivity and higher rates of implantation, pregnancy, and live birth along with reduced chances of miscarriage when the uterus has normal *Lactobacillus* microbiota. Many midwives have found that probiotic supplementation throughout pregnancy reduces the incidence of GBS (a bacteria that causes neonatal respiratory infection) at term, and a clinical study on this practice is currently underway. Taking an *L. rhamnosus* supplement orally over time will ensure ample colonization throughout the digestive, reproductive, and urinary tracts. Because probiotic supplements contain live beneficial bacteria, they must be kept refrigerated. You can also build your systemic microflora by eating foods that are high in *Lactobacillus* species, such as yogurt, kefir, raw kraut, and kimchi. Additionally, if you have been treated for a vaginal infection, or if you experience itching, odor, or abnormal genital discharge, even if it comes and goes over time, taking an oral supplement with *L. rhamnosus* at a dose of at least 10 CFU per day for at least two months is highly recommended, while vaginal application of *L. rhamnosis* is effective for immediate recolonization of beneficial microflora after treatment for a vaginal infection.

GOING OFF TESTOSTERONE TO CONCEIVE

Most of the time, ovulation does not occur while on testosterone (although sometimes it does, which makes it ineffective as a method of birth control). Stopping testosterone is often the first step in regaining fertility. This can bring physical changes such as fat redistribution, loss of muscle mass, and changes in the texture of skin and hair. Genital changes include increased internal lubrication and the resumption of menses. On the other hand, if your voice got deeper on testosterone, that will most likely remain unchanged. If you have had hair loss while on testosterone, it typically will not grow back; however, changes in facial hair and body hair will most likely stop where they are at or even start to revert. If you had genital growth while on testosterone, that will stay. Most people simply feel different on and off of testosterone, and this can be exacerbated by the shifts in mood as you begin to cycle again.

If you went through puberty before starting testosterone, then your egg-producing organs should regain function just fine after you stop. Up to 80 percent of the time, cycles resume within six months, and for some, it can happen as soon as one month after discontinuing hormone therapy. The data we have so far indicates that transgender hormone therapy does not affect egg health or pregnancy rates. You are just as likely to conceive with your own eggs as any other egg-producing human of the same age, whether that is through sex, insemination, or IVF. The data does not support the use of medications to shorten the time to pregnancy in healthy people, whether they have a history of testosterone therapy or not. There has been no demonstrated risk from having been on testosterone prior to becoming pregnant, so you can fully expect to have a healthy pregnancy—and taking good care of your body through this process can help ensure it.

Sperm Health

TESTICULAR HEAT

The testes are outside the body so that the organs that make and store sperm cells can maintain a constant temperature. When the body heats up, the testes drop, and when the outside environment is cold, the testes rise. This is part of how a sedentary lifestyle can contribute to lowered fertility parameters—a lot of sitting increases testicular heat and restricts proper temperature regulation. If you have a desk job, get up and walk around for ten minutes every hour, or try to use a standing desk. Avoid hot tubs and saunas, and opt for loose-fitting underwear. For trans women and nonbinary folks who tuck, look for ways to offset the time you spend tucking with time spent in loose-fitting undergarments. It's also important to pay attention to the type of exercise you are doing and how it affects the temperature of your reproductive organs. For instance, cycling more than five hours per week is associated with a lower motile sperm count. Make sure that your physical activities do not restrict your testes from descending away from the body as your core temperature increases.

MEDICATIONS TO AVOID

Sometimes doctors overlook the effects of certain medications on fertile function, either because they don't realize a person might be trying to conceive, or the benefits of the medication are thought to outweigh risks to fertility. The following are categories of medications to investigate and reconsider, especially if your semen parameters are abnormal (see Chapter 3):

- Antibiotics
- Antifungal medications
- Blood pressure medications
- Steroid medications
- Hormones
- Narcotics
- Prostate and hair loss medications
- Psychotherapeutic medications
- Chemotherapy
- Other medications, including spironolactone, cimetidine, nifedipine, cyclosporine, allopurinol, sulfasalazine, and colchicine

SUPPLEMENTS

The primary way sperm cells are damaged is oxidative stress, which is why antioxidant activity is necessary for reproductive health. Antioxidants are naturally present in seminal fluid to keep the balance in check, and taking antioxidant supplements can help support that process. If you are over age forty-five, antioxidants are especially important for mediating the DNA damage that occurs with age.

ACES + Zn (with selenium): To reach the therapeutic dosage that has demonstrated benefit in the research, take four capsules instead of two (vitamin C, 1,000 milligrams; vitamin E, 600 milligrams; zinc, 30 milligrams; and selenium, 200 micrograms). Zinc and selenium are utilized in the formation of sperm cells, and vitamins A, C, and E work synergistically with the high-potency antioxidants NAC and CoQ10, below.

NAC (N-acetyl cysteine): NAC is therapeutic at 600 milligrams daily. Sperm count, motility, and morphology are improved when NAC is combined with the supplemental nutrients listed above, along with CoQ10.

CoQ10 (ubiquinol): CoQ10 is best absorbed as the ubiquinol form, taken in a dose of 200 to 300 milligrams daily. One study showed that CoQ10 taken together with a combination of L-carnitine and acetyl-L-carnitine (see page 53) resulted in better progressive motility and higher pregnancy rates, significantly better than without supplementation and at a higher rate than either supplement alone. Similar results were found in a study combining CoQ10 with vitamins C and B_{12}, folic acid, zinc, and selenium.

L-carnitine and acetyl-L-carnitine: Most L-carnitine supplements come in a 250- or 500-milligram capsule, and acetyl-L-carnitine comes in a 500-milligram capsule, so make sure you are taking enough to reach the therapeutic dosages: L-carnitine, 2,000 milligrams; and acetyl-L-carnitine, 1,000 milligrams.

Omega-3: Benefits are reached at 1,800 to 2,000 milligrams daily. A proper balance of omega-3 to omega-6 fatty acids has been shown to enhance sperm parameters.

Vitamin D: Take enough to get your serum vitamin D level above 30 ng/mL at a minimum, which depends on your sunlight exposure. Many in the Pacific Northwest need to take 4,000 to 6,000 IU daily, while those in the Southwest may not need a supplement at all. Vitamin D levels have been found to influence sperm motility and morphology.

GOING OFF FEMINIZING HORMONE THERAPY TO CONCEIVE

While some are still able to produce reproductive gametes while on gender-affirming hormone therapy, most of the time, sperm counts are drastically reduced. The best-case scenario is to conceive or bank sperm prior to initiating hormone treatment. Androgen blockers usually put a pause on sperm production, but once you start taking estrogen, the chance of being able to regain your fertility goes down over time, especially after the first six months. The only way to know if you will be able to regain fertility is to discontinue hormone therapy and wait three to six months for new sperm cells to be created. You can certainly attempt to conceive during that time; however, a semen analysis (see Chapter 3) can be done after three months to get a sense of where you are at. Once you discontinue hormones, many physical attributes will revert, such as skin changes, fat distribution, and facial and body hair. However, any breast development you have achieved will remain, which is reassuring if you are planning to induce lactation.

GUIDANCE FOR CARE PROVIDERS

The information provided in this chapter is based on current evidence for lifestyle factors and fertility. Some prospective parents will come to you wanting to know what more they can do to support their fertility. In this case, it is important to remember that no supplement can take the place of good nutrition, regular exercise, ample sleep, and stress reduction. Please do not overlook the importance of these elements of preconception care. Before offering additional herbs, supplements, treatments, or medications, make sure the families you serve are aware of how the way they live day to day affects their efforts to conceive.

Pay attention to the societal injustices and barriers to health your clients may be experiencing as you make recommendations. If major lifestyle changes are indicated to support fertile health, this can require an investment of time, money, and energy that not everyone will have available to them. Be sure to provide options for incremental change, and phrase the advice you give in a way that helps people understand the reasoning behind your recommendations rather than a list of ideals that may or may not be attainable. People are resourceful, especially when faced with oppression. Your job is to help prospective parents find ways to care for themselves given the circumstances, which ultimately instills a sense of confidence and empowerment that will serve as the foundation for parenthood.

The most impactful, long-lasting interventions you can provide to support fertile health are education and support for living a fertile lifestyle. If you do not have the time or training to provide these elements of care in your practice, please have educational resources (such as this book) available for your clientele, along with referrals to other professionals in your community or online who can.

Resources

Safe Fish Guides

US Food and Drug Administration: www.fda.gov/food/consumers/advice-about
  -eating-fish

Environmental Working Group: www.ewg.org/research/ewgs-good-seafood-guide

"Clean 15" and "Dirty Dozen" Fruits and Vegetables

Environmental Working Group: www.ewg.org/foodnews/clean-fifteen.php

Body-Positive Healthy Cooking

Simply Julia: 110 Easy Recipes for Healthy Comfort Food by Julia Turshen

LAB TESTS AND
FERTILITY EVALUATIONS

Conceiving a child with planning and intention means that you have the opportunity to take steps to ensure that you are in optimal health. You may be reading this as a person who plans to carry a pregnancy with your own eggs, a person planning to provide eggs for a partner or surrogate to carry, or as a person planning to carry a pregnancy conceived with your partner's egg or with a donor egg. You may be producing sperm as a prospective parent or as a donor. Regardless of your role in the constellation of queer family building, this chapter will walk you through the lab tests and fertility evaluations you can access in preparation for conceiving and/or carrying a pregnancy.

Accessing Preconception Health Care

Many trans and nonbinary people avoid accessing medical care whenever we can because we still face marginalization in health care contexts, from inattentiveness to using appropriate names and pronouns, to providers who perpetuate stigma in outward displays of discomfort or even instances of providing substandard care, all within a health care system that often has no place for us on medical forms and/or insurance billing codes that are binary specific. Clinics in some areas refuse to care for members of our community, and those who do invite us to enter care may not invest any resources toward ensuring queer and trans sensitivity. While the coming years will hopefully bring about substantial changes in fertility medicine, as indicated in recent guidelines published by the American Society for Reproductive Medicine, until that change occurs, you will need to be selective about the providers you turn to for fertility care and consider taking a fertility doula or other advocate with you to appointments.

Whether or not you experience disparities related to your gender, most queer people entering fertility clinics find them to be deeply cis/heteronormative. We may be denied certain services or be required to pay for services we do not need. For instance, many clinics will not work with families who are conceiving with a known sperm donor due to cis/heterocentric FDA regulations as well as a general distrust in people's ability to discuss and maintain safer sex practices in order to prevent transmission of STIs during sperm donation. Many require a paid visit with a mental health professional for "psychological evaluation" by a provider who knows little about queer family building. And because fertility clinic protocols are designed around treating heterosexual infertility, the highly medicalized (and expensive) approach in fertility clinics may be more than you need.

Ultimately, how this baby is being conceived, and your role in the conception, will determine the type of preconception health care you need and what sort of provider you will seek. If you are a known egg donor or a gestational surrogate, you will need to follow certain guidelines for testing through the fertility clinic chosen by the intended parents—however, this chapter may provide some insight about the tests that are being performed. The same goes for families conceiving via IVF or reciprocal IVF—you will need to access care at a fertility clinic, but you may want more information about what it all means, which is provided here.

On the other hand, if you are conceiving via intercourse or insemination, you can access preconception care through a variety of care providers, many of whom can also provide IUI services. It is still important, however, to advocate for care that is appropriate for you. For instance, your primary care physician is likely to overlook many important aspects of preconception health that are relevant to donor conception because of a lack of training and experience. Even gynecologists, midwives, nurse practitioners, and naturopaths who specialize in reproductive health may be ill-informed about the nuances of providing preconception care for queer and trans families utilizing donor conception. This is why this book exists, and why this chapter covers lab tests and fertility evaluations in depth enough for you to feel confident in asking for the tests you need, and declining or delaying any that you decide you don't. If you love your care provider, but they know nothing about fertility care or donor conception, pass them a copy of this book! You can also find a list of queer/trans-competent care providers with training in donor conception on the MAIA website or access care with MAIA via telemedicine.

Health History and Physical Exam

The physical exam screens for a variety of health conditions that are important to note prior to pregnancy, such as high blood pressure, enlargement of the thyroid gland, abnormalities in the appearance of breast or chest tissue, hair or skin patterns that are indicative of androgen excess, indications of genital infections, and the presence of pelvic masses. If your body makes sperm, you can go directly to the section later in this chapter on semen analysis—however, if your semen analysis results are abnormal, the next step is to get a physical exam to help identify and potentially treat the cause. If you are a prospective parent planning reciprocal IVF with your egg, or if you are planning to be an egg donor, it is better to see a fertility specialist for your physical exam so that it can include ultrasound evaluation of your ovaries. The same goes for those planning to carry a pregnancy with a partner's egg, or those planning to carry a pregnancy as a surrogate, so that your exam can include ultrasound evaluation of the uterus.

A preconception health history investigates how any underlying health issues may affect your reproductive function. If you are going to be carrying the pregnancy, you'll get guidance for managing your health and well-being throughout gestation and postpartum recovery. This includes questions about your overall health, anything you see a doctor or take medications or supplements to treat, past surgeries or major illnesses, mental health issues, family health history, symptoms of endocrine dysfunction, history of prior pregnancies, menstrual problems, gynecological issues, any current medications or supplements that may be diminishing reproductive function or may need to be discontinued once you are pregnant, and fertility inhibitors such as smoking, alcohol, drug use, and environmental exposures. An evidence-based approach will also include questions about nutrition, exercise, and sleep, as well as quality-of-life indicators such as stress and sexual health.

Be aware that many providers take an overly simplified approach to discussing body weight and BMI. These factors are easily measured and correlate with a variety of health conditions, making them readily identifiable for research. As a result, health care providers and researchers often take the data at face value, especially given that it falls so neatly into the pervasive outlook that fatness is itself a problem. Chances are, if your BMI is over twenty-five, most providers will probably tell you to lose weight. Some may even instruct you to lose 10 percent of your body weight before even attempting to get pregnant. Not only is this attitude hurtful and disparaging, it completely overlooks the variety of factors that contribute to large body size, the lifelong psychological impacts of anti-fat bias, and the fact that this approach means refusing care or providing substandard care because of a person's fatness. While you can ask around in your community or access online provider directories such as Plus Size Birth, your options may be limited if there is not a size-friendly provider in your area. However, you will find a number of helpful ways to reframe recommendations about weight loss and/or to maintain confidence in your ability to care for your body and grow a healthy pregnancy throughout this book. (See Chapter 7, specifically.) The bottom line is that you have every right to try to conceive when *you* are ready, at any size, period.

Preconception Lab Tests

If you are conceiving on your own at home with a known donor, partner, or coparent who can provide sperm, you may be tempted to skip preconception lab tests. After all, if you can insert some sperm and get pregnant, why not just go for it? The answer is that preconception care is optimal health care for those who plan to get pregnant, and there are some lab tests that are an important aspect of that care. Lab tests can identify nutrient deficiencies, blood sugar irregularities, and thyroid issues—all of which can be treated, increasing your chances of conception and providing optimal care for the best pregnancy outcomes. Rather than viewing preconception lab work as just another hoop that queer and trans folks have to jump through in order to get pregnant, think of it as an opportunity to support the health of your pregnancy—an opportunity that is all too often overlooked by cis/het couples who typically do not receive care until they are already pregnant.

In addition to health tests, there are tests that are important for donor selection, as well as preventive health tests that you will want to take care of before getting pregnant. If you are planning to do IUI, your provider may require some of these tests as well as screening for sexually transmitted infections. Depending on your age, your provider may recommend ovarian reserve testing—however, your age is still the most important predictor of your ability to conceive.

While some providers are happy to order whatever tests you ask for, some will be reluctant to order some of the following tests if they do not understand the value of preconception health tests and the added benefit of these tests for people conceiving with donor sperm. If this is the case for you, give your provider a copy of this book when you ask them to order your lab work. If your provider does not typically provide pregnancy-related care, or if they don't understand the FDA guidelines for donor conception, they may not know how to advise you. Your ob-gyn who does not provide infertility care may not be aware of current guidelines for ovarian reserve testing, and they may order more tests than are needed. A fertility clinic that is set up for infertile cis/hetero couples may simply provide an infertility workup and STI screening, which is more than you need if you are not experiencing infertility, and less than you need for optimal preconception care. You can use this chapter to understand your options so that you can make well-informed decisions about your preconception health care.

BLOOD TYPE AND ANTIBODY SCREEN

If you browse a sperm donor catalog, you will notice that each donor's blood type is listed. This may seem extraneous—after all, cis/het people couple up and have kids without giving a second thought to their blood type, so why should we? Because we can. Here are two common types of blood group incompatibilities that can affect pregnancy.

RH INCOMPATIBILITY

If you have an Rh-negative blood type (A negative, B negative, AB negative, or O negative), this means that your body will make antibodies to Rh-positive blood if exposed to it through blood transfusion or pregnancy. If you are Rh-negative and you use a donor who is Rh-positive, your baby could inherit the Rh-positive blood type from the donor. Because the baby is living and growing inside your body, you could be exposed to the baby's blood through any known or unknown source of bleeding between the placenta and the uterine wall at any time during pregnancy. The most common time for blood exchange to happen is during childbirth, so the routine practice is to give Rh-negative pregnant parents an injection of Rh immune globulin in the third trimester of pregnancy and again after birth. However, this does not protect the baby in your current pregnancy— it only protects future pregnancies. If your baby's blood happens to mix with yours early in this pregnancy, your body can mount an antibody response that attacks the baby's red blood cells, causing hemolytic disease of the fetus and newborn. While this may be rare, if it happens to you, the consequences can be devastating.

ABO INCOMPATIBILITY

In a similar but much less severe situation, a pregnant parent whose blood type is different from the baby's blood type can create antibodies to the baby's blood. This happens almost exclusively in pregnant parents with type O blood, affecting babies with type A, B, or AB blood. ABO incompatibility is much less severe than Rh incompatibility. Babies who are affected develop jaundice in the first twenty-four hours of life and must receive phototherapy.

Knowing your blood type can inform your donor selection, and adding the antibody screen to your blood work identifies red blood cell antibodies you may already carry from a previous pregnancy or blood transfusion. If you have an Rh-negative blood type, it is ideal to select an Rh-negative donor. If you have type O blood, it is best to select a type O donor. However, this is not always possible for a variety of reasons. If you find yourself in this situation, read more about these conditions and discuss the implications with your care provider as you finalize your donor selection.

CBC AND FERRITIN

The CBC, or complete blood count, measures various indices of red blood cells, white blood cells, and platelets. It can reveal abnormalities in the shape, size, and number of red blood cells, which can indicate iron-deficiency anemia, B_{12} or folate deficiency, hemoglobin synthesis disorders (thalassemia), and sickle cell anemia. Ferritin is a measure of your stored iron, which is the earliest indication of iron deficiency.

Iron is super important for growing a healthy baby, and your red blood cells contain most of your body's iron. Once you are pregnant, your blood volume expands so much that there is 50 percent more blood circulating through your body by twenty-eight weeks of pregnancy. As your blood volume increases, the body does everything it can to build new red blood cells, including slowing down your digestion so that you can absorb more iron from the foods you eat, shifting the way iron is absorbed by your cells, and utilizing your iron stores (which become fully depleted by the end of pregnancy). Iron deficiency can cause you to feel tired and mentally sluggish, and if it continues or worsens during pregnancy, it can affect your baby's brain development and overall growth patterns.

Even if you are not currently anemic, if your stored iron (ferritin) is low, you will most surely develop iron deficiency anemia during pregnancy. This is why the best approach is to test both CBC and ferritin levels before you get pregnant, so you have a chance to build more reserves if needed. Ferritin levels are considered normal above twelve, but it is ideal to start pregnancy above twenty so that you have some leeway in case you have nausea, vomiting, and food aversions in early pregnancy that keep you from being able to eat iron-rich foods or keep supplements down. If you have abnormal red blood cell values or low ferritin, you will want to follow up with your care provider for additional tests to identify the cause and discuss treatment before becoming pregnant.

TSH AND THYROID ANTIBODIES

Thyroid hormones play an important role in the reproductive system. They directly impact ovarian function as well as pituitary hormones such as GnRH (gonadotropin-releasing hormone). At least one out of ten people assigned female at birth will have a thyroid disorder at some point in their lives, often resulting in irregular cycles and impaired fertility. During pregnancy, low thyroid hormone levels can cause miscarriage and preterm birth, and high thyroid levels can cause preeclampsia, small for gestational age babies, preterm birth, and congenital malformations.

Fortunately, testing is easy and treatment is available. Current guidelines support routine testing if it has taken more than a year to conceive; however, due to the resources involved in donor insemination and the compounded grief of pregnancy loss for our families, I highly recommend testing for thyroid conditions prior to conceiving. Furthermore, if you are at increased risk due to an autoimmune condition, a family history of autoimmune thyroid disease, or a BMI over forty, the data supports testing your thyroid function. You should also have your thyroid checked if you have symptoms of hypothyroidism (irregular cycles, weight gain, depression, fatigue, cold intolerance, muscle or joint pain, dry hair or skin, enlargement of the thyroid gland, or constipation) or hyperthyroidism (irregular cycles, weight loss, anxiety, irritability, rapid or irregular heartbeat, heat intolerance or sweating, hand tremors, enlargement of the thyroid gland, or eyes that appear overly prominent). Keep in mind that biotin supplements can interfere with test results, so be sure not to take biotin within twenty-four hours of a thyroid blood test.

TSH

The most basic test for thyroid function is thyroid-stimulating hormone (TSH). Because the role of TSH is to stimulate thyroid hormone production, abnormally low TSH indicates thyroid hormone levels that are too high (hyperthyroidism), and abnormally high TSH indicates thyroid hormone levels that are too low (hypothyroidism). You may have had your TSH tested in the past and been told it was fine; however, when it comes to reproductive function, the target range is 0.3 to 2.5 mU/L, which is more narrow than for general health (and equivalent to the normal range for TSH in the first trimester of pregnancy).

THYROID ANTIBODIES

There are two types of thyroid antibodies, Anti-Thyroperoxidase (TPOAb) and Anti-Thyroglobulin (TgAb), which can cause the thyroid gland to attack itself, resulting in autoimmune hypothyroidism. Up to 17 percent of pregnant people have thyroid antibodies, and this has been shown in multiple studies to double the risk of pregnancy loss, even when TSH values are classified as normal. If you have thyroid antibodies, it is important to test your TSH levels during pregnancy to make sure they are staying in the optimal pregnancy range per trimester.

TREATMENT AND FOLLOW-UP FOR THYROID CONDITIONS

If your lab work indicates hyperthyroidism (TSH under 0.3 mU/L), you should receive a full endocrine workup. For hypothyroidism (TSH over 4.0 mU/L), levothyroxine should be administered to bring TSH into the target range (under 2.5 mU/L). Opt for synthetic levothyroxine rather than desiccated thyroid hormone during pregnancy because desiccated thyroid supplements do not deliver adequate amounts of thyroid hormone to the fetal brain.

Research has still not pinned down the best approach for those with mildly elevated or "subclinical" hypothyroidism, defined by TSH that is higher than the target range but still under 4.0 mU/L. However, since subclinical hypothyroidism is associated with miscarriage and preterm birth, many providers opt to treat with levothyroxine, especially when the level of thyroid antibodies is very high, or when the person is over age thirty-five, has diminished ovarian reserve, or has experienced recurrent miscarriage.

Iodine is vital for the production of thyroid hormones. The recommended total intake is 250 micrograms before and during pregnancy as well as during lactation. Dietary sources include iodized salt and seafood, although poultry, eggs, meat, and commercial dairy products may contain iodine from supplemented feed. Your prenatal vitamin should have at least 150 micrograms of potassium iodide, or up to 250 micrograms if you lack sources of dietary iodine. More iodine is not better, which is why kelp supplements are not recommended—they can actually shut down thyroid function due to abnormally high levels of iodine.

HEMOGLOBIN A1C

The A1c is a simple way to screen for diabetes or prediabetes. Glucose circulating in the bloodstream attaches to hemoglobin on red blood cells and remains there for the lifetime of the cell (about 120 days), which means your A1c is a reflection of your average blood sugar level over the past three to four months. Type 1 or type 2 diabetes presents a wide range of serious concerns during pregnancy and will need to be followed by a physician. However, a more common concern is prediabetes (A1c 5.8 to 6.4 percent), which is a result of insulin resistance, a major risk factor for gestational diabetes.

PREVENTING GESTATIONAL DIABETES

Gestational diabetes mellitus, or GDM, is more common in those of Hispanic, African, Native American, South or East Asian, or Pacific Islander descent; those with a family history of diabetes; BMI above thirty; age above twenty-five (!); and history of GDM or a large baby in a previous pregnancy. Risks of GDM include preeclampsia, which is dangerous for both the pregnant person and the baby, as well as growing a larger-than-average baby, which increases the chances of induction of labor, birth injury, and cesarean birth. Babies exposed to high blood sugar levels during pregnancy have a difficult transition to life outside the womb, including an increased risk of respiratory distress, jaundice, and hypoglycemia, and a higher chance of developing diabetes and metabolic syndrome later in life. Those who develop GDM during pregnancy are seven times more likely to develop type 2 diabetes later in life.

Finding out you have elevated glucose before pregnancy affords you the opportunity to address insulin resistance (see the PCOS Care Plan in Chapter 7) and get your blood sugar under control before you conceive, which lowers your risk of developing gestational diabetes. The recommended changes in nutrition and exercise may feel overwhelming now, but given the lifelong implications of insulin resistance, the new habits you develop will support your health for years to come. Getting your blood sugar into the normal range will help shorten the time to pregnancy once you start trying to conceive, and the nutrition and exercise changes will need to continue throughout your pregnancy in order to prevent a GDM diagnosis. If you do end up developing GDM, it's still possible to have good outcomes with "diet-controlled" GDM, which means using a glucometer to help give you feedback about how the foods you eat affect your glucose levels, along with increasing your exercise. The big picture here is that if you have elevated blood sugar, you will need to adjust your eating habits and increase exercise sooner or later, and the sooner it happens, the better your experience during pregnancy will be. It can help you remain low risk, which has enormous implications for the health of your pregnancy as well as your experiences during pregnancy and birth.

If you have a large body size, many providers will treat you as if you have GDM, and you may be tested for GDM early in pregnancy. While this practice definitely carries undertones of anti-fat bias, the data suggests that both having a large body size and having GDM are independently associated with the same risks. A very large data set called the HAPO (Hyperglycemia and Adverse Pregnancy Outcome) Study showed an increased risk of preeclampsia, growing a large baby, and cesarean birth with either large body size *or* GDM. However, having a large body size *and* GDM presents an even higher level of risk. This means that if you are a large person, it's even more important to get your blood sugar under control prior to pregnancy. It also emphasizes the need to have a fat-positive care provider, or at least a provider who is discerning enough to take your glucose levels into account and have respectful discussions with you about your actual level of risk.

VITAMIN D

Vitamin D is vital for regulating the immune system, keeping inflammation in check, mediating insulin sensitivity, producing reproductive hormones, creating a receptive uterine environment for implantation, allowing ample nutrient exchange through the placenta, growing a healthy baby, and providing ample vitamin D in human milk. In addition to being implicated in PCOS and endometriosis, during pregnancy, vitamin D deficiency is associated with preeclampsia, low birth weight, and GDM. While vitamin D supplementation is recommended in all pregnancies as discussed in Chapter 2, testing your vitamin D level can ensure that you are taking a high enough supplemental dose. While vitamin D levels are considered to be sufficient above 30 ng/mL, insufficient from 20 to 29.9 ng/mL, and deficient below 20 ng/mL, levels up to 100 ng/mL are considered to be normal, and toxicity is not shown until vitamin D rises above 200 to 300 ng/mL. For reproductive health, it is ideal to bring your vitamin D level up to 50 to 60 ng/mL to ensure you remain in the ideal range.

CYTOMEGALOVIRUS (CMV) IGG

CMV is a relatively common viral respiratory infection. More than half of all adults have been exposed to CMV at some point in their lives, usually during childhood or while caring for young children. CMV is typically a mild or even asymptomatic infection; however, if CMV is contracted during pregnancy, the virus can cause hearing loss and delayed cognitive development in offspring. Because of this, the FDA requires all sperm donors to be tested for CMV. If a donor has an active CMV infection (IgM antibodies), their samples will be destroyed. Samples from donors with evidence of a past CMV infection (IgG antibodies) are allowed to donate, and you will see their status in the donor catalog as "CMV positive." This ultimately is very confusing, because you are being notified that the donor has past exposure, and therefore immunity, to CMV, which poses no risk to you. In fact, IUI-ready samples offer additional protection because the part of a sample that could even potentially carry the infection is removed in the wash process.

So why is CMV even an issue? The simple reason for this is that testing for CMV used to be less accurate than it is now, and FDA regulations have not yet been changed to reflect current, more accurate testing methods. However, most clinics still require you to test yourself for CMV and to select your sperm donor according to your own status. If you have evidence of immunity (IgG positive), then you can use donors who are CMV positive or negative. If you do not have evidence of immunity, you may be required to only use a donor who is CMV negative. Your CMV result can be reassuring if you have immunity. If you find that you lack immunity to CMV, it is important to prevent contracting it while you are pregnant by avoiding people with respiratory infections; thorough handwashing after contact with diapers or children's oral or nasal secretions; not kissing kids on the mouth or cheek; not sharing food, drinks, or utensils with young children; and keeping toys and surfaces disinfected. The highest rates of CMV occur in day care workers and in parents who have an infected child.

GENETIC CARRIER SCREENING

Genetic carrier screening is ideal for anyone planning a pregnancy, although many people do not opt for this if they are planning to conceive with a partner. This test identifies genetic variants that do not affect you but are carried in your DNA and may affect your offspring. These are called autosomal recessive conditions. Unless you have a relative who is affected, or unless there is a relative who has been tested and informs you that a certain condition may run in your family, you would not otherwise know you carry the gene for that condition.

Both the sperm cell and the egg cell must carry a genetic variant in order for a child to be affected by the disease or to become a carrier themselves. Sperm banks refuse donors who are carriers of the most common genetic conditions, but they may include donors with rare conditions. In this case, the bank will provide you with this information about the donor, and it is advised that you be tested to make sure you don't carry the same variant. If you are using a known donor, test yourself, and if you find that you are a carrier for a genetic condition, you can then have your potential donor tested to make sure they don't carry the same variant.

Spinal muscular atrophy, cystic fibrosis, and fragile X syndrome are the most common conditions included in genetic carrier screening panels; however, some labs now test for up to five hundred genetic conditions. There are conditions that are more common in certain ethnic populations, such as those of Ashkenazi Jewish descent. No matter what your heritage is, talk to your care provider about conditions you may be at higher risk for passing to your offspring, or opt for the full range of tests. Private labs often include the entire panel for the same cost as smaller panels, so be sure to ask about this as you weigh your decision.

If you are using a sperm bank, have your genetic screening performed by the same laboratory the sperm bank uses so that you will be tested for the same variants the donor has been tested for. With a known donor or a partner, do both tests with the same lab. If you find that you are a carrier of an autosomal recessive condition, you will benefit from a consultation with a genetic counselor, which is often included in the cost of the test.

While you may consider some heritable conditions more important to know about than others—for instance, conditions that greatly impact quality of life or cause death in infancy or childhood versus conditions that are mild and don't show up until adulthood—it is important to make an informed decision about whether or not to get this testing done before you conceive.

IMMUNITY TO RUBELLA AND VARICELLA

Even if you received all of your childhood vaccinations, the immunity provided through vaccines can wear off over time. This is especially a problem for illnesses that can affect babies in utero if they are contracted during pregnancy, such as rubella and varicella. However, if you contracted the actual disease, as is often the case with varicella (better known as chicken pox), then your body will mount an immune response that lasts throughout your lifetime.

You can test for immunity to rubella and varicella with a simple lab test. If you are not currently immune, you can get the vaccine—but you must wait at least thirty days after receiving the vaccine to become pregnant. Some providers recommend testing for varicella immunity even if you had the disease during childhood. Some providers opt to test for immunity to the entire MMR series (measles, mumps, and rubella) to see if a booster shot is needed, even though it is rubella that presents the direct concern for pregnancy—this is because any disease that causes a high fever can be harmful to the fetus, and these diseases still exist in the general population.

SEXUALLY TRANSMITTED INFECTIONS

Infections such as HIV, hepatitis B, hepatitis C, HTLV, syphilis, gonorrhea, and chlamydia are all sexually transmitted, although many of these can also be passed by other routes of exposure to body fluids, including insemination with fresh sperm samples, tattoo or piercing tools, blood transfusions, non-sterile medical equipment, IV drug use, and needle-stick injuries in the health care professions.

Testing for STIs is required by many IUI providers, and it is a routine part of prenatal care. Screening for these infections prior to pregnancy allows you to seek treatment ahead of time. For instance, HIV can be treated with antiretroviral medications. Hepatitis B requires close management during pregnancy, but transmission to the baby can be prevented with hepatitis B immune globulin and hepatitis B vaccine at birth. There is no treatment available for transmission of hepatitis C to the baby during pregnancy, so the best strategy is to identify and treat it prior to conception. Syphilis rates have been increasing in recent years, and if you test positive, it can be treated with antibiotics prior to pregnancy. One thing to note is that pregnancy is notorious for causing false-positive syphilis results, so if you have a negative result prior to pregnancy and no possible route of exposure, you might feel more reassured if you do happen to get a false-positive test result during pregnancy. Gonorrhea and chlamydia are both treatable and can cause infertility and pelvic inflammatory disease if left untreated. The majority of those who have a chlamydia infection do not exhibit symptoms, so it is especially important to have this test completed before doing IUI, which can carry the bacteria into the upper reproductive tract. Additional tests for HTLV (human T-lymphotropic virus), West Nile virus, and Zika virus (for those who have been in geographical exposure areas) are required under FDA regulations for donors.

While HIV-positive donor conception is prohibitively complicated, conceiving with a partner who is HIV-positive is possible. Research indicates that an HIV-positive person who has an undetectable viral load (less than 200 copies/milliliter) cannot transmit the virus. If a pregnant person is HIV-positive, antiretroviral therapy during pregnancy reduces vertical transmission rates (to the baby) to 1 to 2 percent if viral loads are kept below 1,000 copies/milliliter. Serodiscordant couples where the sperm-producing partner is HIV-positive and the carrying partner is HIV-negative can limit the possibility of transmitting the virus to the pregnant person by having the sperm-producing partner reach an undetectable viral load, providing the carrying partner with PrEP (pre-exposure prophylaxis), and using barriers for sexual activity except for timed intercourse to conceive. Assisted reproductive techniques such as modified sperm washing and IUI or IVF with ICSI (see Chapter 8) are additional options for protecting the pregnant person and the baby, although accessing care typically requires maintaining a viral load below 200 copies/milliliter for six months preceding treatment. It is worthwhile to note that the HIV virus can diminish ovarian function, and the virus as well as antiretroviral therapy can affect semen parameters and sperm DNA. Given that the fertility industry is reticent to provide care with fresh samples from a known donor in any case, let alone with a donor who is HIV-positive, accessing care may be nearly impossible. (Certain clinics in the state of California may be the only option, see page 114.)

Herpes simplex virus (HSV) is not on the list of FDA-required tests for gamete donors and is not typically included in preconception lab tests. However, HSV-2 can cause miscarriage or birth defects if it is contracted during the first trimester of pregnancy, and it can cause serious illness if it is passed to the baby during birth. (If you know you have genital herpes, be sure to discuss this with your prenatal care provider once you are pregnant.) HSV is transmitted through shedding of viral particles, which is a consideration for conception if the infection is in the genital area of your sperm-producing partner, coparent, or donor. If you are conceiving with a partner who has genital HSV-2 and you have not yet contracted the infection, you will need to exercise utmost caution to prevent it during pregnancy. Likewise, if your known donor or coparent is found to be positive for HSV-2, you will need to avoid the risk of contracting the infection through viral particles that could shed into the seminal fluid during sample collection. While transmission can be mitigated by having them take medication (acyclovir or valacyclovir) to reduce the likelihood of shedding and refraining from sample collection during an active lesion, some opt instead to have samples washed and cryopreserved in accordance with sperm bank protocols, which are thought to be effective at preventing transmission of HSV.

PAP AND HPV SCREENING

If you are not up to date on your Pap and HPV screening, get this done before you are pregnant. These gynecological screening tests are done to identify and treat reproductive cancers, and pregnancy does not offer any immunity from these conditions. In fact, some cancers are even more prolific during pregnancy, so make sure you are all clear beforehand. Also, make sure you are keeping up with monthly self-chest/breast exams, which help you become familiar with your body so that you can more successfully identify any changes that may need follow-up.

MEASURES OF "OVARIAN RESERVE"

The term "ovarian reserve" is misleading, because there is no test that can tell you how many eggs you have left, nor is there a test that can predict your likelihood of successfully conceiving with your own eggs. Simply put, your age is the most important factor in determining the likelihood that your eggs will be able to contribute to conception. So, if you are planning to conceive via insemination or intercourse, you don't need ovarian reserve testing at the outset. How long to try without seeking medical assistance, based on your age, is covered in Chapter 1.

On the other hand, what ovarian reserve can predict is how your body is likely to respond to fertility medications. If you have had trouble conceiving and you seek evaluation at a fertility clinic, this testing will help inform your care plan. If you are looking to use your eggs for conception via IVF, either as a prospective parent, an egg donor, or a traditional surrogate, your ovarian reserve will be an important part of your initial assessment because medications will be used to stimulate your ovaries during the IVF process. This testing may also be useful if you and your partner both have eggs, and you need help deciding whose eggs to use for IVF.

The gold standard for assessing ovarian reserve is a blood draw for serum AMH (anti-Mullerian hormone) and an AFC (antral follicle count) ultrasound. Together, these tests reflect the relative size of your remaining pool of eggs, as well as the actual number of egg follicles your body selects in preparation for ovulation at the beginning of your cycle. The fewer eggs you have left, the lower your AMH level will be, and the fewer eggs your body will recruit for ovulation each month. You are looking for your AMH to be above 1 ng/mL (ideally above 2), and your AFC to be at least 10 (ideally around 20).

Avoid at-home finger prick or saliva test kits that say they can measure your ovarian reserve. Not only are they less accurate than serum values from a blood draw, they typically include hormones other than AMH that are no longer standard of care. The same goes for test kits that include progesterone in the same sample as other hormones, because these hormones fluctuate throughout the cycle and need to be drawn on the appropriate cycle days. None of these at-home tests actually tell you how many eggs you have left, they don't predict your ability to get pregnant, and getting the tests done does not improve out-comes—but they do increase your financial expense.

PROGESTERONE

Progesterone testing is for confirming ovulation. Some people worry that they might have low progesterone and want to get this hormone tested. However, progesterone is a pulsatile hormone, meaning that it fluctuates throughout the day. A single progesterone result may be from the peak or the trough of a pro-gesterone pulse, or somewhere in between. This means the results are essentially meaningless. A progesterone test cannot tell you whether or not your progester-one is high enough, and there is no evidence that treating low progesterone with pills or suppositories increases live birth rates (unless your cycle was managed with gonadotropin medications or you conceive via IVF or embryo transfer). The single meaningful reason to test your progesterone is to confirm that ovulation occurred, and in this case, it should be drawn about a week after ovulation, typi-cally on cycle day twenty-two or later if you suspect ovulation occurred later than cycle day fifteen. You can also confirm that ovulation is occurring by tracking your basal body temperature (see Chapter 6).

Assessment of the Uterus and Fallopian Tubes

If you are planning to carry a pregnancy, there are a couple of ways to assess the size and shape of the uterus while also checking to see that the fallopian tubes are clear (which means that sperm cells can make it to the egg). Abnormal growths such as fibroids or polyps can also be identified, as well as structural abnormalities such as a bicornate uterus or a uterine septum. The HSG (hysterosalpingogram) involves injecting a dye into the uterus and viewing the structure of the uterus and spillage through the fallopian tubes with an X-ray. The SIS (saline infusion sonogram) is very similar, although saline solution and ultrasound are used. Which test is performed typically depends on physician preference and clinic setup; however, if the results of one test are inconclusive, the other method is often performed as a follow-up.

These tests are part of an infertility workup, but those who want to have every possible screening test performed before attempting conception may opt for this type of investigation. If your tubes are blocked, you could be saving yourself thousands of dollars in futile IUI cycles—dollars that could otherwise have been spent on IVF. If polyps or fibroids are identified that may interfere with implantation, you can increase your chances of pregnancy by having these removed. Some variations in uterine structure present increased risks for pregnancy complications, so you may wish to make an informed decision prior to conception if this is the case for you. At one time, it was thought that doing the HSG procedure might actually help "clear" the fallopian tubes, and some studies showed increased pregnancy rates during the first few cycles following HSG. However, further studies did not replicate those results, so this procedure is not reliable for improving your chances of conception.

The physical discomfort involved with these tests is a valid deterrent. Please know that many care providers minimize the experience of getting an HSG or SIS, but reports of extreme pain and cramping, including nausea and vomiting, are common. Some people even faint or pass out. If you opt to have this test done, you can take an ample dose of ibuprofen or Tylenol before the test, or you can request a prescription for Valium as a stronger alternative, especially if you have a history of trauma or negative experiences with pelvic exams. Because of the pain and discomfort of this test, many people decline it unless they are having difficulty conceiving. On the other hand, conceiving with donor sperm can be quite expensive, so some people opt to have this test performed before spending money on conception attempts. The choice is ultimately yours.

Semen Analysis

The semen analysis is the only test needed to screen for fertile function in a body that makes sperm. Conception is a trial-and-error process, but a basic level of expected fertility is a vital starting point. While some families will simply try to conceive and not look to any further testing unless attempts have been unsuccessful, those who are selecting a known sperm donor will want to ensure that the person they choose to help them conceive is fertile.

Because sperm cells can live for a short time outside the human body, they can be examined with a microscope, and inferences can be made about the fertility of the body they came from by evaluating the quantity and quality of those cells. The semen analysis is used to analyze the qualities of the seminal fluid as well as the sperm cells in a given sample. After a two- to five-day period of abstinence, a sample of ejaculate is self-collected via masturbation and given to the lab for evaluation. The lab measures how many cells there are, how many of those cells are moving, how quickly they are moving, and how many of them are normally shaped.

SEMEN PARAMETERS

Volume: The total amount of seminal fluid

Count: The total amount of sperm cells in the sample

Concentration: How many sperm cells are in 1 milliliter of fluid (count divided by volume)

Motility: The percentage of sperm cells that are moving

Progressive motility: The percentage of sperm cells that are getting somewhere versus just twitching or swimming in circles

Morphology: The percentage of cells that are normally shaped

pH: The chemical property of the seminal fluid from acid to base

Round cells: Either immature sperm cells or white blood cells

The chart on the next page can be used to give you an idea of the range of values you might expect to see on an analysis. The fifth percentile reflects the lowest cutoff for "normal" values, while values up to and beyond the fiftieth percentile are commonly seen among healthy donors in my practice.

Normal Semen Values

	5th Percentile (Low Cutoff)	50th Percentile (Average)
Volume	1.5 milliliters	3.7 milliliters
Count	39 million	255 million
Concentration	15 million per milliliter	73 million per milliliter
Motility	40%	61%
Progressive motility	32%	55%
Morphology	4%	15%

INTERPRETING SEMEN ANALYSIS RESULTS

The cutoff values for a "normal" semen analysis are set by the World Health Organization (WHO). They are based on a data set of people who successfully contributed to a pregnancy within twelve months' time. That data is arranged by percentile. The fifth percentile means that 5 percent of the people who caused a pregnancy had those values. The fiftieth percentile means that 50 percent of the people who caused a pregnancy had those values. The WHO consensus is that anything above the fifth percentile is considered "normal." This does not mean that someone whose values fall below the fifth percentile can't contribute to a pregnancy, it just means it's relatively rare. Most fertility specialists are reassured by values that are above the fifth percentile, because these values are reasonable assurance that you will be able to conceive within a year's time, meeting the cis/heterocentric definition of normal fertility.

The most important factor is the total motile sperm count (TOMO), which is calculated by multiplying the total count by the percentage of cells that are motile.

COUNT X MOTILITY = TOMO

In fertility medicine, a minimum TOMO of 10 million is considered adequate, which is why most sperm banks guarantee a minimum of 20 million per milliliter (which calculates to 10 million per 0.5-milliliter vial).

WHAT TO DO IF YOUR SEMEN PARAMETERS ARE BELOW NORMAL

If your semen analysis shows results below the fifth percentile, repeat the test after about thirty days to make sure the results are accurate. If you get similar results the second time, you will want to investigate the cause. In the human body, many health problems can affect the reproductive system, which makes this test akin to a "canary in the coal mine," meaning that if there is a problem with your overall health or your reproductive health, this may be reflected in a semen analysis. If your semen analysis is abnormal, you should see your physician to investigate the following:

Urinary tract infections and sexually transmitted infections cause high numbers of white blood cells to flood the reproductive system, creating massive amounts of oxidative stress. While this immune response may protect your overall health, it can wreak havoc on your reproductive function.

Chronic nonbacterial prostatitis accounts for the vast majority of cases of increased oxidative stress in semen fluid, and it occurs in 10 percent of people who produce sperm.

Testicular issues include varicocele (enlargement of the vessels in the scrotum); cryptorchidism (undescended testicle), even when surgically corrected early in life; and testicular torsion.

Chronic diseases include diabetes, kidney disease, hemoglobinopathies, and MTHFR.

Vasectomy reversal is sometimes followed by infertility due to inflammation and oxidative stress—this is one of the reasons that reversal may not be effective.

Whether or not you are able to identify and treat a specific culprit, you will want to focus on rebuilding your fertile health while removing fertility inhibitors (see Chapter 2). The things you do to support your overall health can improve the number, shape, and function of your motile gametes. While new sperm cells are being made all the time, it takes about two to three months for each new sperm cell to develop, so plan to get another semen analysis performed about three months after any treatments or fertility support.

Lab Tests and Fertility Evaluations for Every Body

Test/Evaluation	Carrying a Pregnancy	Providing Eggs	Providing Sperm
Physical exam	✓	✓	For abnormal semen analysis
AMH and AFC	For infertility workup/IVF/ ovarian stimulation	✓	
HSG or SIS	For preconception screening or infertility workup		
Progesterone	If ovulation is in question		
Genetic carrier screen	If conceiving with own eggs	✓	✓
Blood type and Rh	✓	✓	If pregnant person is Rh-negative
RBC antibody screen	If Rh-negative		
CBC	✓		
Ferritin	✓		
Hemoglobin A1c	✓		
TSH and thyroid antibodies	✓	✓	
25-hydroxy vitamin D	✓		
Varicella immunity	✓		
Rubella immunity	✓		
CMV IgM/IgG	✓		✓
STI tests (HIV-1/2, hep B, hep C, T. pallidum, gonorrhea, chlamydia)	✓	✓	✓
HSV-2	If sperm source is positive		✓
HTLV-1/2 (FDA required for sperm donors)			✓
West Nile virus/Zika virus as indicated by location and time of year	✓	✓	✓
Pap/HPV	✓		
Semen analysis			✓

Resources

Fat-Positive Provider Lists

Plus Size Birth: PlusSizeBirth.com

Health at Every Size: HAESCommunity.com

Fat-friendly health professionals list: FatFriendlyDocs.com

Queer/Trans-Competent Preconception Care Provider Referrals

MAIA Midwifery & Fertility Services: MAIAMidwifery.com

GAMETE DONORS

When making a baby requires a gamete (sperm or egg) from an outside source, there are two ways to go: someone who is known to you, or someone who is not. There are various medical, legal, ethical, and social implications to consider when selecting the type of donor that is right for you. Accessibility is also a factor, whether that is a matter of finances, geography, or even the existence of the type of donor you would like to help build your family in an ideal world. All of these factors make donor gamete selection a complex issue. This chapter breaks down the issues and considerations to assist you in looking at these choices from all angles so that you not only feel informed, but you feel solid in the decisions you make. The first part of this chapter addresses issues that often come up related to the concept of donor conception, followed by considerations for known donors, and then donors who are unknown to you.

Donor Selection as an Aspect of Family Formation

The genetic factors involved in bringing your baby into the world are important, but they may not be everything. While some donor attributes may be nonnegotiable, such as race or ethnicity, many other attributes, such as being artistic or sporty, may represent qualities you would like to instill in your child but may or may not prove to be genetically expressed. Keep in mind that your influence as a parent may have a greater impact on how your child develops and grows, and regardless of all the contributions along the way, ultimately, your child will be their own unique self. While the initial decisions you make may feel overwhelming, once your child is here, it will all fade into distant memory as your child unfolds into the unique being they truly are, nurtured in your loving care.

PARTNER DYNAMICS IN DONOR SELECTION

When we must go outside of our relationship in order to access the gametes we need to conceive a child, the decisions we make are never simple. They often requiring interacting with a fertility industry that definitely wants our money but makes little effort toward sensitivity and appropriateness to our needs. Many of us navigate our choices within a society that requires additional hoop-jumping in order to secure legal parentage of the offspring we go to such great lengths to bring into the world. At every step of the way, every choice we make, and the ways we go about making those choices, present opportunities to offset cultural marginalization with self-defined expressions of normalcy and affirmation.

For instance, queer parents often field insensitive questions like, "Who is the real mom/dad?" Extended family members may view a parent who is not genetically related to the child as extraneous, perhaps not out of malice but certainly out of a blindingly heterocentric worldview. Even if granted parental status by the laws in your own state or province, parents who are not biologically related still have to adopt their own children in order for the legal integrity of the family unit to remain intact in other states or outside of your country. (Be sure to consult an attorney about this.) Nonbiological parents may be engaged in a constant mental reframing of their role as this baby's parent, because the primacy of genetic connection is so deeply ingrained within the dominant culture.

As one queer parent whose partner carried their baby through pregnancy remarked in early parenthood, nongestational/nonbiological parents can experience "a special kind of loneliness." It pays for parents in this situation to seek care providers who look to you as a full participant in the formation of your family as well as in the gestation and birth of your child. If your care provider never looks you in the eye, or if they dote on your pregnant partner or coparent exclusively, seek care with a more insightful care provider who understands the emotional needs of nonbiological/nongestational parents.

Although there are countless ways to affirm your role as a parent once your baby arrives, during the donor-selection process, there is not yet an actual baby. Be aware of any feelings that are coming up for you during the donor-selection process as a nongenetic parent, and be sure to articulate your experience to your partner. How you each navigate this experience will be different, but communicating your feelings and needs openly will allow you to stay connected as you make this important decision. You may need to come up with creative ways to reflect each parent's central role in the formation of your family. Some families opt to have the nongenetic parent select the donor as an avenue for expressing genetic influence, while others simply allow that parent to carry more weight in the decision or to have the final say. For others, it feels right to have the nongenetic parent take on all tasks related to accessing donor gametes. You may not know at the outset what will feel best to you, but pay attention to your feelings as you go through the process and be ready to make adjustments accordingly.

If there is disagreement among partners regarding donor selection, or even the choice to use an unknown versus a known donor, this is worthy of careful consideration. If you use a known donor, that person will be in your life in some way forever. If you use an unknown donor, you may never have the opportunity to know the person who contributed half of your child's DNA. Once your child is conceived, there is no going back. However, as you process this decision, keep in mind that parenting is a complex, lifelong experience. While the selection process makes the donor's role in your life loom large at the outset, over time, this aspect of the process will fade in comparison to your lived experience raising your child. We may have a lot in common with those whose genes we carry, but we are shaped by those who raise us. Love is a powerful force. Make the choice that most allows love to flow through your family, even if that means something different than you would have chosen as an individual. This is the meaning of family—and family is what you are creating.

TALKING TO KIDS ABOUT BEING DONOR CONCEIVED

In queer communities, donor conception is normalized, which is a major advantage for our kids. Telling your child about how they came to be, in age-appropriate ways, from the time they are very young, gives you many opportunities to figure out exactly how you want to talk about it. Some parents tell their child their arrival story every year on their birthday so that the story can evolve and contain greater detail as the child grows and is better able to understand it. What we are communicating when we share a child's origin story is that they are wanted, they are loved, and they belong. You are not only affirming how they came to be, you are also affirming their sense of family. While their donor may have provided a special and necessary gift, your child's worldview is made up of the day-to-day experiences of who cares for them, who feeds them, who makes sure they are safe, and who tucks them into bed at night. While the language used in the broader culture may conflate familial relationships with genetics, we know this is not always the case. This is but one of the many reasons to be engaged in community with other queer families, so that both you and your child are able to see reflections of yourselves and experience the freedom and validation that comes with not having to explain your very existence. Make sure your child also has access to books and media that represent many different types of families, including books on human conception that are affirming to all routes to parenthood, such as *What Makes a Baby* by Cory Silverberg.

Known Donors

Whether you are in need of sperm or egg, there is something special about knowing the person who will contribute to half your child's DNA. Maybe your chosen donor is your partner's genetic relative, so your child will be biologically related to both of you. Maybe you always knew you would ask your best friend from college to be your donor. Maybe you are going to share child-rearing with another queer couple (which makes them not donors at all, but coparents). Or maybe you don't know anyone (yet) but you are certain that you want to know your child's gamete donor personally.

Any way you look at it, the known donor relationship is just that—a relationship. Some relationships are easy, and some are complicated. As with any relationship, we get to choose how close we want to be, what level of complexity we are up for, and if and when we want the relationship to end . . . except that with a known donor, you are in it for life. The ways in which you set up this relationship, and the intention you put into it, will support you and your family for years to come. The truth is, human beings change over time, and relationships evolve. The donor relationship is no different. Your relationship with your donor will undoubtedly evolve in some way. In this regard, using a known donor involves aspects that bring a greater level of control, such as knowing the person and creating agreements with intention, along with aspects that may be outside your control, because it is a relationship between human beings.

There are valid reasons for choosing a known donor as well as risks, and steps to take to mitigate the risks. Keep in mind that while using a known donor may seem simpler and less expensive than going through a sperm or egg bank, some of the protections that are offered by a bank are not there. This means that you will be doing your own search to find a donor who will be a good match for what you want for your family, you will be funding screening tests for the donor as well as other medical costs associated with gamete donation, and you will need to take some additional legal steps to keep your family secure. Any way you go about it, using a gamete donor takes time, money, and emotional energy. With a donor who is known to you, the investment you make up front to ensure everyone is on the same page will pay off in how smoothly the process goes over time, and it will ultimately create a positive experience for everyone, including your child.

Before diving more deeply into this topic, some clarification is in order. The term "known donor" is commonly used to describe gamete donors who you actually know, as well as donors who you do not know personally but who are willing to have their identity disclosed when the child turns eighteen (called "open identity" or "willing to be known"). But these two situations are vastly different! In this book, I am using the term "known donor" to refer to someone you actually know, and who you choose because you know them personally, and you want that person, specifically, to donate the gamete you need to conceive your child. There are a few reasons for differentiating the term this way.

One is that choosing someone you know to help build your family is uniquely queer. Not that cis/het families don't ever choose this option, but historically, this was the only way queer and single parents-to-be could choose to build their families. There was a time, not so long ago, when we were prohibited from accessing donor gametes from a bank. This is the very reason why The Sperm Bank of California was founded in 1982, and at the time, it was the only bank in the United States allowing access to donor sperm for prospective parents of all orientations and family structures. The known donor in a queer family constellation holds a special place in our hearts, not only for the gametes they have gifted to us but by allowing us to celebrate the extended family relationships we form in our communities. For many, a known donor means so much more than having access to a donor's name and contact information. It's an expression of the many ways we choose to build our families upon a foundation of intention and love.

By contrast, a person you connect with on a known donor website, app, or social media, with whom you have no prior relationship and whom you do not actually know personally, does not provide that level of confidence and trust— and the repercussions of that sort of vulnerability can be harrowing. In the case of sperm donation, if there is no health care provider involved with the insemination and no contract, you also have no way of protecting yourself should the donor (or their parents) seek custody or visitation rights someday. It is also the equivalent of having unprotected sex with a stranger, given that you do not actually know this person and you only have their word to go on regarding their safer sex practices during the time they are providing samples for you. A single STI test result is only accurate at a given point in time, and any future exposure puts you, your partner(s), and your baby at risk.

Building a family with help from a donor you know and trust means that you have the opportunity to discuss your vision for your family and where a donor fits into that vision for you. It allows the donor to weigh the decision and to provide their wholehearted consent for what you are proposing. And most importantly, it allows for mutual trust if your chosen route to conception puts either or both of you in a legally vulnerable position or presents potential risks to anyone's physical health.

WHAT ARE YOU REALLY LOOKING FOR IN A KNOWN DONOR?

Some reasons that people give for wanting a known donor include:

- I have someone who is chosen family to me and whose body makes the type of gamete I need to conceive a child.
- I want to use a gamete from my partner's genetic relative.
- I want a donor that matches my partner's racial background.
- I want to have a sense of who the donor is as a person.
- I want my child to have access to their donor when they choose.
- I want sperm that is cheap, effective, and readily available.

These are the most common reasons people give for desiring a known donor, although there are endless reasons that someone might choose this route. However, if your reasons for choosing a known donor include having someone to help you raise the child, to assist with decision-making for your child, or to refer to as one of the child's parents, you are actually looking for a coparent, not a donor. The difference must be clearly defined for all parties involved. If an individual is genetically related to your child and they refer to themselves as the child's parent/father/mother, or if you or the child refers to them in those terms, then you are vulnerable to having to share physical or legal custody of your child or having to allow for visitation rights. This goes for the donor as well as their parents, who can sue for grandparent rights. If this is not what you had in mind, be very clear from the beginning that you are not looking for another parent, and be firm and up front about the terms that will need to be used to describe the place the donor holds in the child's life.

On the other hand, if there is a person in your life who you would like to form a coparenting relationship with, go for it! But keep in mind that a genetic relationship is not necessary for a person to be a full, active parent in a child's life. If you find that your chosen coparent has impaired fertility, this need not prevent you from creating a family together. There are many advantages to building a family with someone you are not romantically involved with, and there are many drawbacks as well. It would take another entire book to cover the topic adequately. If you plan to create family in this way, I cannot stress enough the need to have a family therapist to guide you along the way. Plan to keep this professional in your life for the duration of the years you are raising a child together so that you have assistance as you forge your unique path. It takes a lot of work, and the rewards can be immense if it is all done with a great deal of intention.

CLARIFYING YOUR VISION FOR YOUR FAMILY

It is imperative to get clear on your vision for your family first, before talking to any potential donors. Are you simply wanting a donor who is willing to be contacted when your child is old enough to ask about them? Do you want someone who is willing to get together once a year? Once a month? Once a week? Are you wanting an "uncle" or "auntie" figure? If so, what does that look like, and what does it mean to you? Be specific. Would you want this person to show up at birthdays, recitals, sports games, bar/bat mitzvah, quinceañera, graduation, etc.? Are you looking to solidify a relationship with someone from your chosen queer family? And if so, is a genetic connection to your child required for that type of intentional family building? What does that say about your partner who is not going to be genetically related to your child? What does it say about this person's parents, who may view your child as a grandchild and want to be involved in their life?

As you begin to clarify your values, explore the emotions that come up for you. Are your true feelings in alignment with your stated values, or are you noticing emotions that seem to come out of nowhere because they are in conflict with your ideals? These types of questions are important to ask yourself, to explore, to journal about. Talk about your feelings, articulate them to your partner, your therapist, your best friend. These are big decisions. The process of becoming a parent will clarify your values and your truths in many ways. Your best guide as a parent is always going to be your gut feeling about what is right for you and for your child. Remember this.

The work of clarifying your vision for your family is a necessary step in the donor-selection process. If you skip this step, you may be tempted to compromise for the sake of maintaining a potential donor's interest and involvement. Be clear from the outset about what you are looking for, not only so you are more likely to end up with what you want for your family but also so that your donor can be clear about what they are consenting to and what they are not.

CHOOSING A PARTNER'S GENETIC RELATIVE TO BE YOUR DONOR

This can be a great situation, and it can also be very tricky. One of the first questions to ask yourself is: Why are genetics important to me? Make sure you consider the possibility that this person may not work out to be your donor for one reason or another. If you have focused on a genetic connection in order to validate your role as a parent, how does this change if you end up using a different donor you are not related to? What does being a parent really mean? Don't forget to consider how your extended family members will view this arrangement. Will they honor and uphold you and your partner as the baby's parents, or will they refer to the donor relative as the baby's "father" or "mother"? If you don't feel your family will understand or honor your wishes, you may be tempted to keep it a secret. But consider how it would feel to keep such a secret in your family, especially as your child gets older and wants to know who their donor is. Another consideration is that, in bringing another family member into the process, you may end up being out to your whole family about trying to conceive a lot sooner than you otherwise would have been. Extended family members might be curious or concerned, and this may end up feeling like additional pressure, especially if conceiving ends up taking a while. Keep in mind as well that if you are going to be inseminating with fresh samples, you will need to discuss safety and risk from the standpoint of their safer sex practices, which may not be something you want to know about your relative.

CHOOSING A DONOR WHO MATCHES YOUR PARTNER'S RACIAL BACKGROUND

For many reasons, including racism, colonization, and the history of enslavement and medical abuse of BIPOC communities (with a heavy dose of white privilege determining who can most easily access expensive reproductive services), Black donors and other donors of color are often hard to find at sperm banks, and finding one at an egg bank can be nearly impossible. The sperm bank with the largest number of Black donors, Xytex in Atlanta, won't release samples directly to recipients (they will only work with clinics and health care providers), which increases costs and may expose conceiving families to racism in the process of accessing health care from a predominantly white fertility industry. Matching a donor to your partner's mixed-race heritage may be like trying to find a needle in a haystack. Donors of some racial backgrounds are next to impossible due to sperm bank requirements, such as Filipino donors who are often shorter than program donor height specifications. Even the very idea of choosing a donor from a bank may reek of a colonialist mindset. If you find yourself in the situation of choosing a known donor by default, because a gamete bank donor is not an option for you and does not meet the needs of your family, it is important to take the additional steps of ensuring that the donor of your choice is a good donor for your family in every other way. Make sure you don't compromise your vision for your family for the sake of a particular donor, even if your pool of potential donors is small.

CHOOSING A DONOR FOR WHO THEY ARE AS A PERSON

For people who have this priority, there is typically a sorting through the mental files of who you know who could possibly be a donor. Is there someone in your life now? A close friend? An acquaintance? A coworker? Is there someone from way back, such as a childhood friend or an ex? With an ex, consider the reasons this person is no longer in your life, and remember how it felt to be in a relationship with them. Are they a good communicator? Honest? Do you still carry feelings for them? It is not uncommon to begin to romanticize or become sexually attracted to a gamete donor. How much room is there in your marriage or partnership for these feelings, whether or not you act on them? Be open, honest, and intentional around this issue if you are partnered. Find ways to keep your partner fully involved in the conception process, which may mean that they take care of all of the communication with the donor; it may mean that you never go to clinic appointments without them; or if you are inseminating, it may mean that they, rather than you, always pick up the sample from the donor. It also may mean that you need to have a ritual, altar, or other concrete way of affirming and reaffirming your roles as this baby's parents.

SEEKING GAMETES THAT ARE CHEAP, EFFECTIVE, AND READILY AVAILABLE

Aren't we all? The truth of it is, just because you know someone and don't have to pay exorbitant prices for donor gametes doesn't mean there are no costs involved.

Part of what you are paying for at a sperm or egg bank is thorough screening to provide the utmost level of assurance that the gametes will be reasonably viable for conception. It is easier to test the fertile potential of a sperm donor than an egg donor, but in either case, it benefits you to have your donor do fertility testing up front so that you don't waste everyone's time, emotional energy, and money on conception attempts without this baseline data about the donor's capacity to help you conceive. While you may save on some costs by using a gamete donor who is voluntarily providing their genetic material to you, keep in mind that the operative aspect of your relationship is that their gametes are needed for conception. Be careful not to lose sight of this as you navigate the heart-centered, relational aspects of your venture.

FINDING A KNOWN DONOR

Once you decide to look for a known donor, make a list of all possible people you might ask. Go big. Your donor need not live in the same community, or even within driving distance (more on distance donors later in this chapter). After your initial brainstorm, go over your list more carefully. While you might be tempted to narrow it down based on looks or personal interests, keep in mind that you are looking for something beyond what you could pick off a list of donors at a sperm or egg bank. You are specifically looking for someone you know to play a certain role in your and your child's life, which means you are looking for some level of relationship. Even if you are not intending to spend much time with this person after the child is conceived, the conception process is quite involved, and you will want to make sure that your donor is clear about what they are signing on for and what they are not. The donor relationship is based on trust and open, honest communication. For this reason, I encourage you to assess each potential donor based on two vital criteria that make for a good donor relationship and a positive experience for everyone:

1. Do you trust the person to be completely honest and forthright, and to stand by their word?

2. Does the person have clear communication skills, even during hard conversations?

THE ASK

When you propose the idea to a potential gamete donor, you want their honest answer. Getting an initial yes and then later having the person back out is an extremely disappointing experience. Ironically, sometimes potential donors say yes because they don't want to disappoint you; however, there are many valid reasons to not want to be a donor. One way to avoid this dynamic is to put the idea out to prospective donors in a way that lets them know you are looking but that allows them to initiate contact with you if they are interested in pursuing the idea further. You might say, "I/We want to let you know that I/we am/are thinking about having a baby sometime in the next year. Of course, I/we am/are missing some vital genetic material to accomplish that, and I/we am/are exploring the possibility of having someone known be the donor instead of going through a bank and finding an anonymous donor. I/We don't want to put any pressure on anyone, so I/we am/are letting a few friends know I/we am/are looking. You are one of those friends. If you are curious to know more, or if you think you might be interested in helping, please let me/us know. I/We am/are hoping to be able to have a more in-depth conversation with a potential donor by the end of next month, so if you're interested, please don't wait to reach out and let me/us know. Otherwise, you won't hear from me/us about this again—no pressure, no questions asked."

This approach lets the person know you are looking for a gamete donor, but it puts them in control to contact you if they are interested. It lets you bring up the idea without putting pressure on them, and it allows them to say no without feeling the need to explain themselves. Being a gamete donor is a huge gift, and it requires forethought and willingness to be involved in the creation of your family. Allowing the donor to come to you means you can be assured that they are actually interested in helping you, and it avoids questioning whether they are only saying yes to avoid disappointing you. Be sure to state clearly what your timeline is for follow-up so they know how long they have to get back to you. Don't make it so far off that it might slip their mind, but make sure you allow time for them to give it some initial thought. Let them know that the next conversation is about exploring the idea further, not about making a final decision.

WHAT TO DO IF . . .

YOUR DONOR IS PARTNERED

If your donor has a spouse or is in a serious relationship, it is vital that
their partner be involved in all discussions at every step of the way,
including the initial ask. Such a momentous decision is likely to bring up
a lot of questions and feelings that your donor and their partner will need
to navigate. Being clear from the very beginning about what you are asking for, and what you are not, will help allay any fears they have about the
donor's place in your life, and it will also create a clear pathway for the
other couple to feel positive and celebratory about participating in your
child's conception. Whether your donor is providing eggs or sperm, there
are going to be times when their physical health and/or sexual habits are
affected by the need to provide gametes for you, which inherently affects
their partner. Ultimately, when you intentionally include the donor's
partner in all your discussions, you will avoid bringing up any feelings
of being left out, which supports them in navigating the effects on their
relationship and keeps everyone feeling connected and consensual.

YOUR DONOR DOES NOT HAVE CHILDREN, OR IF THEIR FAMILY-BUILDING PROCESS IS NOT COMPLETE

This can be tricky territory to navigate. For a donor who does not have
children but wants them someday, being involved in creating a genetic
offspring who is not their child may bring up a certain amount of grief or
longing that could cloud the relationship. For a donor who is still building
their family, sharing gametes with another family may have repercussions
for their own family-building goals. This is especially important for egg
donors, because stimulation and retrieval procedures are not risk free,
including the risk of future sterility.

THE INITIAL CONVERSATION

Once you have a donor who is interested in knowing more, have an initial conversation that addresses the following three topics:

1. Communicating your vision for your family
2. Defining the donor relationship
3. Describing the process

The point of this conversation is clarity. Make sure you have done some thorough soul-searching and that you come to the conversation with a clear vision for your family and the role you are asking the donor to play in it. Reassure the potential donor that the point of this conversation is not for them to give you an immediate answer but for them to make sure they understand clearly what you are asking them for. Guide the conversation through the three separate and distinct parts. For each part of the discussion, let the potential donor know that you are going to describe what you are envisioning, ask them to listen carefully, and let them know they will have a chance to ask questions and repeat it all back to you to make sure they understand clearly.

1. COMMUNICATING YOUR VISION FOR YOUR FAMILY

Be clear, and don't hold back. The more you can clarify your vision and articulate it openly, the more honest the conversation will be, and the more clear your donor can be in agreeing or saying no. This level of transparent, forthright communication is vital. You will in some way be connected to this person for a lifetime, so you owe it to them, to yourselves, and to your child to be as solid and unabashed as you can be from the very beginning. The most important thing to be up front about is who will be a parent and who will not. If you are looking for a donor who will help raise the child, you are not looking for a donor—you are looking for a coparent. On the other hand, if you are not looking for the donor to have any role as a parent whatsoever, you will want to make sure you communicate this clearly from every possible angle. One way to state this is, "I'm not/ We aren't looking for another parent, I/we am/are looking for donor egg/sperm to help me/us have my/our own baby." As you have discussions with a potential donor about what this relationship might look like, you will want to reiterate that you will not be seeking any financial support or assistance with raising the child. You will be making all decisions about health care, education, discipline style, where the child lives, and who is in the child's life. The donor will not be referred to as the child's father/mother/parent, and they will not refer to themselves in that way. Speak these things clearly from the very beginning, even if it is hard and even if you feel you might risk offending the person. It is imperative to be completely honest so that the potential donor can make an informed decision about their involvement in your family building. You might state these desires in ways that affirm your status as a parent, such as, "Of course, since I/we will be the child's parent(s), you will not have any financial responsibility for the child. And since I/we will be the child's parent(s), I/we will have sole discretion about how they are raised, where they live, their education and health care, and who I/we might choose to partner and coparent with in the future. You will not be expected to have any input about any of these things."

2. DEFINING THE DONOR RELATIONSHIP

Come to the initial discussion with your potential donor having given considerable thought to what you want the ongoing relationship to look like. How much contact are you envisioning? If this person is already a close member of your social circle or chosen family, how might your relationship change, and how might it stay the same? If they are someone you only see occasionally, would you want that to be any different after your child is born? Do you want them at birthday parties or special events in the child's life, or does that feel like it's crossing a boundary? Should contact with the donor be initiated by you, should it be initiated by the child, or can it be initiated by the donor? When will you be in contact: Will the donor be at the birth, will you introduce them to the baby soon after, will you wait a year, or will you introduce them after the second parent adoption goes through?

It is extremely important for nongestational parents to weigh in fully on these decisions, because the presence of a known donor with biological ties to the child, within a culture that assumes biology equals parenthood, can sometimes make them feel extraneous or marginalized. This affects how you will talk about the donor's relationship to your family. Will other people know this person is your sperm donor? What will they be called—and are you all on the same page about whether this person will be referred to simply by name, donor, uncle/auntie, etc.? What if the donor moves away? What if the donor moves closer than you intended them to be? Rather than just saying you want an "uncle/aunt"-type relationship, define for yourself what that sort of relationship means to you. Be specific. Although it's impossible to think of every possible scenario ahead of time, give considerable thought to these questions, explore your emotions fully, and if you are partnered, have honest conversations with your partner(s) so that you are clear about what you are looking for ahead of time.

Once you start exploring these ideas, you will soon find that, inevitably, your relationship to this person will change in ways that are not entirely clear to you now. Many families find that their relationship with their donor grows and changes in positive ways, bringing a greater sense of closeness and a lifelong connection. On the other hand, if they are a close friend who you would normally turn to for emotional support, you may find that you can't lean on them in the same way during the conception process, because they are also involved in the process and may have their own emotions to navigate. These are the sorts of things to think about and to be prepared to discuss with your potential donor up front.

While you will need to be prepared to give a clear statement describing your ideal donor relationship, be careful not to get too far into hashing out all the details, because there is still some screening involved in making sure this person is a viable gamete donor. Recognize that this conversation requires a lot of emotional labor on everyone's part, and there may be some aspects that you want to take note of but table for further discussion at a later time. On the other hand, if there are deal breakers or red flags that arise for either one of you, it's important to pay attention to that. Don't sweep anything under the rug, or it is sure to come out to haunt you later. Be clear, stick to your vision, and make notes for future consideration and/or discussion.

3. DESCRIBING THE PROCESS

If the potential donor is still on board after hearing your vision for your family and what the relationship might look like going forward, you will want to give them a sense of what the process will look like. The first thing you will need is to know that they are fertile, and that their gametes can reasonably be expected to be able to help you conceive. Be clear that this screening needs to be done as a first step. If everything checks out fertility wise, then you will need to draw up a donor agreement so that everyone is protected legally. Most families cover all medical and legal costs involved in using a gamete donor, although sometimes the donor can use their own health insurance to cover some tests or procedures.

For sperm donors, fertility screening means that they will need to get a semen analysis, which involves abstaining from ejaculation for two to three days, then collecting a sample via masturbation at a lab or clinic. For egg donors, the fertility assessment involves seeing a fertility specialist to answer questions about their health and their menstrual cycle, an internal pelvic ultrasound to count their egg follicles, and a blood test to assess their ovarian reserve.

The actual donation process is much more involved. For a sperm donor, you have the option of asking for a couple of samples each month until you conceive, or having the donor go to a sperm bank to have samples frozen, which allows them to do all the donating up front. If you opt to have samples stored at a sperm bank, the bank could be close to where they live, allowing you to have those samples shipped directly to you for insemination each month. Or, you may have all the samples transferred to a local storage facility or clinic so that you don't have to deal with shipping individual samples each cycle. There is also an option to have a long-distance donor ship fresh samples to you overnight using a sperm shipping kit with buffer solution that preserves the cells during shipping.

For an egg donor, the process is quite different. They will need to take medications by injection to stimulate as many eggs to grow as possible, and then the eggs must be surgically removed under sedation. The process involves painful injections; mood swings; physical side effects such as nausea, bloating, hot flashes, headaches, chest tenderness, vaginal soreness, cramping, and bleeding after retrieval; and likely missed work for all of the appointments. If the egg donor lives far away, they can undergo treatments at a clinic that is local to them. Egg cells can be cryopreserved at the time of retrieval; however, success rates are higher if they are immediately combined with sperm cells and grown into embryos, which can be genetically tested and then cryopreserved until being transferred to the uterus of the person who will be carrying the pregnancy. If the sperm cells will be coming from you or your partner, you can use a local bank or clinic to freeze those cells and then ship them to the clinic that will be doing the egg retrieval, or you can travel to the clinic and provide fresh samples on the day of retrieval.

MAKING A PLAN FOR FOLLOW-UP

Once you have completed this discussion and these aspects are clearly understood, set a time frame to meet again. Ask the potential donor how much time they think they might need before deciding on the next step, which is to get a fertility evaluation. Allow ample time so if additional questions come up, you will be able to discuss them. Will a month be enough, or do they have final exams or a big project coming up at work? Recognize that if this person ends up saying no, or if they are not fertile enough to be a viable donor, you will be back at square one. If the time they need to make a decision about fertility testing is going to cause you a significant delay, you may want to pursue other options in the meantime so that you can keep your own process moving forward. Be transparent about this and about your own timeline.

GETTING A FERTILITY EVALUATION FOR YOUR PROSPECTIVE DONOR

Sperm donors: If you are not already set up with a preconception care provider who can order a semen analysis for you, your donor can ask their primary care provider for a referral, or in some areas, they might be able to self-refer to a fertility clinic or sperm bank and pay cash for the analysis, which is typically around $200.

Egg donors: Fertility evaluation for a potential egg donor can be done at a fertility clinic or with a midwife or ob-gyn who specializes in fertility. The initial evaluation need not be performed by the provider who will be providing IUI or IVF services, so it is possible to have your potential egg donor see their own provider, if they prefer, for this initial evaluation. On the other hand, it may also be an opportunity for them to see how they feel about the clinic that would be providing their care throughout the donation process. Expect to pay around $500 for the initial assessment. (Potential egg donors may want to reference Chapter 2: Fertile Health for Every Body, Chapter 3: Lab Tests and Fertility Evaluations, and Chapter 8: In Vitro Fertilization and Embryo Transfer.)

ANTICIPATING NEXT STEPS

Once the initial fertility evaluation is performed and you have determined the viability of this person to be your gamete donor, you will be ready to talk further about solidifying your arrangement in a known donor agreement. I highly recommend you complete the fertility evaluation prior to these conversations, because if your donor turns out to have fertility issues, you can save yourself and the donor a whole lot of time and energy. Definitely get a fertility assessment before paying an attorney to advise you and draw up a legal contract, and before providing funds to your donor to secure their own separate legal counsel.

SPELLING OUT THE DETAILS

After assessing the donor's fertility, but before going any further, you will want to have some more in-depth conversations to ascertain that you are on the same page about all the details. Make sure that everyone is involved for reasons that are clear, transparent, and fully agreed upon. Having these discussions will allow any red flags to come up that might reveal hidden hopes or motives on the part of the donor that you are not in agreement with, and vice versa. It also allows for important discussions to take place about your unique relationship with the donor, and how you would want things to go between you in the future. It brings up considerations like what happens if you move away, if you and your partner split up, or if one or both of you becomes deceased. Keep in mind the reality that human beings often go through major shifts in religious beliefs, medical choices, and values around discipline and education—so clarifying who is responsible for these decisions in any possible scenario, even virtually unimaginable ones, is an important distinction to make when defining the role of a donor. What if you split and get remarried, and the donor does not like your new partner? While this would certainly affect your friendship, would the donor have any legal standing to step in if they don't agree with the home life you are creating for the child? Is there any scenario that the donor or their partner could think of where they would want to be consulted or included in decisions that are made for the child? If so, consider and decide if you would be willing to include this stipulation in your agreement or in another legal document such as a will. Your attorney will be invaluable in helping you craft the appropriate legal documents specific to your needs.

DETAILS TO DISCUSS WITH YOUR KNOWN DONOR

- Who will be the parent(s), and who will not?
- Who will name the child? Who will be listed on the birth certificate?
- Who will call themselves the child's mother/father/parent, and who will not?
- Who will have financial responsibility for the child, and who will not?
- Who will have legal custody and decision-making authority for the child, and who will not?
- Who will make medical decisions for the child, and who will not?

- Who will be responsible for religious or spiritual upbringing, and who will not?

- Who will make choices about the child's education, and who will not?

- Who will decide where the child lives, and who will not?

- Who has the authority to choose caregivers for the child, and who does not?

- Who has a say in what discipline style is used to raise the child, and who does not?

- Who will appoint a guardian for the child should the parent(s) become ill or deceased?

- To whom will the donor relationship be disclosed, and when?

- Who will decide when and how the child is told of their genetic origins?

- By what term will the donor refer to their role in the child's life, and what terms are off-limits?

- How will you maintain contact over time?

- How will you communicate with one another in case a hereditary health issue arises for the donor, one of their family members, or for the child?

- Who will pay medical costs related to donor conception?

- Who will pay legal costs?

- How will any legal disputes that arise in the future be addressed?

- How long will the donor be providing gametes to you?

- If you end up with a lengthy conception process, at what point would you want to check in to make sure they are still on board?

DONOR VERSUS COPARENT

If the answers to the previous questions clearly stipulate that the donor will not have any legal rights or responsibilities for the child, no authority for any type of decision-making for the child, and that they in no way will act or be referred to as a parent to the child, then they are a donor. On the other hand, if this person will be participating in raising the child or making decisions for the child, or if they will be referred to as a parent in any way, then you will be vulnerable to having to share legal and/or physical custody of the child.

The distinctions are vital to understand and to be in agreement about. If a potential donor wants to be more involved than you had envisioned, no matter how much you love them as a person, and no matter how excellent their fertile potential might be, do not compromise for the sake of keeping them invested as a donor—because if their desires do not reflect what it means to be a donor, then they are not agreeing to be a donor, and you will ultimately end up with a coparent. (For more guidance about coparenting, review Chapter 1: Making Decisions and Creating a Timeline.)

SPECIAL CONSIDERATIONS FOR USING A KNOWN SPERM DONOR

In contrast to conceiving with an egg donor (which requires IVF managed by a fertility clinic), conceiving with a known sperm donor has the advantage of being relatively low tech. However, there are logistical considerations as well as health risks to consider. This section focuses on known sperm donors, specifically.

LEGAL RISKS OF SELF-INSEMINATION WITH A KNOWN DONOR

Families who conceive on their own with fresh sperm samples from a known donor sometimes attempt to cut costs by forgoing the expense of an attorney. However, doing so can put you as well as your donor at risk. For instance, just because the donor's name isn't on the child's birth certificate does not mean they can't sue for custody—especially if there is no third party such as a midwife or physician who can attest that an insemination occurred, rather than intercourse. (A child conceived via intercourse between two individuals is legally considered to be the child of those individuals, with all the rights and responsibilities of parenthood.) An attorney who specializes in third-party reproduction and family law will have valuable insights and additional considerations for you to think about and include in your agreement, as well as the legal expertise to ensure that your agreement is worded in a way that will hold up according to the laws in your jurisdiction. Just because you have a legal contract defining your agreements doesn't mean you can't also write a cover letter to your child, expressing the love and intention with which you are bringing them into being, with the help of your donor. The legal climate regarding LGBTQ+ families is constantly changing, and how the law affects families varies greatly from state to state. For this reason, it is imperative to seek legal counsel before conceiving with a known donor. Do not make the mistake of using an online known donor agreement template without legal counsel. Costs range from $600 to $2,000 for the donor agreement, but if cost is an issue, seek out local queer organizations that may offer discounted or pro bono legal services for families, or contact the National Center for Lesbian Rights or Lambda Legal for information and referrals.

HEALTH RISKS OF USING FRESH SPERM SAMPLES

Using fresh sperm samples to conceive inherently means exposure to your donor's body fluids. Even if you have the donor tested for sexually transmitted infections, the results only tell you if the donor is currently infected. Some STIs, such as HIV, take a while to show up on a blood test, so a recent exposure may yield a false negative result. And, if you are inseminating with this person on an ongoing basis, you will continue to be at risk beyond the initial STI screen if they are sexually active or if they have exposures in other ways, such as providing health care.

This is why you need to have a frank discussion with your donor about their safer sex practices and potential exposures to transmissible infections. Be clear that you are grateful for their gift, but you need to protect your health, the health of any partner(s) you have, as well as the health of your child. Sometimes a donor is willing to use more precautions during the time they are donating to you, although if this is the case in your situation, make sure you agree on a timeline for this agreement so that it is time limited and clearly defined. It is also important in any situation to have a "time-out with no questions asked" policy, so that if your donor has a potential STI exposure, they can call time-out on donating without also fearing the need to explain why. Some STIs take three months to reliably show up on a test, so expect to wait that long. Safety is the number-one concern, and if taking some time off from donating maintains your safety, it's worth it.

BARRIERS TO CARE WITH FRESH KNOWN-DONOR SPERM

In the United States, there are FDA regulations to guide clinics in the use of donor sperm, and clinics often turn people away or insist on additional requirements for assisted conception with a known donor. However, if you have also inseminated at home on your own with fresh samples from a known donor, the FDA does not even have a category that applies to you. The only categories mentioned in FDA regulations are "sexual partner" or "directed donor." Home insemination with a known donor falls somewhere in between—you don't need a health care provider to self-inseminate with a fresh sample, and the samples have not been frozen at a bank, so they are not really "directed donor" samples. And legally, having sex with your donor makes them not a donor at all, so a donor cannot also be a sexual partner. The only allowance the FDA makes for those who want to inseminate in a clinic with fresh samples from a known donor is to have the donor tested (using more costly FDA-approved tests) within seven days of *each* sample collection. Not only can this be cost prohibitive, the time frame for the testing can be a logistical nightmare if your ovulation varies by a few days and/or if your donor is not always available to go in on a specific day for the blood test. Of course, if you have already been inseminating with your donor's fresh sperm at home, then from a clinical standpoint, you have shared sexual fluids, which presents the same risk as being "sexual partners." Not all physicians are willing to interpret the regulations in this way, and additionally, some fertility clinics have tissue bank certifications that limit their freedom to utilize a more appropriate (and less heterocentric) clinical interpretation of the FDA regulations. So far, only the state of California has laws protecting access to fertility medicine by families conceiving with known donors.

DIRECTED DONORS

The most secure and cost-effective way to circumvent legal and health risks of using a known donor is to have your donor provide samples as a "directed donor" at a sperm bank for cryopreservation. A directed donor's samples belong to you and will not be released to any other family. The donor goes to the bank for an initial analysis and test freeze to make sure their samples are adequate for cryopreservation. Then, they get the FDA-required testing and provide a few samples, the samples are quarantined for three to six months, and then the donor is tested again. If the results are all still negative, the samples are available for you to withdraw as needed. The FDA does not actually require a quarantine for directed donors, so if you are not concerned about STI transmission, you may be able to sign a consent form to have the samples released sooner. If you do want quarantine and retesting, transmissible infections take no more than three months to produce detectable antibodies with currently available tests, so there is no reason to quarantine samples for longer than three months.

Another benefit of cryopreserving known donor samples is being able to have access to your samples over time, meaning that the donor doesn't need to continue to be available for you every month. You can even have extra samples saved for future children. And because you have gone through a clinic, this process also legally establishes this person as a donor. Insemination is a little more involved, because IUI will increase your chances of conceiving with frozen samples, but the trade-off in protection and accessibility is often worth it. Expect to pay around $2,000 to $3,000 plus storage and/or shipping fees.

LONG-DISTANCE SPERM DONORS

If your donor does not live close to you, there are a few ways to access their samples. One is to use the directed donor process, either at a clinic or bank close to where they live or where they can travel and stay for a couple of weeks. Another is to travel to the donor or have them travel to you for each conception attempt. If the donor comes to you, make sure they stay well hydrated on the journey, and that they pay attention to "testicular heat" during their travels, which means getting up and walking around for ten minutes every hour during a long flight or road trip. If you go to them, try not to cross more than one time zone during the days immediately preceding ovulation, as ovulation patterns tend to be affected when traveling so far at ovulation time. It is best to go two to three days before your earliest anticipated day of ovulation, which also allows for more inseminations as ovulation approaches. There is also the option of having your donor ship samples to you overnight using a shipping kit that contains special "test yolk buffer" to keep the cells alive. A long-standing, queer-owned service called Donor Home Delivery provides this service in the United States for about $200 per kit (including shipping). Once you receive the samples, you can either do self-insemination or you can have the samples prepared for IUI. The timing can be a bit tricky, because the sample has to be mailed the day before you anticipate needing it, and it's best to use it the day it arrives. It's also a good idea to have your donor's shipped sample tested to make sure it survives the shipping process in ample numbers to expect conception to occur. Talk to your preconception care provider about ordering this test for you.

FRESH SAMPLE INSEMINATION LOGISTICS

There tend to be a lot of logistics involved with accessing fresh samples, so be sure you discuss these with your donor ahead of time so that everyone knows what to expect.

HOW MANY CYCLES?

Ask your donor to commit to three to six cycles of insemination. This allows your donor to know what to expect in terms of how they are going to alter their habits or support their fertility for you. If you get to your agreed-upon number of cycles without conceiving, you can renegotiate, but having an initial time frame will help keep the process from feeling too overwhelming in the beginning.

WHAT ARE THE POSSIBLE DATES YOU WILL NEED A SAMPLE?

Careful charting will help you identify the potential days that you might ovulate (see Chapter 6). Please do not rely on the predicted day of ovulation calculated by an app, as this can be inaccurate and confusing for both you and the donor. Instead, chart a few cycles and pay attention to the range of cycle days when ovulation occurs for you. While an app might use the same data and average it to predict ovulation day, you and your donor will want to know the full range of days when a sample might be needed, not just the average day. Once your period starts, which is cycle day one, you can look at the calendar and determine the date range when you will need samples. Give your donor these dates so that they can be prepared to hear from you during that time.

HOW DOES YOUR DONOR WANT TO BE CONTACTED BY YOU?

Be sure to ask your donor's preferences for how to be contacted when you need a sample. Some prefer text or a messaging app, and others prefer a phone call. Clarify ahead of time how long you should expect to wait before receiving a reply. This will avoid wondering if you should message or call again, and it will avoid your donor feeling overwhelmed with messages if they happened to be away from their phone during the time you were trying to arrange for a pickup with an impending ovulation looming. Most of the time, there is twelve to twenty-four hours of lead time, so you can also let your donor know how soon you will need to hear from them in order to arrange logistics on your end. Make some agreements, follow them, and then check in afterward, especially if you end up needing to try again. Take the initiative so that you can keep the communication clear and feeling good to everyone.

HOW WILL YOU GET THE SAMPLE?

There are a number of ways to do the handoff of a sperm sample. Be creative about what will work best for you, your partner(s), and for your donor. Here are some ways that families in my practice have handled the production and handoff of the sperm sample:

- One couple had their donor and the donor's partner over to their house to provide the sample together. The donor couple was in one bedroom messing around (and ultimately collecting the sample), while the recipient couple was in the other bedroom doing the same. Eventually, the nongestational parent-to-be met up with the donor's partner in the living room for the sample handoff, which they took back into their bedroom to do the insemination.

- A prospective single parent let their donor know it was the day to inseminate and arranged a time for him to come over to provide the sample. They left a hidden key so the donor could let himself in and waited at the corner coffee shop. The donor called once the sample was ready and he had left the apartment, so they never even saw each other on conception day.

- A poly family lived a few hours away from their donor, so they booked a hotel room in the donor's town. The donor had kids at home, so once the family was checked in and ready for a sample, the donor arranged for some "alone time" and then drove his sample over to the hotel, keeping it warm in his lap for the short drive. The conceiving parent's partners met up with the donor in the hotel lobby for the handoff and then went back upstairs for the insemination.

- Another single parent drove to her donor's house a couple of hours away, letting him know when she was about thirty minutes out. Once she arrived, she knocked on his door, he handed over the sample, and she returned to inseminate in the car using a menstrual cup to keep the sample against her cervix during the drive back home.

Unknown Donors

Conceiving with eggs or sperm from a donor who is unknown to you is more straightforward in a number of ways. While the fact of another human's contribution to conceiving your child is undeniable, the lack of relationship with that person makes accessing the gametes you need from a bank or clinic less complex. The gamete donation process provides you with well-screened donors who meet standards for fertile potential. Cryopreserved gametes are readily available when you need them, and the testing and quarantine process ensures that samples are free from communicable disease. You may be able to sift through a large number of donors to find one who has physical characteristics, interests, or accomplishments that you hope will be passed on to your child, and screen for genetic conditions to protect your offspring from inherited disorders.

However, many families struggle with choosing a donor from a bank. For such an intimate thing as choosing half your child's genetic makeup, the process of selecting a donor can feel strangely impersonal. You may be confronted with values you didn't know you had as you weigh the reasons you are drawn to one donor but not another. In your heart, you may be open to your child being whoever they are meant to be, but how do you balance that with putting your own hopes into the genetic potential you are literally choosing for them? What do you do when your emotions are in conflict with your politics? There is no right answer to such questions, so you may need to take some time to grapple with what is coming up for you before settling on a donor.

WILL MY CHILD BE OK WITH NOT KNOWING THEIR DONOR?

Further complicating the donor-selection process are fears about how your child will feel about their donor-conceived origins. Parents who were themselves adopted may fear that their child will have a similar experience to their own if they are unable to know their genetic ancestors. Sensationalized news stories about kids from the same donor finding each other and lamenting the anonymity of half their DNA can make prospective parents second-guess this choice. Some donor offspring have even formed groups on social media and created websites to express deeply unsettled emotions about their genetic origins. While such concerns are certainly valid, it is important to remember that our own children's stories have the potential to be different in essential and meaningful ways.

In queer communities, donor conception and third-party reproduction are a fact of life. The openness and honesty with which we talk to our kids about how they came to be is just one of the ways we raise our children to have pride in themselves and their families. Unfortunately, this is not the case for many cisgender, heterosexual families who find themselves unable to conceive with their own gametes. Straight parents of donor-conceived children lack the framework of normalcy we experience within queer culture. The cis/heterocentric cultural mindset is that everyone has a mother and a father, and genetics and parenthood are one and the same. However, we know that a mother or father need not be genetically related to their child, and that does not make them any less a parent. Straight parents have historically kept their children's donor conception a secret—often under the advice of a physician—thinking that somehow secrecy offers protection for their kids. However, research has shown that openness about a child's donor origins is key to supporting them in developing a positive sense of self and fostering acceptance of how they came to be.

The lens with which we view the world is at the crux of the debate about unknown gamete donors. If you view queer families as a positive expression of love and belonging in the world, make sure you apply that framework to anything you read about donor conception. So few of us were raised with such a worldview that it can be easy for the societal homo- and transphobic beliefs we were brought up with to creep in and cause us to question the validity of donor conception. Stories of offspring who are upset about their donor origins purport that donor conception is the problem—not the worldview that led their parents to feel that conceiving with a donor was something to be ashamed and secretive about, and not the worldview that makes these donor-conceived kids feel there is something unacceptable about how they came to be or that leads them to believe that a donor should have been their parent.

Raising kids in a cis/heterocentric world means cultivating pride in every aspect of who your child is, who your family is, and how it all came to be. Our children are deeply wanted, and our families are built with a great deal of intention. Once you have kids, rejecting homo/transphobic ideas is not just about you, it's about them. Our work as parents is to foster our child's sense of self, and to nurture and protect their concept of family. We do this actively every time we reframe cultural narratives that don't reflect our reality and the validity of our lives. Remember this if you are struggling with the need to access donor gametes to bring your child into the world. What narrative is playing to make you feel this is anything less than a positive, acceptable, necessary option to support you in creating a life filled with love, belonging, and family? Be cautious and attuned to your internal self-talk, the same way you would be attentive to how your child views themselves and their place in the world.

ANONYMOUS VERSUS
REVEALED-IDENTITY DONORS

Donor sperm is most commonly accessed through a sperm bank, while donor eggs or donor embryos can be accessed through clinics, banks, or agencies. While sperm donors are typically classified as anonymous or willing to be identified when the child turns eighteen, egg donors can be anonymous, willing to be known, or in some cases, even be willing to meet prospective parents prior to being selected. However, the concept of anonymity is increasingly inaccurate now that direct-to-consumer DNA testing and ancestry databases are being accessed by recipient families and donor-conceived offspring. Some parents are even able to identify a donor by cross-referencing details shared in their donor profile with information widely available on social media. Others connect with families who used the same donor through signing up with a donor registry, which adds to the potential for families to become aware of the donor's identity long before the child turns eighteen. Because of this, the donor gamete industry is pulling back from the practice of guaranteed donor anonymity, and the vast majority of donors are now classified as "willing to be known" (or other terms such as "open identity" or "ID release"). This is an important distinction considering that many offspring become curious about their genetic background at some point. Donors who agree to have their identity disclosed are more likely to be open to being contacted, which means your child is more likely to receive a positive response if and when they choose to reach out to their donor.

When comparing banks, clinics, or agencies, keep in mind that they may be the only point of contact for you to locate your donor, and they may be the only place for your donor to receive education and counseling about the prospect of being contacted by offspring. It's OK to ask questions about how donors are provided with this guidance, how the donors are contacted, and how the bank ensures that they are able to locate the donor when the time comes. The Sperm Bank of California was the first bank to institute an Identity-Release Program, and they pride themselves on not only maintaining contact with the donors but also on collecting data to guide best practices in brokering donor/offspring contact.

INFORMATION ABOUT THE DONOR

Sperm banks typically provide basic information such as hair and eye color, height, racial background, ethnic origin, level of education, and personal interests. There is always medical information such as blood type, CMV status, and genetic background. However, banks vary in how they provide additional ways to navigate donor selection, from baby photos to adult photos, handwritten letters to audio or video recordings, and sometimes even matching services that provide donor suggestions based on a parent's appearance. Typically, there are costs associated with accessing additional information about donors. Be sure to take these expenses into account when selecting a bank.

DONOR ETHNICITY

If you are in the United States, if you are white, and if you live in a major metropolitan area that has a local sperm bank or donor egg resources, you may find exactly what you need quite easily. On the other hand, if you are looking for a mixed-race donor, a donor of color, or a donor from a particular ethnic background, you will quickly find your options to be quite limited. If you are trying to match your own or a partner's non-white ethnicity, the lack of available donors presents a huge barrier. Some banks have more Black donors and other donors of color, but those banks may not be in geographical proximity to you, which means additional shipping costs. If there is a local facility that can store your donor gametes for you, you may be able to purchase multiple vials and have them all shipped at once and stored locally rather than shipping individual vials for each conception attempt. Look for local andrology ("male" fertility) labs or contact local clinics to inquire about this.

There may be further barriers if the bank that has a wider selection of donors will not release vials directly to you, and you were not planning to use a clinic to help you conceive. Most sperm banks will release vials directly to recipients with a release form signed by a health care provider (including a midwife); however, Xytex in Atlanta will only ship samples to a clinic. Given that Xytex has the largest number of Black donors, this practice perpetuates barriers to care for Black parents. Other large banks in metropolitan areas include Seattle Sperm Bank, California Cryobank, Fairfax Cryobank, and Cryos International. The Sperm Bank of California is smaller in size; but on the other hand, they also have lower family limits, unparalleled queer inclusivity, and a great deal of guidance for donor-conceived families on their website, including considerations for donor ethnicity.

Sometimes white parents-to-be consider choosing a donor of color, but this is not recommended for a variety of reasons. The simple math is that there is a significant shortage of non-white donors, and every bank has a limit on how many families can conceive with a given donor. This means that, for BIPOC families, it can be next to impossible to find a gamete donor who is racially congruous and also meets other preferences for donor gamete selection. So when a white family chooses a donor of color, they are literally preventing a family of color from selecting gametes from that donor.

Another important consideration for matching your donor with your own (or your partner's) racial background has to do with your child's lived experience. When a child looks different than their parents, others may question "where they came from" or who their "real" parents are. Racism and heterocentrism play an intersecting role in the life of a child of color who is being raised by white queer parents. Research supports selecting a donor who looks similar to you (or your partner) because of the ways that physical appearance communicates kinship to the outside world. Kids who have the same racial background as their parents tend to feel a greater sense of connectedness and belonging, versus having an experience of "otherness." This experience can be exacerbated when a child of color experiences racism in the world yet their parents do not. While it is possible for white parents of kids of color to educate themselves and to create opportunities for connection with communities of color, the lack of shared experience is a shortfall that cannot be remedied. On the other hand, if you are adding a child to a family that is already of mixed race, you may be building a greater sense of connection and cultivating resiliency in your kids by opting for a donor that reflects the racial background of your older child or children. Ultimately, the decision of donor ethnicity may be complex, but it is always worth thorough consideration.

Accessing Donor Gametes and Embryos

Since conceiving with a donor egg or using a donor embryo requires the involvement of a fertility clinic and generally has a wider variety of options for contact with the donor(s), selection is done under the guidance of your clinic or surrogacy agency. Donor sperm, on the other hand, can be accessed independently, but sperm donor selection can still be confusing and overwhelming. All of the options are covered in this section, with special attention given to the steps involved in selecting donor sperm.

DONOR SPERM FROM A BANK

1. Start at the sperm bank's home page. How do the images make you feel? If you wince every time you go to the bank's website, this will be a part of your conception process. If this is the bank that has your donor of choice, consider bookmarking a different page of the bank's website so that you don't have to be exposed to aspects that don't feel appropriate or supportive of your family.

2. Go to the donor catalog. Check out the list of available donors. If you have a specific requirement such as ethnicity, this will be your first point of investigation. Next, notice what donor qualities you gravitate toward: Height? Eye color? Educational background? Hobbies or interests? Something else?

3. Find out what additional information you can get about donors. Does the bank offer baby pictures? Voice recordings? Videos of the donor? An essay written by the donor? What type of information is important to you?

4. Check the costs. How much does this bank charge for a vial of washed, IUI-ready sperm? What extra fees do you have to pay to get background information on selected donors? Are there additional fees in the selection process that may start to add up?

5. Make sure you can get information about each donor's success in the program. Have there been pregnancies with the donor's samples? If not, and it's not a new donor, you may want to select a different option.

SELECTING THE APPROPRIATE TYPE OF VIAL

Most banks have two or three types of vials: ICI, IUI, and ART. Some even have "premium" vials with higher sperm counts. The main thing to know is that conceiving with frozen sperm is most successful with IUI, and the more sperm cells in a vial, the better. If you are doing IUI, you will need to opt for the IUI vials, and make sure they have at least 20 million motile cells per milliliter. IUI vials have been "washed," which means the sample has been processed to remove the seminal fluid, isolating the sperm cells and putting them in a carrier solution for placement in the uterus. This mimics what happens in physiological conception, where seminal fluid acts as a buffer for placement of sperm cells in the acidic environment of the vaginal canal, and the motile cells leave that fluid behind when they enter the uterus. The wash procedure does this for you so that the sperm cells can be placed directly inside the uterus and closer to the egg. For self-insemination, you can use either ICI or IUI vials. Unless you are purchasing sperm for an IVF procedure, avoid the ART vials because they are low count and only intended for IVF.

HOW MANY VIALS TO BUY

Some families select a specific donor and purchase enough vials to conceive with that donor. On average, it takes four cycles to conceive with frozen donor sperm; however, if you want to be on the safe side, plan for a total of eight to twelve cycles—especially if you hope to have enough for an additional child. You will use one vial for each insemination, and ideally, you will just do one insemination per cycle. However, if your ovulation pattern varies from month to month, or if you are not able to pinpoint your ovulation accurately, you can cover more time by doing more than one insemination per month. Alternatively, some people opt to switch donors if the first few cycles are not successful, in which case you would only want to buy one to three cycles' worth at a time.

If you want to secure your access to a specific donor, you must purchase the vials all at once. (The bank will store the vials for you until you are ready to use them.) In this case, be sure to research your options for unused vials. Will you save additional vials for a second pregnancy? What are the storage fees? Would you want to sell back unused vials? What is the reimbursement rate? What if you want to pass them on or sell them to someone else—what are the bank's policies? Make sure you know what your options are before buying more vials than you may need if you conceive on the first try. On the other hand, if you plan to purchase your vials one cycle at a time, you will need backup options in case your first-choice donor runs out. Make sure you have a plan B, and even a plan C, donor.

HOW THE VIALS GET TO YOU

Your vials will come in a tank charged with liquid nitrogen to keep them frozen until ready for use. Most tanks last up to a week; however, some banks will provide a two-week tank. Your cycle charting will inform you about the range of cycle days when you may ovulate, and the more cycles you have charted, the more accurate this prediction will be. Order the tank to arrive or be picked up at least one day before you will possibly need it, and make sure the life span of the tank will cover your latest possible day of ovulation. If your range of potential ovulation days is more than a week and your bank does not provide two-week tanks, you will want to ensure there is a way to recharge your tank. Talk to your clinic or insemination provider to find out what options there are in your community, and keep in mind that this may be a reason to use a local bank instead of one from out of town.

DONOR EGGS

If you are in need of donor eggs, the availability and cost will depend on whether you or your partner are carrying the pregnancy or you are using a surrogate. Some fertility clinics have their own egg donation program, and they may even require that you use one of their program donors. Others are more flexible in allowing you to choose your donor from an outside source. Many surrogacy agencies match intended parents with egg donors as well as gestational surrogates, which provides an enhanced level of support in the selection process, but that also comes with a higher price. Going through an egg bank is the least expensive option in terms of the cost of the gametes; however, that expense may be canceled out by the lower rate of success in IVF with frozen eggs versus eggs that are fertilized at the time of retrieval. The range of cost for a batch of donor eggs is $15,000 to $40,000, depending on whether they are frozen or fresh, or accessed through a bank, clinic, or agency. You will want to start by talking with your agency or the clinic that will be managing conception. They will provide guidance about what donor egg options your clinic is willing to work with, and from there, you can start to sort through the available donors.

DONOR EMBRYOS

Many fertility clinics have donor embryo programs (also called embryo adoption), which are a very cost-effective option worth considering under a variety of circumstances. Embryos become available for donation when families go through the IVF process and end up with extra embryos. The cost for a donor embryo cycle is $2,500 to $4,000, which is about $10,000 less than the cost of an IVF cycle. If you conceive with a donor embryo, you do not need to go to the expense of a full IVF cycle, because the in vitro fertilization has already been done. Your costs are therefore limited to the transfer of a frozen embryo. The identity of the donors can be open or anonymous, depending on the wishes of the donating family. If knowing your child's gamete donors is important to you, open embryo adoption is one way to achieve this. Using a donor embryo is especially worth looking into if you are in need of both donor egg and donor sperm, as the costs are significantly less.

GUIDANCE FOR CARE PROVIDERS

If you work with conceiving queer and trans families, conversations about donor selection are inevitable. This book provides key information; however, you will find that over years of practice, you will have a nuanced understanding of all the ways this decision-making process can play out in family constellations. You may find that the families you serve want counseling, guidance, and facilitation of decision-making, or conversely, you may find that families contact you just because they need a provider to sign their sperm bank release form. But you are so much more than a signature on a form! The need to have a health care provider sign a release form in order to access donor gametes may in some ways feel like yet another barrier for queer parents. However, as much as each family deserves agency as well as privacy in the process of conceiving their child, the use of donor gametes presents the opportunity for screening and the mitigation of risk in a way that conceiving via intercourse with an intimate partner does not. The fact that you are involved because you are a health care provider means that you must uphold your responsibility to provide health care, even if that care merely consists of providing informed consent for available testing that some parents may ultimately decline. However, you will find more often than not that once parents understand why certain preconception tests are recommended, and once they have a full understanding of the clinical considerations in donor selection, they will make more nuanced choices about this aspect of their care.

While the clinical aspects of donor selection may be relatively straightforward, the psychosocial landscape is complex. If you are a midwife, you may have the training and expertise to hold both. In fact, if you are a queer midwife, you may be the only provider in your community who has counseling skills, awareness of the donor conception process, and an identity that is culturally congruent with the clientele you serve. This is part of why queer midwives are so very needed, and why serving families in the conception process is such a vital and unique aspect of midwifery practice. Although you may need to access additional training or engage in self-directed learning in order to serve your community well, you will gain expertise over years of practice if you utilize your counseling skills, allow time for families to share their experiences with you, and hold space for your community as they navigate family formation.

Assisting families who have a known gamete donor requires special care and consideration of social risks, legal risks, and health risks. Providing information and guiding families through informed decision-making are vital aspects of care. This is yet another area of preconception care that is well served by the midwifery model. Rather than denying care for families who choose to conceive with a known sperm donor, midwives have the training and expertise to provide a thorough, informed decision-making process as well as education for mitigation of risks. This is a major advantage given that most clinics deny access to care when families have a donor who is known to them. If you feel confident in your ability to provide clinical guidance and informed choice, yet you are limited in your ability to provide counseling to families who are considering conceiving with a known donor, make sure you have a reliable referral to a mental health care provider who is well versed in LGBTQ+ family building and can provide this expertise as families navigate known donor relationships.

If you provide insemination services for families who are conceiving with fresh sperm samples from a known donor, it is imperative that you provide thorough informed consent for the risk of STI transmission, as well as reviewing guidelines for donor testing recommended in your jurisdiction (see page 114). If your client wants you to order STI testing for their donor, be very clear that a single test does not ensure they are protected from infection. A recent infection may not show positive on a test, and any ongoing exposures that occur after the test will continue to put them at risk. The FDA guidelines for donors providing fresh sperm samples are to have testing completed for specific infections within seven days of each donation, using FDA-approved tests, which cost upwards of $1,000 per cycle.

More often than not, you will find that your clients have already considered their risk for STIs from donor sperm samples. Donors can be trusted friends or relatives in monogamous relationships. They can be asexual, abstinent, or between partners (and willing to stay that way during the conception process). Your role as a clinician is to educate your clients about the risks, provide information about how to mitigate those risks, and document your informed consent discussions accordingly. Make sure you include the entire range of options, including referral to a fertility clinic or sperm bank for government-sanctioned testing and directed donor gamete cryopreservation, quarantine, and retesting, or in the United States, completing FDA-approved testing within seven days of each sample collection.

You must decide the level of risk you are willing to take as a provider when clients are seeking assisted conception services using fresh samples from a known donor. Are you willing to circumvent federal guidelines that do not account for the existence of families who inseminate at home with known donor sperm? Do you want a copy of the known donor agreement they filed with an attorney? Do you want to screen the donor and assess their STI risk yourself? Do you want to document the trusting relationship your clients have with their donor and their reasoning for feeling safe using fresh samples on an ongoing basis? What if they don't actually know the donor but they connected online or through an app—do you consent to providing assisted conception services under this circumstance? Be clear about the boundaries you have and be prepared to state them up front so there is no confusion, especially if there are circumstances in which you wish to refrain from providing services.

To understand the marginalization and lack of sensitivity many LGBTQ+ people experience in fertility clinics, see the video series "Scenes from a Fertility Clinic" available on Vimeo. Of particular concern is the requirement for prospective parents and their donor (and the donor's partner if they have one) to complete psychological evaluations and receive counseling from an in-house mental health provider. In a best-case scenario, these sessions can be useful for advising families on how to talk to their child about their donor-conceived origins and helping families and donors make sure their expectations are clear. However, the most common experience for queer and trans families is that the required mental health appointments are reminiscent of being pathologized for being queer or transgender, the mental health providers at fertility clinics rarely have more than a surface-level understanding of the needs of queer and trans parents, and the required visits represent an additional barrier to a process that is already wrought with barriers to care.

As you provide information to the families in your care, carefully navigate how you provide information about legal matters if you are not also an attorney. Laws vary from country to country and state to state. Not only do laws change all the time, case law is evolving constantly. Even if you are generally aware of some of the processes and requirements of family law in your jurisdiction, refrain from giving specific recommendations other than to consult directly with an attorney. State clearly for your clients that you are not a legal professional and cannot give legal advice. They will be much better served in the legal arena by a specialist who is current and experienced in caring for the legal aspects of family building.

Resources

Legal Support

California AB 2356—Equal Access to Fertility Medical Care: www.nclrights
.org/wp-content/uploads/2013/09/AB_2356_fact_sheet_individuals1.pdf

National Center for Lesbian Rights: www.nclrights.org/our-work
/relationships-family

Lambda Legal: www.lambdalegal.org/issues/marriage-relationships-and
-family-protections

Donor Insemination Information and Services

Donor Home Delivery sperm shipping service: DonorHomeDelivery.com

USFDA Donor Testing Guidelines: www.fda.gov/vaccines-blood-biologics
/tissue-tissue-products

Health Canada Directive for Sperm and Ova Donors: www.canada.ca/en
/health-canada/services/publications/drugs-health-products/technical
-directive-sperm-ova-donors.html

Talking to Kids About Donor Conception

The Sperm Bank of California: TheSpermBankofCA.org

What Makes a Baby by Cory Silverberg

SURROGACY

Having someone outside your relationship carry your baby through pregnancy is complex in many ways. A simple desire to become a parent, and a surrogate's simple desire to provide the gift of pregnancy to a family that needs it, can unfold into considerations for physical and mental health, legal protection, finances, and special insurance coverage for surrogacy. The village it takes to bring a child into the world via surrogacy is an intricate web to navigate, yet any steps that are skipped can put your family and/or your surrogate in jeopardy. The need for intentionality at every level is something that cannot be overlooked.

The Village It Takes to Make a Child via Surrogacy

Attorneys for:

- Parents
- Gamete donor
- Surrogate

Medical providers for:

- Gamete retrieval and IVF
- Embryo transfer
- Pregnancy and birth

Mental health providers for:

- Setting up surrogacy agreements
- Support for your surrogate
- Support for you

Health insurance carriers for:

- Gamete donor
- Surrogate
- Baby

Qualities That Make a Good Surrogate

On the surface, surrogate pregnancy can appear transactional, given that there are so many expenses and protective mechanisms involved in the process. However, the desire to be a surrogate comes from the heart. The best qualities to look for in a surrogate (and what is required by agencies who screen surrogates) is someone who has already carried at least one pregnancy, someone who is finished building their own family (because of the risks to future fertility that come with any pregnancy), someone who has a robust support system, someone who is not in a place of financial need, and someone who is in good health and is in a BMI category that represents low pregnancy risk. A surrogate must live in a state where surrogacy is legal, and they must pass medical and psychiatric evaluations. Although you may not feel this level of scrutiny is necessary when someone you know is going to be your surrogate, agencies will also perform a criminal background check, review past tax returns, and even secure a copy of the surrogate's driving record.

Choosing the Right Surrogate for You

While these aspects of determining whether or not a person would make a good surrogate are important, which person would make a good surrogate for *you* is a personal matter. One of the most important aspects of matching a surrogate with parent(s)-to-be is the personality fit. In fact, many families have found that they connected with their surrogate based on a gut feeling, or a sense that it was going to be a good fit, only to find out later that they shared different political ideologies, made different life choices, and had different ways of walking through the world than their surrogate. The uniqueness of the connection between a surrogate and a parent-to-be is that it is centered around bringing your baby into the world. This means that love is present in that relationship, which is a greater force of connection than the differences that would otherwise hold you apart.

Because of the profound nature of such a relationship, in many families, the connection continues for years to come. Surrogates and parents who live in different parts of the country or different parts of the world may travel to see one another on vacation, and surrogates sometimes attend important events in the child's life such as birthdays or graduations. The surrogate's partner may also be involved in the connection you all share, because the gift of surrogacy is so all-encompassing to the surrogate's life and those who love and care for them.

Costs of Surrogacy

Legal expenses in surrogacy are multifaceted. Laws regarding surrogacy vary across jurisdictions, including whether or not surrogacy is outlawed outright, whether or not a surrogate can receive payment, and whether one or both parents will need to go through an adoption process to secure legal parentage of their own child. Legal expenses include attorneys for the parents, the surrogate, and any gamete donors who are involved. Add to that the medical and insurance expenses of conception, pregnancy, and birth; travel costs for a surrogate who does not live close to you; the cost of mental health professionals to guide everyone through the relational aspects of the surrogacy process; and surrogacy fees that compensate for the physical and emotional labor of pregnancy and cover lost wages. It is no wonder that the typical cost of a surrogate pregnancy can be anywhere from $100,000 to $200,000.

SURROGACY AGENCIES

Many readers may be overwhelmed already by this brief listing of considerations and providers needed to help a surrogacy arrangement go well. Luckily, surrogacy agencies exist to help navigate all aspects of the process. While this can make up $25,000 to $40,000 of the overall price tag, it provides for the expertise needed to navigate insurance, medical, and legal systems; the many practical tasks that need to be completed; and the emotional labor you would otherwise be incurring while wading through the process yourself. If you were doing a home remodel or planning a wedding that cost that much, you would most likely hire a contractor or a wedding planner, especially if you don't have those skills or expertise yourself. A surrogacy agency is similar. Surrogacy agencies provide education about the process, access to screened gamete donors and surrogates, connections to vetted professionals, anticipatory guidance through a medically complex process, and advice that is grounded and informed as experienced navigators of all aspects of surrogacy. For instance, considering the legal process alone, a surrogacy agency knows what states are surrogacy friendly and in what scenario (queer, hetero, married, unmarried, country or state of origin), while the attorney in your local jurisdiction may only be an expert on the laws (and the judges) in your own state. You need both, but at the outset when you may be involving a surrogate who lives in a different jurisdiction than you, you will benefit by having the guidance of a professional who is in the know.

Surrogacy agencies typically offer a free interview, so there is nothing to lose in making contact, getting a feel for the agency, and learning more about the services they provide. Some surrogacy agencies focus on serving LGBTQ+ families, such as Growing Generations and Circle Surrogacy. They provide an established process that is primarily based on making each step as streamlined as possible. Other agencies, such as Heart to Hands, take a more holistic approach and emphasize careful matching and relationship facilitation between intended parents and surrogates. No matter what agency you choose, you are paying to be guided through the process by someone who is familiar with it, knows the pitfalls, knows how to prepare you for what's ahead, and knows how to talk with you about all the potentialities. Surrogate pregnancy is not simple—it involves human beings, human bodies, and a clinical process with no guarantees. In the midst of it all, you are building a creation story for your family, which means the process matters.

NAVIGATING FINANCIAL DISPARITIES

There are organizations that provide financial assistance for some of the medical aspects of the process, although the only funding source specifically available for surrogacy in our community is the Men Having Babies Gay Parenting Assistance Program, which caters to cisgender gay men. However, cisgender women and nonbinary and transgender parents-to-be are at an even greater level of economic disparity. The cost of surrogacy is unattainable for many of us, and intersectional factors such as systemic racism and disability injustice make matters even worse. When the only funding program for queer families focuses so exclusively on the needs of cisgender gay men, prospective parents who do not fall in this category bear the burden of marginalization from within our own community. However, another benefit to working with an agency is their knowledge of funding sources that are appropriate for queer and trans families, so it may be worthwhile to pursue this option for support in navigating the finances. Alternative options include taking out a loan, borrowing from a retirement savings account, or asking family members for help.

Types of Surrogacy

Some people attempt to circumvent the costs of surrogacy by asking a friend or family member to carry a pregnancy for them via insemination. Because the baby is conceived with the surrogate's own gametes, this is known as *traditional surrogacy*. While this option may seem more simple, there are pitfalls at every turn, and the result can be anything but simple. If things don't go as anticipated, the relational fallout can be insurmountable, especially if the surrogate is a family member, and especially if there has been a lack of guidance in setting up agreements at the outset. A surrogacy agency that provides services for traditional surrogacy can be invaluable in this situation. It can be difficult to find a clinic that will work with a traditional surrogacy because of the high potential for litigation over parental rights. In fact, it can be difficult to find an attorney who will work with traditional surrogacy, because an attorney's job is to protect you from legal risk, and traditional surrogacy is inherently legally risky. Your legal vulnerability in a traditional surrogacy means that a judge may be the one to decide who the baby's parents are after the baby arrives. If you want to avoid this legal ambiguity and the fallout that could occur if your surrogate changes their mind or if a judge does not agree to grant you legal parentage, the best option for you is gestational surrogacy.

Gestational surrogacy involves a person who carries a pregnancy that is conceived via IVF with gametes that do not belong to them. You could potentially have someone you know carry the pregnancy for you, called a compassionate carrier, which is typically done without financial compensation. There are still many expenses involved in the process, including donor gametes, IVF, embryo transfer, mental health screenings, legal expenses, medical expenses, and surrogate health insurance. If you think you might know someone who could carry a pregnancy for you, put the notion forward, and then let the potential surrogate come to you if they are interested (see Chapter 4 for more specifics). This avoids having someone who cares about you saying yes because they feel they can't say no. It's also important to realize that your relationship with this person will change irreversibly. If they are part of your support system, their ability to support you objectively will shift because they will be personally involved. And from here on out, they will be the person who carried your baby for nine months. Questions will arise about what place this person holds in your life, in your child's life, and in your family. If the pregnancy doesn't go as planned, if there is a pregnancy loss, or if the surrogate's ongoing health, well-being, or future fertility is affected by the pregnancy, this will be a part of the fabric of your relationship. All of this might seem to fit perfectly within the relationship you have with a known surrogate, but that still doesn't mean you can safely skip the process of creating written agreements.

If you don't have someone in your life who might want to carry a pregnancy for you, a surrogacy agency can help you locate a surrogate. Matching intended parents (the term used in the surrogacy world to signify the parent(s) of a child who is being carried by a surrogate) with surrogates is a very important part of the role of an agency and requires special skill for assessing aspects of relational compatibility such as personality, communication style, and sense of humor.

Navigating the Surrogate Relationship

Once you identify a potential surrogate, there are a number of tough conversations to be had. This is another area that can be tricky with someone you know; however, if done well, it will serve all of you in the end. Surrogacy is an arrangement among human beings, and humans are complex. There are many emotions involved on both sides. There is a need to have honest, transparent conversations with all parties involved and to create a solid and thorough written agreement. It is highly recommended to have a mental health professional who is experienced in third-party reproduction to guide you in making sure your expectations are in alignment. This is typically done by meeting with each of you separately, and then bringing everyone together to facilitate a discussion. Some of the things that are covered include:

- Making concrete agreements about finances at every step of the process
- Establishing preferred modes of communication
- Determining frequency of communication at various stages in the process
- Choosing the model of care for pregnancy and birth
- Deciding who will attend prenatal visits, ultrasounds, birth
- Noting indications for termination of pregnancy and who decides
- Setting expectations and boundaries around nutrition, supplements, and self-care
- Planning for the surrogate to lactate and provide milk, and if so, for how long
- Outlining expectations for ongoing contact
- Planning for how disagreements or misunderstandings will be addressed

This type of honest, forthright communication ultimately provides the foundation for a healthy relationship between a surrogate and intended parent(s). After all, written contracts are simply a way to record the things you have discussed and the decisions you have all agreed upon, which provides clarity for your ongoing connection. At its core, the relationship between parent(s)-to-be and their surrogate is about the gift of life, brought forth with intention and love. Setting things up well in the beginning allows the relationship to unfold unhindered by things left unsaid and questions left unanswered. It opens the pathway to share empathy and understanding for what each of you is going through. Beyond this heartfelt emotional connection, intended parents can also provide outward expressions of support for the person carrying, such as sending gift certificates for pregnancy massage, restaurant meals, or books; comfort items such as a body pillow, soft blanket, plush robe or slippers; and self-care supplies such as bath salts, body oil, and candles.

A NOTE ABOUT TWINS

It's important to consider the potential for multiple pregnancy and what that would mean. Many intended parents prefer twins, in hopes that a single surrogate pregnancy could fulfill the totality of their family-building goals. However, the best chance of a full-term, live birth and a healthy baby is a singleton pregnancy. The fact is that multiple pregnancy presents increased risk of major health issues, including mortality, for both the carrier and the babies. You can't always ensure that a pregnancy will result in only one baby, because splitting can occur even in single embryo transfer, so you will want to make agreements ahead of time about how this will be handled. Will you transfer one, and then leave it be if the embryo splits? Will you do a selective reduction if multiple pregnancy occurs? Will the pregnancy be terminated? A mental health professional who understands these processes can be invaluable in guiding you through these decisions and mediating agreements with your surrogate.

Going to a Clinic That Has a Surrogacy Program

Some fertility clinics have their own surrogacy program, and if one of these exists in your area, you can often go directly to them instead of working with a surrogacy agency. However, if you do not have your own compassionate carrier in mind, you will still be referred to an agency for surrogate matching. Such clinics typically have someone you can talk to about their process up front, and those who work with queer families will have given some level of attention to this in terms of the questions they ask, the forms they use, and the language they use to discuss your family-building goals. If your clinic manages the surrogacy process, this involves having your potential surrogate forward their medical records to the clinic for preliminary review. They will then be educated on the process of frozen embryo transfer and go to the clinic for a medical evaluation. Legal contracts will be signed under separate representation, and both the intended parents and the surrogate (and their partner) will need to complete psychological screening and counseling.

Build a Strong Foundation for Your Baby's Arrival

There are unique considerations for surrogate pregnancy that apply to parents versus surrogates. Eventually, you will be navigating the pregnancy of your child, but the body that carries your child will belong to your surrogate. Take the time and invest in setting everything up as well as you possibly can so that the arrival of your baby can be all about love and connection, and the gift of life.

GUIDANCE FOR CARE PROVIDERS

If you are an independent practitioner who provides insemination services, you may be approached from time to time by families who are pursuing pregnancy with a traditional surrogate. However, keep in mind that surrogacy is a complicated labyrinth of relationships, legal concerns, and health care needs that are underscored by financial considerations and the need to navigate health insurance systems that apply uniquely to surrogacy. If you do not have a care team of legal and mental health providers and expertise regarding surrogate pregnancy, I encourage you to refrain from providing conception services, because the implications for any oversight or mistake you make could be legally or financially calamitous to the intended parents as well as to the surrogate. Instead, refer inquiries to a surrogacy agency that serves families seeking traditional surrogacy, or a clinic in your area if there is one. Alternatively, if you want to build a practice that includes surrogacy services, consult with an attorney who specializes in surrogacy and expect to continue to access legal counsel on an ongoing basis as you provide care.

Resources

Surrogacy Agencies

Growing Generations: GrowingGenerations.com

Circle Surrogacy: CircleSurrogacy.com

Heart to Hands Surrogacy: HearttoHandsSurrogacy.com

INSEMINATION METHODS
AND TIMING

In order to inseminate at the appropriate time, *you must know when you are ovulating.*

Sperm and egg have to be in the same place at the same time for conception to occur. While fresh sperm can live in the cervix and fallopian tubes for up to three days, frozen sperm is only viable for twelve to twenty-four hours. The egg cell is only viable for twelve to sixteen hours, and if there are no functional sperm cells awaiting its release or appearing shortly after ovulation, conception will not occur.

Fresh sperm is most successful at conception when insemination or intercourse is timed twenty-four to forty-eight hours before ovulation, but if you are using frozen sperm, timing needs to be much more precise due to its shortened life span. In fact, if you are using frozen samples, you will double your chances of pregnancy by doing IUI (intrauterine insemination) as opposed to self-insemination, but IUI is most effective when performed within twelve hours of the release of your egg. Given that many of us are spending more than $1,000 per cycle on a vial of frozen sperm and an IUI procedure, finding the right day to inseminate, and the best hours of that day to inseminate, is absolutely worth the effort—and totally doable.

Inseminating at the Right Time for the Sperm You Have

	Sperm Life Span	Best Time to Inseminate
Fresh sperm	Up to three days	Twenty-four to forty-eight hours before ovulation
Frozen sperm	Twelve to twenty-four hours	Within twelve hours of ovulation

The methods of identifying ovulation and timing inseminations in this chapter are based on available scientific evidence, but you will likely find a great deal of conflicting information on the internet, social media, ovulation tracker apps, package instructions on ovulation predictor kits, and even from your doctor or fertility clinic. This is because common knowledge, as well as medical education about reproductive function, is deeply cis/heteronormative. It often erroneously applies what is known about conception via intercourse to donor insemination, which is completely different—especially if donor samples have been frozen. It also overlooks the individual differences that are inherent in the human body. For more than thirty years, myself and other providers at MAIA Midwifery & Fertility Services have relied on an individualized approach to insemination timing. This means observing the real-time physiological signs of ovulation and timing inseminations accordingly, rather than blindly relying on a standardized approach that may work for some but is not appropriate for all. An individualized approach requires taking time to educate conceiving families, trusting people to play a central role in their conception, and using each person's observations of ovulation to create an appropriate timing plan. Ultimately, it puts people at the center of managing their reproductive care, which means the conception experience is participatory, embodied, and empowering.

As you read through this chapter, keep in mind that taking the extra steps to get the timing right could save you a great deal of expense on multiple levels. Repeating insemination cycles that are unsuccessful due to poor timing can be financially draining and emotionally exhausting. Fertility clinics have IVF at the ready if insemination does not result in conception, but if this is not your preferred route to pregnancy, it will serve you well to make sure you've got the timing right. Fortunately, identifying your signs of ovulation is not expensive. With a few basic tools, and about fifteen minutes in the morning and evening for about a week mid-cycle each month, you can accurately identify your ovulation pattern and time your inseminations successfully, to within a few hours of the release of your egg.

Physiology of Ovulation

A new cycle begins on the first day of your period. During the first few days of your cycle, while menses is occurring, your body is selecting a pool of egg follicles to develop during that month. This is why the first half of your cycle is called the "follicular phase." Estrogen and progesterone are both low as the cycle begins, but soon, under the influence of follicle-stimulating hormone (FSH) from the pituitary gland, estrogen starts to rise.

By the end of the first week of your cycle, a few dominant egg follicles are chosen, and over the next few days, those follicles start to become more and more robust, filling with follicular fluid and preparing to respond to the signals that tell the chosen follicle to release an egg. Meanwhile, estrogen continues to rise, thickening the lining of the uterus in preparation for receiving an embryo if conception occurs. You might sense this with a heavy or bloated feeling in your lower abdomen, or cramping that can occur as ligaments stretch with the increased weight of the uterus and ovaries. You may also notice that your genital fluid becomes more copious, clear, and watery.

Sometime near the end of the second week of your cycle (this can be anywhere from cycle day eleven to seventeen, and sometimes even later), there is a final crescendo of hormonal events that result in the release of your egg. FSH takes a sharp drop and then rises again, selecting one dominant follicle. Estrogen levels start to peak, triggering the release of luteinizing hormone (LH) from the pituitary gland. As LH surges through the bloodstream, it is picked up by the ovary, and the dominant follicle responds to this chemical message by preparing to release the egg. LH is also secreted in your urine, which is what causes an ovulation predictor kit (OPK) to turn positive.

During the lag time between the LH surge and the release of the egg, the chromosomes inside the egg are lining up on their spindle, completing the first stage of meiosis 1. With estrogen levels at their highest, you may find clear, stretchy, or even egg-white consistency fertile fluid on your underwear or when you wipe after using the bathroom (although as we age, it sometimes isn't so obvious). Libido increases, and there may be a number of notable changes in your mood, appetite, and sleep. Finally, anywhere from a few hours to a couple of days after LH has reached the ovary, the follicle erupts, and the egg cell comes flooding out in a pool of follicular fluid. The fimbriae at the end of the adjacent fallopian tube sweep up the egg cell and move it toward the inner part of the tube where it awaits the arrival of motile, hyperactivated sperm cells.

Once the egg is released, estrogen levels diminish slightly, causing the genital fluid to lose its stretchy quality and shift to a creamy or tacky consistency. Within a day or two, the empty follicle, now called the corpus luteum, begins secreting high levels of progesterone. This is why the second half of the cycle is called the "luteal phase." Progesterone takes over the function of maintaining the uterine lining, and it raises body temperature slightly (think of this as making a cozy nest). If conception occurs, the fallopian tubes gently move the embryo down into the uterus, where it nestles itself into the rich uterine lining to connect with the pregnant person's blood supply. Sometimes a little bit of blood is released as this happens, so you may get "implantation bleeding" about six to eight days after conception. Estrogen levels rise, as do levels of human chorionic gonadotropin (hCG), which cause the positive reading on a urine pregnancy test. If conception has not occurred, progesterone levels drop (as does basal body temperature), and within a day or two, the uterine lining begins to shed, starting a new cycle all over again.

THE OVULATION CYCLE

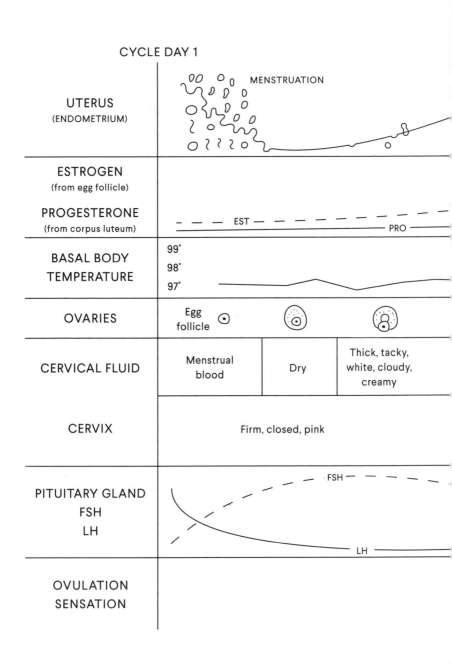

CYCLE DAY 1

UTERUS (ENDOMETRIUM) — MENSTRUATION

ESTROGEN (from egg follicle)

PROGESTERONE (from corpus luteum) — EST — PRO

BASAL BODY TEMPERATURE — 99° 98° 97°

OVARIES — Egg follicle

CERVICAL FLUID — Menstrual blood | Dry | Thick, tacky, white, cloudy, creamy

CERVIX — Firm, closed, pink

PITUITARY GLAND FSH LH — FSH — LH

OVULATION SENSATION

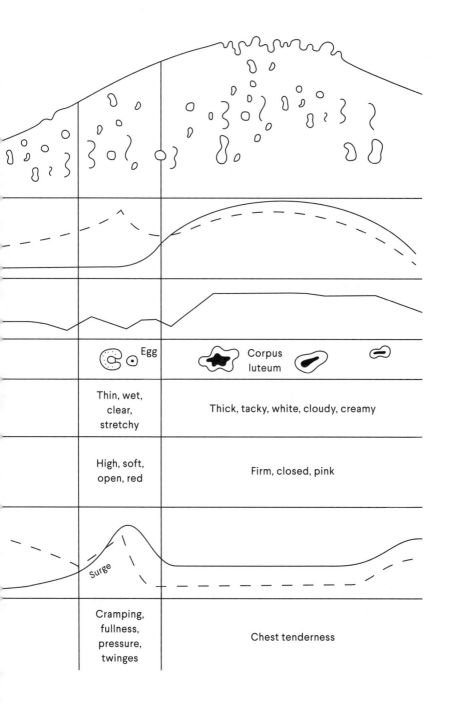

Egg

Corpus
luteum

Thin, wet,
clear,
stretchy

Thick, tacky, white, cloudy, creamy

High, soft,
open, red

Firm, closed, pink

Surge

Cramping,
fullness,
pressure,
twinges

Chest tenderness

How to Know When You Are Ovulating: Track Estrogen and LH

You can get a general idea of when you are ovulating by mapping your symptoms of high estrogen. Estrogen symptoms increase until the egg is released, and then they go away. The day those signs are strongest is the day you release your egg. With fresh sperm, you can inseminate during the high estrogen days leading up to ovulation, knowing that your body will harbor the sperm for a few days awaiting the release of the egg. Understanding this can be revolutionary, and it's why Toni Weschler's *Taking Charge of Your Fertility* has become so popular with cis/het women who want to welcome or avoid pregnancy.

However, if you are conceiving with frozen sperm, you will need to take it one step further, so that your insemination can be scheduled with precision—within twelve hours of the release of your egg. You can do this by using a urine ovulation predictor kit, or OPK, alongside tracking your symptoms of high estrogen. The OPK detects the onset of the surge in luteinizing hormone, or LH, that precedes ovulation. The LH surge tells your ovary to prepare the egg for fertilization, and when that process is complete, it ovulates. Meanwhile, until your egg is released, your estrogen keeps rising, which gives you all the symptoms of high estrogen listed below. Noting the length of time from the onset of the LH surge (as signified by the first positive reading on the OPK) to your strongest signs of high estrogen will help you determine what the OPK positive means for *you*. How long after the LH surge do *you* ovulate?

IDENTIFYING SYMPTOMS OF HIGH ESTROGEN

The symptoms of high estrogen are unmistakable once you realize what to look for.

Fluid: Estrogen changes the cellular structure of all secretions from mucus membranes in the body. The genital fluid produced by the cervix (the opening to the uterus) becomes clear and stretchy, often in copious amounts.

Cervix: The cervix becomes very soft, and the os (opening to the cervix) enlarges in order to allow for the passage of sperm.

Abdominal sensation: The uterine lining becomes very thick by this time, and many people notice a feeling of fullness in the lower part of the abdomen. High estrogen levels also affect the mucosa of the large intestine, causing gas, bloating, and even rumbling noises. The ligaments that hold the uterus in place and connect the ovaries can start to pull and stretch, and they might even cramp or twinge repeatedly under the added weight and activity of the reproductive organs.

Libido: High estrogen levels have a marked effect on libido, and sex drive increases as ovulation approaches.

Sleep: On the night you ovulate, you may be wakeful or have vivid dreams.

Mood: Mood changes can happen in a myriad of ways, most often presenting as feeling "on," creative, outgoing, or especially productive on ovulation day. Track what you experience, and see what patterns occur for you.

Appetite: The body is doing a lot of work to manufacture hormones at ovulation time, which you may observe as food cravings or just generally feeling hungrier than usual.

There are a few simple tools you can use to help you observe signs of high estrogen. You can use your own fingers to detect fertile fluid, as well as changes in the consistency of the cervix from firm to soft. Or, a good-quality plastic speculum, along with a flashlight and a mirror, can help you view the changes in your cervix. Detailed instructions are provided later in this chapter. If you are planning to inseminate with frozen sperm, it is very important to track your estrogen symptoms twice daily—so that you pinpoint ovulation within twelve hours. If you monitor the physiological signs of peak estrogen twice daily, in the morning and evening, you will find that the body will often tell you what time of day you are releasing the egg. You will know your estrogen levels have peaked (and therefore stopped rising) once they begin to go away. This is important for learning what to predict in future cycles, which will help you time your inseminations.

UNDERSTANDING THE LH SURGE

The onset of the LH surge signals that ovulation is approaching, but it doesn't tell you exactly how far away ovulation is. To find out your body's pattern of ovulation in relation to your LH surge, you will test your urine twice each day (about every twelve hours) as ovulation approaches. The first positive OPK reading (when the test line is equally as dark as the control line) indicates the onset of the LH surge. The onset of the LH surge is the benchmark you will use to predict when your ovulation will occur. This means you can stop testing with the OPK once you have noted a positive reading.

As you get your OPK positive, track your peak estrogen symptoms closely. If your estrogen symptoms tend to peak twelve hours after the onset of your LH surge, then that means you ovulate twelve hours after your OPK positive. If they peak twenty-four hours later, then you ovulate twenty-four hours after your positive. If they peak thirty-six hours later, you ovulate thirty-six hours after your positive. If you find that by the time you get an OPK positive, your estrogen symptoms are peaking, and they go away twelve hours later, your ovulation is already occurring by the time you get a positive on your OPK. In any case, IUI should happen as closely as possible to the release of your egg, so knowing the timing of your ovulation in relation to the OPK positive will help you achieve the right timing for your body.

Use the MAIA Cycle Chart to Track Your Observations

The MAIA Cycle Chart (see page 142) is an ovulation detection tool that allows you to record your signs and symptoms of ovulation twice daily during the fertile window, which is necessary to hone in on the twelve-hour window most appropriate for insemination with frozen sperm. At first glance, the chart may look overwhelming—but look a bit more closely. Even though the chart contains space to track a forty-day cycle, you will only be tracking fertile signs for about a week, mid-cycle. Also note that the first page of the chart has three lines that are repeated for tracking the most important fertile signs twice each day. Turn the chart sideways to write vertically in the space provided. Limit your notes to the most important and descriptive terms, which will assist you in interpreting the chart more easily.

The MAIA Cycle Chart has space for the most distinct fertile signs on page one, with corroborating signs and a large basal body temperature chart on page two. If you print the chart single-sided and record your temp line in pen, you can put page two behind page one and hold it up to the light to see the changes in temperature as a backdrop to your record of your peak fertile signs. Low-tech genius!

Keep in mind that you will be identifying ovulation by noting three things clearly on your chart:

1. The onset of the fertile window

2. The peak of the fertile window

3. The end of the fertile window

You will need to start tracking early enough to catch the onset of your fertile window. If your cycles are twenty-eight days or less, start tracking fertile signs on day nine. If your cycles are twenty-nine days or more, you can start tracking on day ten or eleven. Once you become more familiar with the range of days you tend to start getting fertile signs, you will be able to hone in on the days you really need to track. In other words, cast your net wide at the beginning, and over time, the charting will get much easier and take less time and effort. In the meantime, enjoy learning some new skills and witnessing the magic that happens in your body each month!

INSTRUCTIONS FOR USING THE MAIA CYCLE CHART

You can either download the MAIA Cycle Chart (see page 184), or you can make a photocopy of the chart in this book. Using the MAIA Cycle Chart will assist you in making sure you don't miss any vital information as you progress through your fertile window.

Month and year, cycle number, cycle length, and days of insemination: You will be keeping charts for a few months, and the information at the top will be important to reference as you look back over the charts to learn your body's patterns. If you are submitting your charts to your care provider for interpretation and assessment, be sure to include your name at the top.

Cycle day, date, and day of the week: Cycle day one is the first day of your period—specifically, your first day of full flow—so if you get some light spotting at the beginning, wait for your full flow and note that as cycle day one. Everything is tracked according to cycle day, which over time allows you to become familiar with the range of cycle days when you tend to ovulate. This can help a lot with planning. Once you get your period (day one) fill out the date and the day of the week across the top of the chart, for as long as you expect your cycle to last. Do this on page two of the chart as well. This is here to help you chart your symptoms on the correct day as you go along.

Conception attempts: Record any time your body is exposed to sperm, whether this is via intercourse, vaginal insemination, or IUI. Be sure to track the method and the time of day for each attempt. You will be able to look back and see what worked or what didn't.

AM fertile signs and PM fertile signs: Notice that there are two identical sections under shaded gray lines, for morning fertile signs and evening fertile signs. These are the fertile signs that should be tracked and recorded *twice per day*. Many people do this in the morning before they go to work and the evening before they go to bed. Tracking these signs will help you narrow down your ovulation patterns to successfully time your IUI within twelve hours of ovulation.

Cervix: The cervix provides the single most direct indication of peak estrogen and the release of your egg. Most people are amazed—even incredulous—at what they can know about their bodies just by looking. *Why aren't we taught this in school?* The cervix gives clear information every single month about when we are ovulating. It is the most straightforward fertile sign we have, and it is right there to be observed, granting you the ability to harness your body's reproductive capacity. Because the cervix is located inside the body, where the vaginal canal meets the uterus, observing its changes requires looking or feeling inside your body. While this can be deeply empowering for some, it can be deeply dysphoric for others. If you are not able to observe changes in your cervix, tracking the other symptoms of high estrogen will become even more vital for identifying the time of ovulation.

Some of the cervix changes are observable by feel, and others require viewing your cervix with a speculum. At some point after your period has stopped, and no later than day nine, start checking your cervix daily until you notice it getting softer and more open. Once these changes start to occur, check twice per day, being careful to note the texture as well as how open the os is. You may also notice that there is a change in position—you might feel the cervix higher (harder to reach) or lower (easier to reach) than it was last time you checked, or maybe you will find it off to the side, or maybe it will become more midline. Everyone is different. Whatever you feel, write it down.

Cervical changes you can observe with your fingers:

- You will find the cervix by inserting your fingers into the vaginal canal and feeling all the way inside, past the ridged vaginal walls, to the very end of the tunnel where there is a round, smooth, donut-shaped cervix. It might be kind of firm or pointy, or it may be soft and mushy, depending on where you are at in your cycle. When you are not fertile, the cervix is firm, like the tip of your nose. As ovulation approaches, it gets softer, like your chin. When estrogen levels are highest, the cervix is very soft, like your lips.

- Try to find the dimple or hole in the cervix, called the os. If it's not immediately obvious, try reaching around to the back, or feel around the sides. Sometimes the cervix is pointed downward or to the side. Take note of this position, as well as how far or "high" you had to reach to feel it.

- As you approach ovulation, you will also note that the os becomes wider or more open, and after ovulation, it closes again. This is easier to see than to feel at first, which is why a lot of people look with a mirror and a speculum to monitor the changes.

- Don't be discouraged if it all seems the same and you can't detect many changes from day to day. It typically takes two or three cycles to start to understand what you are feeling with your fingertips, which is why it pays to start tracking your cycles a few months before you plan to conceive.

Cervical changes you can observe with a speculum and mirror:

- You will be amazed at the changes you observe when you view your cervix through ovulation. The color may deepen to a darker red or even purple. The os may go from being a tight dimple to a wide-open O—or if you have given birth before or had any procedures through your cervix, your os may look like a smile that opens slightly at ovulation time. Using a speculum on your own at home is completely different than having a speculum placed by a health care provider. For one thing, you are in complete control. If something doesn't feel right, you can stop immediately. Once you get the hang of it, it will be quite easy. You can see examples of what the cervix looks like at The Beautiful Cervix Project website or in the Timing is Everything online course on the MAIA website.

- To view your cervix with a speculum, first make sure you have a speculum that is easy to use. A plastic speculum that has a hinge where the handle meets the bills is best. While most people do fine with a size medium speculum, if you don't typically engage in penetrative sex, you might be more comfortable with a size small. You can get a good-quality speculum on the MAIA web store.

- You will also need a flashlight and a medium- to large-size handheld mirror—not a tiny compact mirror. You can either lie down in a semi-reclining position, or place the mirror on the floor and squat over it while you place the speculum inside. If you choose to observe your cervix lying down, use plenty of pillows—two to prop up your head and shoulders, and a couple of pillows to support each of your knees as you relax them open. Otherwise, you may inadvertently be tensing the muscles in your pelvic floor as you hold your knees open, which will make insertion more uncomfortable.

- With your body fully supported on your bed, or squatting over a mirror, place one or two fingers inside your opening. Take a deep breath, sending your breath to the muscles that you can feel surrounding your fingers, and breathe out any tension until you feel the muscles relax.

- Once your opening is relaxed, make sure the speculum is completely closed, and insert just the tip of the speculum, with the handle pointing up and the speculum tilted slightly to the side. The insertion will be more comfortable if you use your other hand to hold the labia open and out of the way—otherwise they can get pulled inside as the speculum is inserted. A little bit of lube on the outside of the bills can help as well.

- Apply slight pressure in and back, toward your tailbone. The angle is the same as if you were inserting a tampon. Once the tip of the speculum passes your opening, it will slide easily into place, all the way until the handles of the speculum are touching or almost touching the outside of your body.

- At this point, take a deep breath before you do anything else. Relaxing your body will help your cervix slide more easily into view once you open the bills of the speculum.

- When you are ready, press the lever on the outside of the speculum to open the bills. You will hear the lever click once or twice as you open it, and then it should stay in place.

- Pick up the mirror and flashlight. Hold the mirror so that you can see inside your body, and point the flashlight into the mirror. The mirror will reflect the light inside, so once you tilt the mirror to bring your cervix into view, the light will be shining right where you need it to be.

- If you see a round, smooth donut with a small hole or dimple (the os), you have found your cervix. You may need to adjust the angle of the speculum to bring the cervix into the speculum bills and center the os. If instead you see something that looks like stretched skin, with no os in sight, you have probably passed the cervix—but it is most likely sitting right on top of the bill of the speculum. Simply close the speculum, pull it out just a bit (not more than a centimeter or two) and open the bills again. The cervix should slide right into view.

- If you can't find your cervix no matter what you do, stop and try again tomorrow. You may find that squatting is more successful than lying down, or vice versa. You might find it helpful to feel for the location and position of your cervix with your fingers before you insert the speculum, so that you know where to go. Is the cervix super high and hard to reach with your fingers? If so, you may need to insert the speculum as far as it can possibly go—you can even try jumping up and down for a bit before you insert the speculum, to relax the pelvic floor and bring the cervix down. Squatting may also be more helpful if your cervix is high. If the cervix is way off to the side, you can angle the speculum toward it as you insert the bills. If the cervix is very low—right inside without having to insert your fingers very far—then you won't need to insert the speculum very far either.

- If you have someone to help you view your cervix, they can use a head-lamp for light, allowing them to view inside the speculum and watch for the cervix to appear as the speculum is inserted. Aiming the speculum toward the tailbone, look carefully through the top bill, watching for the dark dimple of the cervical os to appear. Once you see it, you can open the bills and allow the cervix to slip into place.

- Once the cervix is clearly in view, note the following:

  ◦ Was the cervix high, low, medium, or to the right, left, or midline?

  ◦ Does the cervix seem to be firm, medium, or soft?

  ◦ What color is the cervix? Are there any darker areas?

  ◦ Is the os more open or more closed than last time you looked? You are looking for what is "most open" for you, before the os closes again.

- When you have noted all the pertinent information, you can remove the speculum. Do this very carefully. A speculum is designed to hold the cervix in place, so you will want to release the cervix before pulling the speculum out. This is easily done by opening the speculum an additional click or two, tilting it up or down, pulling it out slightly to bring the tips of the bills off of the cervix, and then closing the bills before bringing the speculum out completely.

- Wash your speculum with soap and water and leave it to dry until it is time to check your cervix again.

With all of the information to be gleaned by observing your cervix, you may feel frustrated that so little space is given to record it on the chart! However, this is intentional, because the information is most useful when it is distilled down to simple, focused terms. On a typical ovulation day, the cervix is high, soft, and open, which can be recorded as "HSO" or simply "OPEN" in all caps. Days leading up to ovulation might read "opening" or "more open" as well as "softer" in consistency. If your cervix tends to change positions, you can note this with an "R" or "L" for right or left, or "forward" or "back." Color change can be noted by "pink" or "red." After ovulation, you can note "closing" or "closed."

Fluid: You can check your fluid with your fingers, which works fine for many people. However, many people don't ever find their fertile fluid until they view the cervix with a speculum. Any way you go about it, intentionally looking for your fertile fluid is much more accurate than haphazardly waiting to find fertile fluid on your underwear or toilet paper. To check with your fingers, first make sure they are clean. Insert a finger or two as far as you can reach, then bring your fingers back out and note the consistency of the fluid as you pinch your index finger and thumb together and apart. With a speculum, you can view your fluid at its source—the cervix. Fertile fluid can be seen glistening at the cervical os and/or flowing out into the bills of the speculum. You can check to see how stretchy the fluid is after you remove the speculum—take a bit on your fingers, and see how far it stretches. Some people think they don't have fertile fluid until they start looking with a speculum—only to find that it was there all along.

When estrogen levels are high, the fertile fluid becomes clear and sometimes stretchy—it may even stretch to four centimeters or more! Some people note a raw egg-white consistency. Any day you note clear, stretchy, or egg-white fluid is a potentially fertile day. Take note of the fluid becoming more copious or stretching longer. After ovulation, you will see the fluid return to a non-fertile consistency, which is creamy, sticky, or tacky—think of various stages of drying Elmer's glue. You never need to use more than one or two words to note the consistency of your fluid on the chart—use the words that are most descriptive, especially noting any "clear" or "stretchy" fluid, even if it is interspersed with creamy or white.

OPK and fertility monitor: This is where you will track indicators of LH in your urine. To get an accurate reading, you will need to allow at least three hours for urine to accumulate in your bladder before testing. Twice each day, morning and evening, catch some urine in a cup and dip the reagent strip, or you can just hold the strip in your urine stream. As the urine is absorbed into the reagent strip, one line shows up to tell you the kit is working (the control line), and a second line starts to appear when there is LH in your urine (the test line). Note when a light test line appears, and continue to take note as the test line becomes darker over time. The first time you see a test line equal to or darker than the control line is your OPK positive, indicating the onset of your LH surge. *After you record a positive reading, stop using the OPK.* Any continued secretion of LH in your urine is meaningless in determining the release of your egg (even though some brands say otherwise). Instead, keep a close eye on your estrogen symptoms after noting the onset of the LH surge, which is a much more accurate method. If you find that your estrogen symptoms peak within twelve hours or less of the OPK positive, you may need to use those darkening, almost-positive readings for a bit more heads-up to schedule your insemination. In addition to a morning and evening test, some people do a midday test as well. This may be especially important if you tend to ovulate soon after your OPK positive. Whatever you decide, be consistent so that your timing plan will be congruent with the data you collect.

Ferning: This refers to the phenomenon that occurs in saliva and vaginal fluid in response to high levels of estrogen; when observed under a microscope, these secretions form a crystalline, fernlike pattern. If you don't own or have access to a microscope, you can purchase an inexpensive pocket microscope designed for this purpose. To observe ferning, place a thin layer of saliva on the slide. This can be done by wiping a clean, dry finger under your tongue or inside your lower lip, and then wiping it across the slide. Allow the sample to dry. Then, bring the sample into focus while shining the microscope light through. You may see no ferning, partial ferning (such as one or two areas of ferning on the slide), or full ferning (the entire slide is covered with ferns). For some, full ferning is a consistent sign of ovulation. For others, ferning appears for a handful of days, which does not narrow down the ovulation window at all. Still others get no ferns at all. If you want to give it a try, ferning might just work for you—plus, it can be fun!

Ovulation sensation: There are a variety of sensations that people may feel in association with ovulation. However, don't assume that mid-cycle cramping or twinges are the actual release of your egg—ovulation sensation can happen before ovulation occurs, as the egg is being released, or after ovulation has already passed. You might feel pressure, fullness, or bloating in the lower abdominal area, or you may have gas or hear stomach noises. Cramping is common, which can take many forms, from menstrual-like cramps to a pulsing sensation to twinges that come and go. Some people even get one strong cramp that can be a bit painful.

Because ovulation sensation can happen before, during, or after ovulation, it is important to write down what you feel and when you feel it. Be as specific as possible. Note when the sensation begins, when it changes, and when it goes away. If there is a specific period of strong cramping or twinges, be sure to note what time frame this occurred. Once you have tracked your ovulation sensation carefully on your chart, you will be able to see how it lines up with other fertile signs. Then, you will know what your ovulation sensation means for you.

Fertility medications and ultrasound: The bottom line on side one of the chart is a place to note any fertility medications you are taking that cycle (such as Clomid or letrozole), which may change your pattern of fertile signs. Note what medication you are taking and the dose. You can also track the size of your follicles if you are observing their growth via ultrasound in a clinic—note the size and which side they appear on. If you did an hCG "trigger shot," record that here as well. You can also write down the day of your progesterone draw and the result, as well as any days you used supplemental progesterone, including method and dose.

Bleeding and menstrual cramps: At the top of page two, you can track your periods. Some people notice changes once they start supporting their fertile health, and it can feel rewarding to note this on your chart. Some people draw little dots for spotting, a small x for a light flow day, or a large X for a heavy flow day. Others shade in the box partially or fully depending on the amount of flow. Be as creative as you like and do what works for you. You can also track any menstrual cramps you experience. This is one area where you will really see your efforts toward improving your fertile health pay off. When the body is getting everything it needs, it can function more effectively. When it's not, it struggles. A uterus that cramps painfully each month might be doing so for a number of reasons; however, most people notice that when they regulate their blood sugar, or stop drinking coffee, or start exercising, their menstrual cramps improve, sometimes drastically. Note this on your chart.

Basal body temperature: Tracking changes in your body temperature at rest (your basal temperature) requires a special basal body thermometer that is more precise than a typical thermometer, but you still use it by placing it under your tongue. Take your temperature as soon as you wake up in the morning, before sitting up, turning over, talking, or doing anything other than reaching over to get the thermometer and putting it in your mouth. Don't snuggle up to your bedmate or pet your dog while you are waiting for the thermometer to beep—just lie still for this short time. If you already have a baby or a toddler, just do what you can, and skip this piece if parenting makes collecting basal body temperature impossible.

If you have purchased a thermometer with a memory function, you will be able to put the thermometer down and record the reading later, when you are more awake. If you sometimes wake up early and then go back to sleep for a couple of hours before getting up for the day, be sure to take your temp the first time you awaken. If you sometimes wake up to use the bathroom during the night, check the time first and take your temperature before you get up if you know you won't have another three hours to sleep.

It is *not required* to take your temperature at the same exact time every single day. The chart includes space to record the time that your temperature was taken. If it's the weekend and you sleep later than usual, that's OK. Just take your temperature when you wake up, and note the time you took your temp. You don't need to sacrifice the ability to sleep in for the sake of conceiving. In fact, sleep now, while you still can! Once your baby comes, you won't have this option again for quite some time.

Track your BBT every day throughout the cycle. To record your reading on the chart, find your temperature on the left-hand side and follow that row over to the column for the cycle day you are on. Fill in the square, or make a little dot over the number for that day. Connect the dots each day so that a line appears. At the end of your cycle, you will draw a "cover line" to help you see that ovulation occurred, and to confirm when ovulation occurred.

To draw the cover line, take a blank piece of paper and place it at the bottom of your BBT chart. Slowly begin moving it upward until it starts to cover some of the lower temps you recorded in the first half of your cycle. Keep moving it up until all the temperatures on the left-hand side are covered up, and you are left only with temperatures on the right-hand side. Stop moving the paper here, and draw a line on your temp chart by using the edge of that paper as a guide. This is your cover line.

If you ovulated, you will clearly see higher temperatures throughout the second half of your cycle. This is because the release of the egg causes a rise in progesterone, which makes the body slightly warmer. You can also confirm approximately when ovulation occurred, because BBT rises within a day or two after ovulation.

As long as your sleeping conditions are relatively consistent, your BBT can be an important tool for assessing the strength of your ovulation and the adequacy of your progesterone. Distinct signs of ovulation followed by a BBT rise that occurs one to two days later and goes straight up by a few tenths of a degree indicate strong ovulation and timely progesterone rise. A weak ovulation has fertile signs that are very spread out and a BBT that doesn't go up right away, or goes up slowly in a stair-step pattern. It is also ideal to have all the luteal phase temps sustained above the cover line, like a tabletop. If your luteal phase temps form a sawtooth pattern, you may need to pay closer attention to your fertile health. Additionally, sometimes a hypothyroid condition can be detected by tracking BBT—if your temps don't ever rise above 97.3, even after ovulation, be sure to get your thyroid hormones checked.

Mood changes: Shifts in mood occur quite commonly around ovulation. Track yours and find out what happens for you. It is most common for people to feel really great, "on," creative, or especially outgoing on the day they ovulate. Others have a series of mood shifts before, during, and after ovulation. You won't know your pattern until you track this sign. One client found that she always felt really depressed the day before ovulation, followed by happiness and relief the next day. When compared with her physiological symptoms of high estrogen, the lift in her mood clearly and predictably lined up with ovulation. This person also had a very short fertile window and didn't always get a positive OPK, so the mood drop ended up being the sign she used to make arrangements for insemination the next day.

Sex drive: It's no wonder that sex drive increases as ovulation approaches. In fact, because the body is designed to keep sperm alive for a few days awaiting the release of an egg, sex drive tends to go up a few days before ovulation occurs. You might notice a day of really high libido, or there might be a day when your sexual desires are more visceral or you desire something different than usual. Pay attention to this when it happens around ovulation time, and track it on your chart.

Breast and chest changes: The chest may look or feel different during and especially after ovulation. The nipples might be more erect, the areolas might be darker, and the area might feel more sexually sensitive. You might also notice the tissue feeling more full, or even tender or achy. This happens more commonly after ovulation, but track it to see what the pattern is for you.

Increased appetite or food cravings: Due to the massive hormonal fluctuations that happen at ovulation time, it's common for appetite to increase. The need for protein and healthy fat increases—remember that if you are craving sugar, your body actually needs more protein. Remember to feed your body well during this important time, and also note the cravings you are experiencing on your chart.

Sleep changes or dreams: It's common for people to wake up in the middle of the night or to have very vivid dreams on the night of ovulation or just before. Keep track and see if this is a predictable pattern for you.

Intuition: Sometimes people "just know" that ovulation is happening, and this may or may not occur in alignment with your other fertile signs. One client had a strong sense that ovulation was happening, and she scheduled an IUI even though she did not have an OPK positive yet. A few days later, the OPK turned positive, and she assumed that the insemination had been too early. However, her period never came, and she got a positive pregnancy test! We sometimes know more about what is happening in our bodies than even science can measure. If you are having a strong intuitive sense that ovulation is occurring, listen to your body—and track this valuable information on your chart.

Herbs and supplements: Some people like to use this line to track that they have taken their fertility-boosting herbs or supplements each day. Use this line if you want to!

Exercise: Same with exercise—some people like to keep a record of the days they exercise and/or what type of exercise they did. Give yourself a gold star on these days if you like!

Stress, alcohol, travel, and illness: These occurrences have an effect on the endocrine system, and they may explain variations in your typical pattern of fertile signs. If you have a day that is particularly stressful, note this on your chart. If you have enough alcohol to feel buzzed or intoxicated, be sure to include this on your chart. Travel might be fine if it's a short trip and you don't cross time zones, but overseas travel definitely has an effect, as does cross-country travel. You might even find it useful to note vacations or other trips, as a way to remember what was going on in your life during a particular cycle. Sleeping in a different space or a different bed than usual can also affect BBT, so this is important to note. If you are ill or you receive a vaccine that causes a notable immune response, be sure to record this on your chart because the immune system will nearly always take precedence over the reproductive system, and you will most likely see differences in your cycle as well as your fertile signs. Some people choose to call off an insemination if they are very ill prior to ovulation, especially those who need extra fertility support to begin with.

MAIA midwifery & fertility

NAME:

MONTH: **YEAR:**

CYCLE DAY	1	2	3	4	5	6	7	8	9	10	11	12	13	14	15
DATE															
DAY OF THE WEEK															
CONCEPTION ATTEMPTS METHOD & TIME OF DAY															

AM FERTILE SIGNS

CERVIX high / med / low right / left soft / med / firm pink / red opening / +open / OPEN / closing / closed															
FLUID clear / white / yellow / brown dry / sticky / wet / slippery fertile / egg white (EW) Stretchy: How many inches/centimeters?															
OPK / FERTILITY MONITOR neg (-) / light line / darker / pos (+) Brand used: _____															
FERNING: none / partial / full															

PM FERTILE SIGNS

CERVIX high / med / low right / left soft / med / firm pink / red opening / +open / OPEN / closing / closed															
FLUID clear / white / yellow / brown dry / sticky / wet / slippery fertile / egg white (EW) Stretchy: How many inches/centimeters?															
OPK / FERTILITY MONITOR neg (-) / light line / darker / pos (+) Brand used: _____															
FERNING: none / partial / full															
OVULATION SENSATION TODAY? What did you feel? (cramp, twinge, pressure, fullness, gas) Which side? When did it start/stop?															
FERTILITY MEDS / ULTRASOUND which medications / follicle size / L or R															

CYCLE NUMBER: **CYCLE LENGTH:**   **DAYS OF INSEMINATION:**

16	17	18	19	20	21	22	23	24	25	26	27	28	29	30	31	32	33	34	35	36	37	38	39	40

CYCLE DAY	1	2	3	4	5	6	7	8	9	10	11	12	13	14	15
DAY OF THE WEEK															
Bleeding x = light day / X = heavy day / • = spotting															
Menstrual Cramps															

Basal Body Temperature: Mark your temperature on the graph each day, then connect the dots to make a line.

What time did you take your temp?

	1	2	3	4	5	6	7	8	9	10	11	12	13	14	15
98.9	9	9	9	9	9	9	9	9	9	9	9	9	9	9	9
98.8	8	8	8	8	8	8	8	8	8	8	8	8	8	8	8
98.7	7	7	7	7	7	7	7	7	7	7	7	7	7	7	7
98.6	6	6	6	6	6	6	6	6	6	6	6	6	6	6	6
98.5	5	5	5	5	5	5	5	5	5	5	5	5	5	5	5
98.4	4	4	4	4	4	4	4	4	4	4	4	4	4	4	4
98.3	3	3	3	3	3	3	3	3	3	3	3	3	3	3	3
98.2	2	2	2	2	2	2	2	2	2	2	2	2	2	2	2
98.1	1	1	1	1	1	1	1	1	1	1	1	1	1	1	1
98.0	0	0	0	0	0	0	0	0	0	0	0	0	0	0	0
97.9	9	9	9	9	9	9	9	9	9	9	9	9	9	9	9
97.8	8	8	8	8	8	8	8	8	8	8	8	8	8	8	8
97.7	7	7	7	7	7	7	7	7	7	7	7	7	7	7	7
97.6	6	6	6	6	6	6	6	6	6	6	6	6	6	6	6
97.5	5	5	5	5	5	5	5	5	5	5	5	5	5	5	5
97.4	4	4	4	4	4	4	4	4	4	4	4	4	4	4	4
97.3	3	3	3	3	3	3	3	3	3	3	3	3	3	3	3
97.2	2	2	2	2	2	2	2	2	2	2	2	2	2	2	2
97.1	1	1	1	1	1	1	1	1	1	1	1	1	1	1	1
97.0	0	0	0	0	0	0	0	0	0	0	0	0	0	0	0
96.9	9	9	9	9	9	9	9	9	9	9	9	9	9	9	9
96.8	8	8	8	8	8	8	8	8	8	8	8	8	8	8	8
96.7	7	7	7	7	7	7	7	7	7	7	7	7	7	7	7
96.6	6	6	6	6	6	6	6	6	6	6	6	6	6	6	6
96.5	5	5	5	5	5	5	5	5	5	5	5	5	5	5	5
96.4	4	4	4	4	4	4	4	4	4	4	4	4	4	4	4
96.3	3	3	3	3	3	3	3	3	3	3	3	3	3	3	3
96.2	2	2	2	2	2	2	2	2	2	2	2	2	2	2	2

	1	2	3	4	5	6	7	8	9	10	11	12	13	14	15
Mood Changes anxious, depressed, content, creative, ecstatic, happy, irritable, "on," voluptuous, or anything else notable around ovulation															
Sex Drive increase or decrease in libido															
Breast / Chest Changes tender, full, areola darkening, nipples more erect or sensitive															
Increased Appetite / Food Cravings															
Sleep Changes / Dreams waking up in the night, vivid dreams															
Intuition internal sense that ovulation is happening															
Herbs / Supplements															
Exercise															
Stress / Alcohol / Travel / Illness															

16	17	18	19	20	21	22	23	24	25	26	27	28	29	30	31	32	33	34	35	36	37	38	39	40

Mark your temperature on the graph each day, then connect the dots to make a line.

16	17	18	19	20	21	22	23	24	25	26	27	28	29	30	31	32	33	34	35	36	37	38	39	40
9	9	9	9	9	9	9	9	9	9	9	9	9	9	9	9	9	9	9	9	9	9	9	9	9
8	8	8	8	8	8	8	8	8	8	8	8	8	8	8	8	8	8	8	8	8	8	8	8	8
7	7	7	7	7	7	7	7	7	7	7	7	7	7	7	7	7	7	7	7	7	7	7	7	7
6	6	6	6	6	6	6	6	6	6	6	6	6	6	6	6	6	6	6	6	6	6	6	6	6
5	5	5	5	5	5	5	5	5	5	5	5	5	5	5	5	5	5	5	5	5	5	5	5	5
4	4	4	4	4	4	4	4	4	4	4	4	4	4	4	4	4	4	4	4	4	4	4	4	4
3	3	3	3	3	3	3	3	3	3	3	3	3	3	3	3	3	3	3	3	3	3	3	3	3
2	2	2	2	2	2	2	2	2	2	2	2	2	2	2	2	2	2	2	2	2	2	2	2	2
1	1	1	1	1	1	1	1	1	1	1	1	1	1	1	1	1	1	1	1	1	1	1	1	1
0	0	0	0	0	0	0	0	0	0	0	0	0	0	0	0	0	0	0	0	0	0	0	0	0
9	9	9	9	9	9	9	9	9	9	9	9	9	9	9	9	9	9	9	9	9	9	9	9	9
8	8	8	8	8	8	8	8	8	8	8	8	8	8	8	8	8	8	8	8	8	8	8	8	8
7	7	7	7	7	7	7	7	7	7	7	7	7	7	7	7	7	7	7	7	7	7	7	7	7
6	6	6	6	6	6	6	6	6	6	6	6	6	6	6	6	6	6	6	6	6	6	6	6	6
5	5	5	5	5	5	5	5	5	5	5	5	5	5	5	5	5	5	5	5	5	5	5	5	5
4	4	4	4	4	4	4	4	4	4	4	4	4	4	4	4	4	4	4	4	4	4	4	4	4
3	3	3	3	3	3	3	3	3	3	3	3	3	3	3	3	3	3	3	3	3	3	3	3	3
2	2	2	2	2	2	2	2	2	2	2	2	2	2	2	2	2	2	2	2	2	2	2	2	2
1	1	1	1	1	1	1	1	1	1	1	1	1	1	1	1	1	1	1	1	1	1	1	1	1
0	0	0	0	0	0	0	0	0	0	0	0	0	0	0	0	0	0	0	0	0	0	0	0	0
9	9	9	9	9	9	9	9	9	9	9	9	9	9	9	9	9	9	9	9	9	9	9	9	9
8	8	8	8	8	8	8	8	8	8	8	8	8	8	8	8	8	8	8	8	8	8	8	8	8
7	7	7	7	7	7	7	7	7	7	7	7	7	7	7	7	7	7	7	7	7	7	7	7	7
6	6	6	6	6	6	6	6	6	6	6	6	6	6	6	6	6	6	6	6	6	6	6	6	6
5	5	5	5	5	5	5	5	5	5	5	5	5	5	5	5	5	5	5	5	5	5	5	5	5
4	4	4	4	4	4	4	4	4	4	4	4	4	4	4	4	4	4	4	4	4	4	4	4	4
3	3	3	3	3	3	3	3	3	3	3	3	3	3	3	3	3	3	3	3	3	3	3	3	3
2	2	2	2	2	2	2	2	2	2	2	2	2	2	2	2	2	2	2	2	2	2	2	2	2

Identifying Ovulation Using the MAIA Cycle Chart

Now that you have tracked all this information, how are you going to use it? Well, remember earlier in this chapter, when I highlighted the importance of tracking the onset of your fertile window, the peak of your fertile window, and when your fertile window ends? The onset of fertile signs are your early warning to start looking more closely, tracking LH and estrogen symptoms twice each day. When your estrogen symptoms are strongest, you will have at least three or more fertile signs lining up on the same day. The primary signs to look for are open cervix and clear, stretchy fluid, and these will be accompanied by secondary fertile signs. Once ovulation has passed, your fertile signs will start going away. Pinpointing the onset, peak, and end of the fertile window will accurately identify your best time to inseminate.

PRIMARY SIGNS OF OVULATION:

- Open cervix—may also be soft and high,
  with a position or color change
- Clear fluid—may also be more stretchy
  or more copious than other days

SECONDARY SIGNS OF OVULATION:

- High sex drive, ovulation sensation, mood shift, ferning, appetite
  changes, wakefulness, vivid dreams, intuition

Locate the cycle day and time when your fertile signs were strongest, just before they started going away. This is the time of ovulation. Then, look at when you got your OPK positive. How long was it between your positive reading (the onset of your LH surge) and when your estrogen symptoms peaked? This is what the OPK positive means for you.

CHART AT LEAST ONE MONTH, IDEALLY THREE OR MORE, BEFORE YOU START INSEMINATING

Reading a cycle chart is a retrospective analysis, which means you will need to chart at least one cycle in order to know your body's pattern of ovulation. To increase your confidence, track another cycle or two. If the fertile signs appear in the same way every month, you can rely on them to time inseminations accordingly. If you note that the pattern shifts by twelve hours or more in a given cycle (with no other identifiable cause such as illness, travel, alcohol use, or stress), you may have a different pattern of fertile signs that occur when ovulating from one ovary versus the other, or you may need some fertility support. If this is the case for you, try to come up with a plan that will work for all the ovulation patterns you have observed, or a plan that can be altered based on what is unfolding in real time. You may want to seek assistance from a midwife or other provider who is experienced in reading cycle charts and designing timing plans accordingly. A changing ovulation pattern may mean doing two or more inseminations in a cycle in order to cover any scenario. On the other hand, if you are having difficulty narrowing down the ideal twelve-hour window because you did not track your fertile signs every twelve hours as ovulation was occurring, give yourself another month to collect this data before trying to make a plan.

HOW DO I GET MY CLINIC TO INSEMINATE AT THE RIGHT TIME FOR ME?

Many clinics don't use individualized IUI timing. They tell you to do an OPK once a day, and call to schedule your IUI the day after your positive. While this may end up working for some people, for others, it doesn't. As confident as your doctor might be in their approach, there are no two bodies alike, and a one-size-fits-all approach does not work for everyone. If you have tried a few cycles using the clinic's timing approach without success, take some time to chart your cycles and find out if the inseminations you have had so far have been valid timing for you. If you are ovulating fewer than twenty-four hours after your OPK positive, especially if you may have missed catching the onset of your LH surge by only testing once per day, you may have been inseminating too late by going in the following day. If your clinic insists on scheduling your IUI the day after your OPK positive, you can get around this by identifying the fertile signs that happen the day before your ovulation occurs. Consider these signs your "OPK positive" and call the clinic to schedule when you know you will need IUI the next day.

Pitfalls and Misconceptions about Identifying Ovulation

Most of the information you will find online about identifying ovulation is there because someone is making money from the tools they are selling. Whether it is an app that promises to identify your day of ovulation, one of the various OPKs or fertility monitors on the market, or even a clinic protocol that uses ultrasound to time inseminations, there is no tool as reliable as the signs you can observe in your own body.

USING OPKS AND FERTILITY MONITORS TO TIME INSEMINATIONS

Although the OPK can be very useful, it's not fail proof. Sometimes the kits malfunction. Knowing your pattern of fertile signs can protect you in this scenario. If your body is screaming that ovulation is happening, don't second-guess yourself for the sake of a reagent strip on an OPK. If your fertile signs indicate that ovulation is approaching, and you don't get an OPK positive when you expected to, doubt the kit before you doubt what you are seeing with your own eyes and experiencing in your own body. If your body says "go," don't wait for the kit!

If you test the OPK just once a day, your assessment of the onset of the LH surge could be way off, especially if it occurs just a few hours after you test. This is why fertility monitors that only allow one reading per day are not appropriate for timing insemination with frozen sperm. Additionally, these monitors automatically read "Peak" for two days, which is not true for everyone.

Over the years at MAIA, we have observed many products on the market designed for detecting the LH surge. Spending more on these tools does not necessarily mean increased accuracy or even greater utility for timing inseminations with frozen sperm. For instance, companies that sell OPKs say they can pinpoint your ovulation by using the kit alone, and many clinics rely on the OPK for timing IUIs. The general understanding is that ovulation occurs twenty-four to thirty-six hours after the onset of the LH surge. However, while this may be true for some, scientific research as well as the thousands of cycle charts reviewed in my practice show it certainly is not true for all. This is why you need to track your estrogen symptoms in relation to the positive reading on your OPK.

The *only* thing an OPK can reliably tell you is when the LH surge begins—it cannot tell you when you have reached peak fertility or when you release your egg (any brand that tells you otherwise is just vying for sales). The OPK indicates the onset of the LH surge. Your OPK will help narrow down your ovulation window in a predictable way so that you know when to inseminate, but it does not pinpoint the release of your egg. How many hours after the OPK positive do you get your peak fertile signs? And when do your fertile signs go away (cervix starts to close, fluid is no longer clear or stretchy)? These three pieces of information will determine when you ovulate. The OPK can help you predict your ovulation, but only if you know what the time frame is for *you*.

Steer clear of OPKs that promise to identify your ovulation by taking photos of test strips with an iPhone, especially those who claim the faulty idea that ovulation can be determined by the rise and fall of LH in your urine. Not only can lighting issues and varying dilution of urine impact the reliability of this method, the entire premise that the egg is released when urinary LH peaks is inaccurate for many people. Research shows that individuals can ovulate before, during, or after the peak level of LH. The best use of LH to indicate the time of ovulation is to note the *onset* of the LH surge, which is your first positive reading on the OPK. After you note your first positive reading, stop testing for LH. The onset of the surge is what you were looking for, and what you will measure your peak estrogen signs against.

Some people like to use kits that read positive with a digital smiley face instead of having to compare two lines on a reagent strip. But be warned: over the past few years, we have watched these kits become less consistently reliable—so unreliable that we have seen several instances of the same urine sample resulting in both a negative and a positive reading.

We tested all of the kits on the market in 2020 in preparation for the publication of this book, and we found that the most basic, individually wrapped LH reagent strip OPKs were the most consistent and reliable. However, some are harder to read than others, and some include instructions that are inaccurate and confusing (such as continuing to test after the onset of the LH surge is observed). Because OPKs are such an important aspect of getting the timing right with frozen donor sperm, we are committed to continuing to provide our community with consistent, reliable OPKs. Just as we have over the past thirty years, we will continue to keep you informed as the products on the market change over time. Check our website for updated information about OPK brands and accuracy, and find approved kits available for purchase in our web store.

WHY APPS DON'T WORK FOR TIMING INSEMINATIONS—ESPECIALLY WITH FROZEN SPERM

Ovulation rarely occurs on the same cycle day from month to month, so you will need to know the pattern of your body's ovulation signs and time your insemination based on the pattern that occurs for you. This is why apps that try to predict your ovulation can be incorrect, and they certainly aren't precise enough for timing with frozen sperm. Apps that predict your ovulation day based on your periods alone can be way off—they don't even track your ovulation signs! If your app also tracks your basal body temperature, it still won't be accurate, because BBT goes up *after* ovulation occurs. In fact, unless an app records OPK readings and estrogen symptoms twice a day, it won't be accurate enough for timing IUI with frozen sperm. This means that there is currently no app on the market that can be used to time your IUIs with precision.

Also, your body is not a computer. Ovulation patterns can fluctuate from month to month based on stress, travel, life events, or simply being human. There is enough nuance to the human body that you can't simply put it all into a computer program and end up with certainty. However, with a little knowledge about how to identify signs of ovulation in real time, and a little time and effort in tracking those signs, your human brain can do a much better job of knowing when ovulation will occur. And while it may seem convenient to track your fertile signs in an app, you risk putting too much faith in the computer, or even not being able to interpret the information you have recorded when it is reduced to color-coded symbols. It's also a real bummer if your data is lost during a system update.

For all of these reasons, I recommend you track your fertile signs using the MAIA Cycle Chart—yep, a paper chart. For over thirty years, this simple tool has helped countless families conceive by timing their inseminations with precision. The most accurate information you can get about when you are ovulating comes from your own body, in real time, as long as you know what to look for and what the pattern looks like for you. For many people, this realization is revolutionary. How can a paper chart be more accurate than an app or an ultrasound machine? Although ultrasound can be used to view your developing egg follicles (if you can afford it), it can't tell you exactly when those follicles are going to release the egg.

USING ULTRASOUND TO TIME INSEMINATIONS

If your fertility doctor has told you that you don't need to track ovulation because they can time insemination by using ultrasound and a trigger shot, it's important to know that while this method can sometimes be effective, it can also fail you. Meanwhile, you could be flushing thousands of dollars of sperm down the drain and end up with a costly IVF cycle because you thought IUI didn't work for you.

Using ultrasound to time inseminations requires going in for an ultrasound sometime after your period ends but before ovulation occurs, typically around cycle day ten to twelve. (If you end up ovulating early, before your ultrasound, this means you have missed your opportunity to inseminate that month.) A follicle scan is done using an internal vaginal probe, and if there are one or more follicles that appear to be large enough to ovulate, a "trigger shot" is given. If the follicles are not yet large enough to trigger, you may need to go back in for additional scans. The trigger shot is an injection of hCG, which mimics LH and causes the dominant follicle to rupture and the egg to release. It is believed that ovulation will occur twenty-four to thirty-six hours after the shot.

However, there are a couple of faults to this method. One is that while your follicles may appear large enough, they may not have actually reached full maturity, and you could theoretically be inducing ovulation before your egg is ready. Another error in this method lies in the assumption that once ovulation is triggered, the egg will release in twenty-four to thirty-six hours. If your body was just about to ovulate on its own when you got the shot, it still will—the shot won't make it wait. If you release your egg soon after the shot is given, but your IUI doesn't happen until the next day, the egg will be gone before the sperm arrive. There are certainly some cases where ultrasound and a trigger shot can be useful tools, such as those who have difficulty ovulating. But if your body ovulates each month, your timing will be much more accurate by simply observing its symptoms and timing your inseminations accordingly.

Charting Can Be a Gateway for Healing and Personal Growth

After a few unsuccessful cycles of insemination, most people start to wonder, "What is wrong with me?" or "Why doesn't my body work?" However, it could merely be a timing issue. Your doctor will likely suggest proceeding to medicated cycles or moving on to IVF. But if this is not the way you want to conceive, this situation can set the stage for a pregnancy wrought with doubt and concern, culminating in a birth process that is steeped in feelings of distrust in the body and its capabilities, which can easily transfer over into lactation and the early days of parenting your newborn. As a midwife, I want something entirely different for you. I want you to enter new parenthood feeling strong, empowered, and self-assured. Because new parenthood is inherently vulnerable, I want you to start with the most solid foundation possible. The process of building confidence in your body's reproductive process starts at the very beginning, as you prepare to conceive your child. This is why I recommend getting to know your body, becoming familiar with how it works, and taking full accountability for your role in getting this baby in there, as preparation for being fully embodied during pregnancy and empowered through the process of bringing new life into the world.

Charting is not always easy. We all have histories stored in our bodies, and the reproductive system is certainly no exception. Our genitals may contain legacies of cultural shame, or trauma from sexual assault. For those with transgender experience, the genitals may represent a bodily betrayal of who you know yourself to be, and for some, detachment from this part of the body may be necessary to sustain emotional health. Even experiences of fat-shaming, insinuations that small bodies are weak or incapable, and other messages of bodily insufficiency or wrongness come up as we enter the very physical experience of engaging with fertility, conception, and pregnancy.

Every one of the feelings that come up for you in the process of engaging with your body at this level is valid. The invitation is to let these things come up and to work through them so that you can begin to transform your bodily experience. Your body is becoming the fertile ground for growing your child. You are cultivating the physical and emotional environment that your baby will grow in. Once your child is born, they will inherit their sense of themselves, and their own body image, by first viewing the world through your eyes, and listening to the ways you talk about yourself, and the ways you talk to them about their body. Any residual shame, discomfort, or fear that you hold will not be missed by your child as they keenly observe your pauses and vocal inflections as you teach them about their own body. Working through any body issues you have is foundational, and it will serve you well in your parenting.

You might get the hang of charting right away, or it may take a few months to get the information you need. If you are noticing reluctance, use this for self-reflection. Tap into why you are not looking at your fertile fluid, or why you forgot your OPK test. Is there something getting in the way? Something you need to make a priority? Something that you need to take some time to talk through with your therapist, your partner, or a friend? A trauma that needs time to heal and be integrated so that you can move into this next phase of life? Do you simply need some support? This is useful, important work. Value the messages your body is giving you, and take the time you need to fully prepare for pregnancy and parenthood.

No matter how busy you are, it is worth some time and effort to make sure you have the information you need to time inseminations accurately. To put this into perspective, ask yourself: How much time will it take to care for a baby? How much time does it take to earn the money for a vial of sperm? What other costs are you shouldering to make the most of your chances? It all adds up, which means that the ten to fifteen minutes you spend at the beginning and end of your day, for a week or less each month, are incredibly valuable.

What Does the Science Say about Insemination Timing and Success Rates?

Scientific evidence that applies to fertile people conceiving via donor insemination is very limited. Most studies are conducted to solve problems of infertility in heterosexual couples. Of the studies that have been done on donor insemination or unmedicated IUI, conclusions cannot be made on a single approach for how to time inseminations in relation to a positive OPK. If you have read the first part of this chapter, you can probably guess why—people ovulate at different times in relation to the onset of the LH surge! In addition to my own clinical experience, I have done a deep dive for scientific research that applies to healthy people in natural, unmedicated cycles. If you are feeling skeptical about my approach because it differs from what is practiced in fertility clinics, please take a look at the studies included in the references section at the end of this book. The evidence is there; it's just that fertility medicine overlooks the needs of queer and single people conceiving with donor sperm, in favor of the needs of heterosexual people with infertility. This is precisely why I do the work I do, and why this book and the approach it describes is needed.

SCIENTIFIC EVIDENCE ABOUT IUI

- With frozen sperm, IUI doubles the success rate over vaginal insemination.

- A single, well-timed IUI results in a 17 percent chance of live birth overall; however, the pregnancy rate for IUI with frozen sperm is strongly affected by age: 18.5 percent under age thirty-five; 11.9 percent for ages thirty-five to forty; and 5.4 percent for those over age forty.

- Aside from age, timing is the most important factor for IUI success.

- Egg cells are able to be fertilized for only twelve to sixteen hours after ovulation.

- Pregnancy rates are higher when IUI is performed as close to the release of the egg as possible (just before or within ten hours after ovulation).

- The time of ovulation in relation to the onset of the LH surge varies from person to person.

- Detection of the LH surge in urine typically happens twelve to forty-eight hours before ovulation; however, in some individuals it can occur after the egg is released.

- The beginning of the LH surge is an excellent predictor of ovulation, but the peak of LH levels can vary in relation to ovulation and are less reliable than the onset of the LH surge.

- Self-observation of peak cervical mucus (clear, stretchy, egg white) in combination with urine LH is more reliable for identifying the day of ovulation than the use of urine LH alone.

- Natural-cycle IUI is recommended as the first-line approach over medicated IUI, because pregnancy rates are higher in unmedicated donor insemination cycles, while the use of ovarian stimulation increases the rate of multiple pregnancy.

- Timing inseminations with the LH surge rather than a "trigger shot" or hCG injection increases the pregnancy rate significantly.

- At-home urine LH kits are just as effective as blood work in identifying impending ovulation.

- The experience of the IUI provider is a determinant of success.

- Success is increased when you lie down for at least ten to fifteen minutes after IUI.

SCIENTIFIC EVIDENCE FOR SELF-INSEMINATION WITH FRESH SPERM

- Pregnancy rates are higher with fresh sperm than with frozen sperm.

- Pregnancy rates are highest with fresh sperm when insemination happens during the days of peak quality fertile fluid.

- Chances of conception are highest when sperm is deposited near the cervix one to two days before ovulation. The day of ovulation is slightly less effective, and there is almost zero chance the day after.

- Some of the sperm cells reach the fallopian tubes within two to ten minutes of insemination near the cervix. Others are harbored within crypts alongside the cervical os.

- With fresh sperm, success rates are higher when two inseminations are done instead of one.

PUTTING THE EVIDENCE INTO PRACTICE

After reading this book, you may know more about timing your inseminations than your provider, even if your provider is a fertility doctor. Fertility doctors don't teach or expect people to make observations of their signs of high estrogen, and they don't typically have experience with timing inseminations in accordance with observable physiological signs of ovulation. The financial reality is that fertility clinics don't really make significant income from IUI, so it's not lucrative to spend much time on this aspect of care. What fertility doctors do best is infertility and IVF. Most fertility doctors I know are caring people (although their experience and training can be deeply cis/heterocentric), and I don't believe they are just out to get your money. However, practically speaking, if you don't have a medical fertility issue making it a challenge to conceive, you are better off making your own decisions about timing, or consulting with a fertility specialist who can provide guidance for a low-tech, individualized approach.

Inseminating with Frozen Sperm

Your knowledge about your ovulation trends will help you know when to have your samples in hand, which can save a lot of stress. Cryopreservation tanks are charged with liquid nitrogen to keep samples frozen for seven to fourteen days (check with your sperm bank to find out how long their tanks last). Always have the tank available at least one day before you expect to use it. Once you have begun an insemination cycle, call the sperm bank to order your tank—do not wait until the last minute. Most sperm banks require at least twenty-four to forty-eight hours' notice to have your sperm samples ready for you to pick up or to be shipped. As an example, if you have identified ovulation in previous cycles to occur on cycle days thirteen to fifteen, call the sperm bank within the first few days of your cycle, and arrange to pick it up or to have it arrive at your home or provider's office no later than cycle day twelve. If cycle day twelve is a Sunday, and the bank is closed or the shipping company does not deliver on Sundays, you may want it to arrive on Saturday, or even Friday, if it is being shipped to a clinic that is only open during the week. That way, you won't be caught empty-handed if your ovulation happens earlier than you were expecting. Also be aware of your latest possible day of ovulation, and make sure the tank will last until then. If this time frame spans longer than the tank will last, ask the bank to provide extra coolant or an option for you to recharge the tank if needed.

TIMING SELF-INSEMINATION OR IUI WITH FROZEN SPERM

You can get pregnant by doing self-insemination with a frozen sperm sample; however, your chance of success doubles with IUI. Regardless of the method of insemination, cryopreserved sperm samples are only reliably viable for about twelve hours, and by twenty-four hours, they are dead. The egg cell is only viable for twelve to sixteen hours after it is released from the ovary. This means that timing is of utmost importance when using frozen sperm—and this is why apps designed for cis/het folks with endless availability of fresh sperm will fail you if you are inseminating with frozen sperm. The limited life span of frozen sperm and the necessity for accurate timing are what make so many queer conceptions more complicated—and it is why this book exists to support you. We are resilient folks who actively manifest our own destiny, and we are prepared to take matters into our own hands when needed. We can use science, including the science of what our individual bodies tell us, for perfect timing with frozen donor sperm.

Since your frozen sperm sample is viable for about the same length of time as your egg, you just need to identify your most fertile twelve hours. Inseminate when your fertile signs are at their peak (most open cervix, most copious clear fluid, plus one or more supporting signs) and about twelve hours before you expect them to wane based on your observations of previous cycles. Determining the length of time between your OPK positive and your peak fertile signs will allow you to time your inseminations perfectly.

SCENARIO A

If you get your most copious fertile fluid and softest, most open cervix at the same time you get your OPK positive (or the closest reading you get, if a full positive does not appear for you), and by twelve hours later, the fluid is gone and your cervix is closing, you will want to inseminate with frozen sperm as soon as you get your positive, or as soon as your best fluid/most open cervix appears—even if your OPK isn't positive yet.

SCENARIO B

If your fertile signs peak at twelve hours after the OPK positive, and they are fading away by twenty-four hours, inseminate with frozen sperm at twelve hours after the OPK positive.

SCENARIO C

If you have clear, stretchy fertile fluid and a soft, open cervix for a good twenty-four hours after your OPK positive, and your fertile signs don't start to wane until thirty-six hours after the positive, you have a broad window to cover. If you are only planning one insemination with frozen sperm, do it around twenty-four hours after the OPK positive. In the meantime, look for any subtle nuances that might help you hone in on your timing: Do you get any cramping or other ovulation sensation? Have you been viewing your cervix to see when it is most open (most open equals egg release)? What does your intuition say?

MAIA midwifery & fertility

NAME: Scenario A

MONTH: SEPT **YEAR:** 2021

CYCLE DAY	1	2	3	4	5	6	7	8	9	10	11	12	13	14	15
DATE	10	11	12	13	14	15	16	17	18	19	20	21	22	23	24
DAY OF THE WEEK	R	F	S	S	M	T	W	R	F	S	S	M	T	W	R
CONCEPTION ATTEMPTS METHOD & TIME OF DAY												IUI 10am			

AM FERTILE SIGNS

	1	2	3	4	5	6	7	8	9	10	11	12	13	14	15
CERVIX high / med / low right / left; soft / med / firm pink / red; opening / +open / OPEN / closing / closed											opening	open			
FLUID clear / white / yellow / brown; dry / sticky / wet / slippery; fertile / egg white (EW); Stretchy: How many inches/centimeters?											wet	clear			
OPK / FERTILITY MONITOR neg (-) / light line / darker / pos (+); Brand used: _____										—	—	darker			
FERNING: none / partial / full															

PM FERTILE SIGNS

	1	2	3	4	5	6	7	8	9	10	11	12	13	14	15
CERVIX high / med / low right / left; soft / med / firm pink / red; opening / +open / OPEN / closing / closed											opening	closing			
FLUID clear / white / yellow / brown; dry / sticky / wet / slippery; fertile / egg white (EW); Stretchy: How many inches/centimeters?											wet	sticky			
OPK / FERTILITY MONITOR neg (-) / light line / darker / pos (+); Brand used: _____										—	light line				
FERNING: none / partial / full															
OVULATION SENSATION TODAY? What did you feel? (cramp, twinge, pressure, fullness, gas); Which side? When did it start/stop?															
FERTILITY MEDS / ULTRASOUND which medications / follicle size / L or R															

CYCLE NUMBER: 5   CYCLE LENGTH: 24   DAYS OF INSEMINATION: 12

16	17	18	19	20	21	22	23	24	25	26	27	28	29	30	31	32	33	34	35	36	37	38	39	40
25	26	27	28	29	30	1	2	3																
F	S	S	M	T	W	R	F	S																

CYCLE DAY	1	2	3	4	5	6	7	8	9	10	11	12	13	14	15
DAY OF THE WEEK	R	F	S	S	M	T	W	R	F	S	S	M	T	W	R
Bleeding x = light day / X = heavy day / • = spotting															
Menstrual Cramps															

Basal Body Temperature: Mark your temperature on the graph each day, then connect the dots to make a line.

What time did you take your temp?

	1	2	3	4	5	6	7	8	9	10	11	12	13	14	15
98.9	9	9	9	9	9	9	9	9	9	9	9	9	9	9	9
98.8	8	8	8	8	8	8	8	8	8	8	8	8	8	8	8
98.7	7	7	7	7	7	7	7	7	7	7	7	7	7	7	7
98.6	6	6	6	6	6	6	6	6	6	6	6	6	6	6	6
98.5	5	5	5	5	5	5	5	5	5	5	5	5	5	5	5
98.4	4	4	4	4	4	4	4	4	4	4	4	4	4	4	4
98.3	3	3	3	3	3	3	3	3	3	3	3	3	3	3	3
98.2	2	2	2	2	2	2	2	2	2	2	2	2	2	2	2
98.1	1	1	1	1	1	1	1	1	1	1	1	1	1	1	1
98.0	0	0	0	0	0	0	0	0	0	0	0	0	0	0	0
97.9	9	9	9	9	9	9	9	9	9	9	9	9	9	9	9
97.8	8	8	8	8	8	8	8	8	8	8	8	8	8	8	8
97.7	7	7	7	7	7	7	7	7	7	7	7	7	7	7	7
97.6	6	6	6	6	6	6	6	6	6	6	6	6	6	6	6
97.5	5	5	5	5	5	5	5	5	5	5	5	5	5	5	5
97.4	4	4	4	4	4	4	4	4	4	4	4	4	4	4	4
97.3	3	3	3	3	3	3	3	3	3	3	3	3	3	3	3
97.2	2	2	2	2	2	2	2	2	2	2	2	2	2	2	2
97.1	1	1	1	1	1	1	1	1	1	1	1	1	1	1	1
97.0	0	0	0	0	0	0	0	0	0	0	0	0	0	0	0
96.9	9	9	9	9	9	9	9	9	9	9	9	9	9	9	9
96.8	8	8	8	8	8	8	8	8	8	8	8	8	8	8	8
96.7	7	7	7	7	7	7	7	7	7	7	7	7	7	7	7
96.6	6	6	6	6	6	6	6	6	6	6	6	6	6	6	6
96.5	5	5	5	5	5	5	5	5	5	5	5	5	5	5	5
96.4	4	4	4	4	4	4	4	4	4	4	4	4	4	4	4
96.3	3	3	3	3	3	3	3	3	3	3	3	3	3	3	3
96.2	2	2	2	2	2	2	2	2	2	2	2	2	2	2	2

	1	2	3	4	5	6	7	8	9	10	11	12	13	14	15
Mood Changes anxious, depressed, content, creative, ecstatic, happy, irritable, "on," voluptuous, or anything else notable around ovulation															
Sex Drive increase or decrease in libido											↑ −				
Breast / Chest Changes tender, full, areola darkening, nipples more erect or sensitive													tender		
Increased Appetite / Food Cravings															
Sleep Changes / Dreams waking up in the night, vivid dreams											yes				
Intuition internal sense that ovulation is happening															
Herbs / Supplements															
Exercise															
Stress / Alcohol / Travel / Illness															

16	17	18	19	20	21	22	23	24	25	26	27	28	29	30	31	32	33	34	35	36	37	38	39	40
F	S	S	M	T	W	R	F	S																

Mark your temperature on the graph each day, then connect the dots to make a line.

16	17	18	19	20	21	22	23	24	25	26	27	28	29	30	31	32	33	34	35	36	37	38	39	40
9	9	9	9	9	9	9	9	9	9	9	9	9	9	9	9	9	9	9	9	9	9	9	9	9
8	8	8	8	8	8	8	8	8	8	8	8	8	8	8	8	8	8	8	8	8	8	8	8	8
7	7	7	7	7	7	7	7	7	7	7	7	7	7	7	7	7	7	7	7	7	7	7	7	7
6	6	6	6	6	6	6	6	6	6	6	6	6	6	6	6	6	6	6	6	6	6	6	6	6
5	5	5	5	5	5	5	5	5	5	5	5	5	5	5	5	5	5	5	5	5	5	5	5	5
4	4	4	4	4	4	4	4	4	4	4	4	4	4	4	4	4	4	4	4	4	4	4	4	4
3	3	3	3	3	3	3	3	3	3	3	3	3	3	3	3	3	3	3	3	3	3	3	3	3
2	2	2	2	2	2	2	2	2	2	2	2	2	2	2	2	2	2	2	2	2	2	2	2	2
1	1	1	1	1	1	1	1	1	1	1	1	1	1	1	1	1	1	1	1	1	1	1	1	1
0	0	0	0	0	0	0	0	0	0	0	0	0	0	0	0	0	0	0	0	0	0	0	0	0
9	9	9	9	9	9	9	9	9	9	9	9	9	9	9	9	9	9	9	9	9	9	9	9	9
8	8	8	8	8	8	8	8	8	8	8	8	8	8	8	8	8	8	8	8	8	8	8	8	8
7	7	7	7	7	7	7	7	7	7	7	7	7	7	7	7	7	7	7	7	7	7	7	7	7
6	6	6	6	6	6	6	6	6	6	6	6	6	6	6	6	6	6	6	6	6	6	6	6	6
5	5	5	5	5	5	5	5	5	5	5	5	5	5	5	5	5	5	5	5	5	5	5	5	5
4	4	4	4	4	4	4	4	4	4	4	4	4	4	4	4	4	4	4	4	4	4	4	4	4
3	3	3	3	3	3	3	3	3	3	3	3	3	3	3	3	3	3	3	3	3	3	3	3	3
2	2	2	2	2	2	2	2	2	2	2	2	2	2	2	2	2	2	2	2	2	2	2	2	2
1	1	1	1	1	1	1	1	1	1	1	1	1	1	1	1	1	1	1	1	1	1	1	1	1
0	0	0	0	0	0	0	0	0	0	0	0	0	0	0	0	0	0	0	0	0	0	0	0	0
9	9	9	9	9	9	9	9	9	9	9	9	9	9	9	9	9	9	9	9	9	9	9	9	9
8	8	8	8	8	8	8	8	8	8	8	8	8	8	8	8	8	8	8	8	8	8	8	8	8
7	7	7	7	7	7	7	7	7	7	7	7	7	7	7	7	7	7	7	7	7	7	7	7	7
6	6	6	6	6	6	6	6	6	6	6	6	6	6	6	6	6	6	6	6	6	6	6	6	6
5	5	5	5	5	5	5	5	5	5	5	5	5	5	5	5	5	5	5	5	5	5	5	5	5
4	4	4	4	4	4	4	4	4	4	4	4	4	4	4	4	4	4	4	4	4	4	4	4	4
3	3	3	3	3	3	3	3	3	3	3	3	3	3	3	3	3	3	3	3	3	3	3	3	3
2	2	2	2	2	2	2	2	2	2	2	2	2	2	2	2	2	2	2	2	2	2	2	2	2

MAIA midwifery & fertility

NAME: *Scenario B*

MONTH: *DECEMBER* **YEAR:** *2021*

CYCLE DAY	1	2	3	4	5	6	7	8	9	10	11	12	13	14	15
DATE	7	8	9	10	11	12	13	14	15	16	17	18	19	20	21
DAY OF THE WEEK	M	T	W	R	F	S	S	M	T	W	R	F	S	S	M
CONCEPTION ATTEMPTS METHOD & TIME OF DAY													IUI 8pm		

AM FERTILE SIGNS

	1	2	3	4	5	6	7	8	9	10	11	12	13	14	15
CERVIX high / med / low right / left soft / med / firm pink / red opening / +open / OPEN / closing / closed											firm, closed	opening	+ open	closing	
FLUID clear / white / yellow / brown dry / sticky / wet / slippery fertile / egg white (EW) Stretchy: How many inches/centimeters?									dry	dry	dry	wet	watery	creamy	
OPK / FERTILITY MONITOR neg (-) / light line / darker / pos (+) Brand used:									–	–	light line	light line	+		
FERNING: none / partial / full															

PM FERTILE SIGNS

	1	2	3	4	5	6	7	8	9	10	11	12	13	14	15
CERVIX high / med / low right / left soft / med / firm pink / red opening / +open / OPEN / closing / closed											softer	opening	OPEN	closed	
FLUID clear / white / yellow / brown dry / sticky / wet / slippery fertile / egg white (EW) Stretchy: How many inches/centimeters?											wet	wet	EW	sticky	
OPK / FERTILITY MONITOR neg (-) / light line / darker / pos (+) Brand used:									–	–	light line	darker			
FERNING: none / partial / full															
OVULATION SENSATION TODAY? What did you feel? (cramp, twinge, pressure, fullness, gas) Which side? When did it start/stop?												full	cramp 7pm		
FERTILITY MEDS / ULTRASOUND which medications / follicle size / L or R															

CYCLE NUMBER: 4   **CYCLE LENGTH:** 25 days   **DAYS OF INSEMINATION:** 13

16	17	18	19	20	21	22	23	24	25	26	27	28	29	30	31	32	33	34	35	36	37	38	39	40
22	23	24	25	26	27	28	29	30	31															
T	W	R	F	S	S	M	T	W	R															

CYCLE DAY	1	2	3	4	5	6	7	8	9	10	11	12	13	14	15
DAY OF THE WEEK	M	T	W	R	F	S	S	M	T	W	R	F	S	S	M
Bleeding x = light day / X = heavy day / • = spotting															
Menstrual Cramps															

Basal Body Temperature: Mark your temperature on the graph each day, then connect the dots to make a line.

What time did you take your temp?

Temp	1	2	3	4	5	6	7	8	9	10	11	12	13	14	15
98.9	9	9	9	9	9	9	9	9	9	9	9	9	9	9	9
98.8	8	8	8	8	8	8	8	8	8	8	8	8	8	8	8
98.7	7	7	7	7	7	7	7	7	7	7	7	7	7	7	7
98.6	6	6	6	6	6	6	6	6	6	6	6	6	6	6	6
98.5	5	5	5	5	5	5	5	5	5	5	5	5	5	5	5
98.4	4	4	4	4	4	4	4	4	4	4	4	4	4	4	4
98.3	3	3	3	3	3	3	3	3	3	3	3	3	3	3	3
98.2	2	2	2	2	2	2	2	2	2	2	2	2	2	2	2
98.1	1	1	1	1	1	1	1	1	1	1	1	1	1	1	1
98.0	0	0	0	0	0	0	0	0	0	0	0	0	0	0	0
97.9	9	9	9	9	9	9	9	9	9	9	9	9	9	9	⑨
97.8	8	8	8	8	8	8	8	8	8	8	8	8	8	8	8
97.7	7	7	7	7	7	7	7	7	7	7	7	7	7	7	7
97.6	6	6	6	6	6	6	6	6	6	6	6	6	⑥	6	6
97.5	5	5	5	5	5	5	⑤	5	5	5	5	5	5	5	5
97.4	4	4	4	4	④	4	④	4	4	4	4	4	4	4	4
97.3	3	3	3	③	③	3	3	③	3	3	3	③	③	3	3
97.2	2	②	②	2	2	2	2	2	②	②	②	②	2	2	2
97.1	①	1	①	1	1	①	1	1	1	1	1	1	1	1	1
97.0	0	0	0	0	0	0	0	0	0	0	0	0	0	0	0
96.9	9	9	9	9	9	9	9	9	9	9	9	9	9	9	9
96.8	8	8	8	8	8	8	8	8	8	8	8	8	8	8	8
96.7	7	7	7	7	7	7	7	7	7	7	7	7	7	7	7
96.6	6	6	6	6	6	6	6	6	6	6	6	6	6	6	6
96.5	5	5	5	5	5	5	5	5	5	5	5	5	5	5	5
96.4	4	4	4	4	4	4	4	4	4	4	4	4	4	4	4
96.3	3	3	3	3	3	3	3	3	3	3	3	3	3	3	3
96.2	2	2	2	2	2	2	2	2	2	2	2	2	2	2	2

	1	2	3	4	5	6	7	8	9	10	11	12	13	14	15
Mood Changes anxious, depressed, content, creative, ecstatic, happy, irritable, "on," voluptuous, or anything else notable around ovulation												ON!			
Sex Drive increase or decrease in libido												++	++		
Breast / Chest Changes tender, full, areola darkening, nipples more erect or sensitive														tender	full
Increased Appetite / Food Cravings												sugar			
Sleep Changes / Dreams waking up in the night, vivid dreams													vivid dreams		
Intuition internal sense that ovulation is happening												X			
Herbs / Supplements															
Exercise															
Stress / Alcohol / Travel / Illness															

16	17	18	19	20	21	22	23	24	25	26	27	28	29	30	31	32	33	34	35	36	37	38	39	40
T	W	R	F	S	S	M	T	W	R															
								•	•															
								X	X															

Mark your temperature on the graph each day, then connect the dots to make a line.

MAIA midwifery & fertility

NAME: *Scenario C*

MONTH: *FEB/MAR*　　**YEAR:** *2021*

CYCLE DAY	1	2	3	4	5	6	7	8	9	10	11	12	13	14	15
DATE	20	21	22	23	24	25	26	27	28	1	2	3	4	5	6
DAY OF THE WEEK	S	S	M	T	W	R	F	S	S	M	T	W	R	F	S
CONCEPTION ATTEMPTS METHOD & TIME OF DAY															

AM FERTILE SIGNS

	1	2	3	4	5	6	7	8	9	10	11	12	13	14	15
CERVIX high / med / low　right / left / soft / med / firm　pink / red / opening / +open / OPEN / closing / closed															*higher*
FLUID clear / white / yellow / brown / dry / sticky / wet / slippery / fertile / egg white (EW) / Stretchy: How many inches/centimeters?															*EW 1"*
OPK / FERTILITY MONITOR neg (-) / light line / darker / pos (+) Brand used:												*light*	*light*	*light*	*light*
FERNING: none / partial / full															

PM FERTILE SIGNS

	1	2	3	4	5	6	7	8	9	10	11	12	13	14	15
CERVIX high / med / low　right / left / soft / med / firm　pink / red / opening / +open / OPEN / closing / closed					!									*opening, firm*	*same*
FLUID clear / white / yellow / brown / dry / sticky / wet / slippery / fertile / egg white (EW) / Stretchy: How many inches/centimeters?										*wet*	*wet*	*wet*	*wet*	*EW 1"*	*EW 1"*
OPK / FERTILITY MONITOR neg (-) / light line / darker / pos (+) Brand used:														*light*	*light*
FERNING: none / partial / full															
OVULATION SENSATION TODAY? What did you feel? (cramp, twinge, pressure, fullness, gas) Which side? When did it start/stop?															
FERTILITY MEDS / ULTRASOUND which medications / follicle size / L or R															

16	17	18	19	20	21	22	23	24	25	26	27	28	29	30	31	32	33	34	35	36	37	38	39	40
7	8	9	10	11	12	13	14	15	16	17	18	19	20	21	22									
S	M	T	W	R	F	S	S	M	T	W	R	F	S	S	M									
	IUI PM																							
+ open	+ HSO	same	less open																					
EW 5"	EW 6"	less fluid	creamy																					
light																								
same	++ open	same	closed																					
EW 5"	EW 6"	creamy	creamy																					
+																								
	PM cramp	AM cramp/ fullness all day	cramps AM/PM	sensation all day					pinching @ 4pm															

CYCLE DAY	1	2	3	4	5	6	7	8	9	10	11	12	13	14	15
DAY OF THE WEEK	S	S	M	T	W	R	F	S	S	M	T	W	R	F	S
Bleeding x = light day / X = heavy day / • = spotting															
Menstrual Cramps															

Basal Body Temperature: Mark your temperature on the graph each day, then connect the dots to make a line.

What time did you take your temp?

	1	2	3	4	5	6	7	8	9	10	11	12	13	14	15
98.9	9	9	9	9	9	9	9	9	9	9	9	9	9	9	9
98.8	8	8	8	8	8	8	8	8	8	8	8	8	8	8	8
98.7	7	7	7	7	7	7	7	7	7	7	7	7	7	7	7
98.6	6	6	6	6	6	6	6	6	6	6	6	6	6	6	6
98.5	5	5	5	5	5	5	5	5	5	5	5	5	5	5	5
98.4	4	4	4	4	4	4	4	4	4	4	4	4	4	4	4
98.3	3	3	3	3	3	3	3	3	3	3	3	3	3	3	3
98.2	2	2	2	2	2	2	2	2	2	2	2	2	2	2	2
98.1	1	1	1	1	1	1	1	1	1	1	1	1	1	1	1
98.0	0	0	0	0	0	0	0	0	0	0	0	0	0	0	0
97.9	9	9	9	9	9	9	9	9	9	9	9	9	9	9	9
97.8	8	8	8	8	8	8	8	8	8	8	8	8	8	8	8
97.7	7	7	7	7	7	7	7	7	7	7	7	7	7	7	7
97.6	6	6	6	6	6	6	6	6	6	6	6	6	6	6	6
97.5	5	5	5	5	5	5	5	5	5	5	5	5	5	5	5
97.4	4	4	4	4	4	4	4	4	4	4	4	4	4	4	4
97.3	3	3	3	3	3	3	3	3	3	3	3	3	3	3	3
97.2	2	2	2	2	2	2	2	2	2	2	2	2	2	2	2
97.1	1	1	1	1	1	1	1	1	1	1	1	1	1	1	1
97.0	0	0	0	0	0	0	0	0	0	0	0	0	0	0	0
96.9	9	9	9	9	9	9	9	9	9	9	9	9	9	9	9
96.8	8	8	8	8	8	8	8	8	8	8	8	8	8	8	8
96.7	7	7	7	7	7	7	7	7	7	7	7	7	7	7	7
96.6	6	6	6	6	6	6	6	6	6	6	6	6	6	6	6
96.5	5	5	5	5	5	5	5	5	5	5	5	5	5	5	5
96.4	4	4	4	4	4	4	4	4	4	4	4	4	4	4	4
96.3	3	3	3	3	3	3	3	3	3	3	3	3	3	3	3
96.2	2	2	2	2	2	2	2	2	2	2	2	2	2	2	2

Mood Changes anxious, depressed, content, creative, ecstatic, happy, irritable, "on," voluptuous, or anything else notable around ovulation															
Sex Drive increase or decrease in libido						⌃1	⌃1					⌃1			
Breast / Chest Changes tender, full, areola darkening, nipples more erect or sensitive															
Increased Appetite / Food Cravings															
Sleep Changes / Dreams waking up in the night, vivid dreams															
Intuition internal sense that ovulation is happening															
Herbs / Supplements															
Exercise															
Stress / Alcohol / Travel / Illness															

16	17	18	19	20	21	22	23	24	25	26	27	28	29	30	31	32	33	34	35	36	37	38	39	40
S	M	T	W	R	F	S	S	M	T	W	R	F	S	S	M									
															::									
															X									

Mark your temperature on the graph each day, then connect the dots to make a line.

emotional " " " " "

↑ ↑

tender " " " " " " " " " " "

WILL IT INCREASE MY CHANCES IF I DO TWO, OR EVEN THREE, INSEMINATIONS?

Although multiple inseminations have been shown to increase success with fresh sperm, if you are conceiving via IUI with frozen sperm, you only need one well-timed insemination. Doing multiple inseminations may benefit you if your timing isn't precise, which often happens for those who are ready to start trying to get pregnant before charting enough to be sure of their ovulation pattern. Or, you may want to do multiple inseminations if your body gives you varied ovulation patterns from month to month and you need a contingency plan for all possible scenarios. In any case, if you haven't been able to narrow down your ovulation to a predictable twelve-hour window, or if your ovulation pattern varies by more than twelve hours from month to month, you can cover more time by doing multiple inseminations.

- With fresh sperm, time inseminations twenty-four hours apart (intercourse or self-insemination first, followed by IUI).

- With frozen sperm, time self-inseminations twelve to eighteen hours apart (or time IUI twelve to eighteen hours after self-insemination).

- With frozen sperm, time IUIs twelve hours apart.

Inseminating with Fresh Sperm

Charting ahead of time can alleviate some of the logistical stress involved in coordinating with a known donor or coparent (or even with a busy partner). Knowing when in your cycle ovulation is likely to occur can help you all plan for conception attempts on those days and helps everyone know what to expect.

TIMING SELF-INSEMINATION WITH FRESH SPERM

Whether through insemination or intercourse, there are many ways to time conception with fresh sperm. This is because there are so many aspects of human physiology that work together to make conception happen, and it is why books, websites, and apps designed for cis/het people are so confident in their methods. If you have the advantage of conceiving with fresh sperm, those sperm cells can stay alive in the conceiving body for two to three days, so your timing does not need to be any more precise than that. The single most important factor for insemination with fresh sperm is the fertile cervical mucus your body makes when estrogen levels are high. The cellular structure of clear, stretchy cervical fluid has long, branched pathways that guide sperm cells into the upper reproductive tract. As long as you inseminate on the days you have your best fertile fluid, your timing will be great.

That being said, don't wait until the last minute if you are self-inseminating with fresh sperm. Conception rates are highest when fresh sperm are present one to two days before ovulation, and the day after ovulation is too late.

Multiple inseminations: If you have many days of fertile fluid each month and a highly available sperm source, you can time inseminations every other day once fertile fluid starts to appear. (See sample chart on page 174.)

One or two inseminations: If you only have sperm available for two inseminations, time them as indicated by your ovulation pattern, with the goal of inseminating a day or two before and no later than the day of ovulation. For instance, if you always get three days of fertile fluid, and your egg releases on the final day, contact your sperm source once the fluid appears, and arrange to start inseminating that day or the day after.

One insemination: If you only have sperm available for one insemination, try to determine the fertile sign that indicates pending ovulation in twenty-four hours, and inseminate once that sign appears. For example, if your LH surge happens the day before ovulation, be sure to inseminate soon after your OPK positive appears.

With fresh sperm, time inseminations at least twenty-four hours apart so that there is time for your donor, coparent, or partner's body to regenerate a sizable sample of sperm cells. The best samples occur between twenty-four to forty-eight hours after the previous ejaculation. After about three days without ejaculation, sperm cells start to break down. Given this physiology, it is ideal to have the person ejaculate one to three days before you think you will attempt to conceive (you can inseminate with this sample or not), and then abstain until a sample is needed for a conception attempt.

TIMING IUI WITH FRESH SPERM

Consider IUI when intercourse or self-insemination has not been successful, or when there is a low sperm count or low motility. The samples will need to be "washed," which is a process that removes the seminal fluid and isolates the sperm cells in a carrier medium so that they can be placed directly inside the uterus. (Placing seminal fluid in the uterus can cause severe cramping and infection, both of which would inhibit conception.) Finding a provider who is willing to provide IUI and washing with fresh known-donor samples can be difficult, so you may need to access this care with an independent care provider who has this capability and is willing to provide the necessary informed consent.

You will want to time IUI with fresh sperm as close to ovulation as possible, so determining the length of time between your LH surge and your peak fertile signs will allow you to make arrangements for this. If you have not charted closely enough to identify the peak twelve-hour window, you may opt to do two IUIs. However, the person providing your sperm samples needs twenty-four hours to regenerate enough sperm cells for a second insemination. If you need to do two IUIs with fresh, start on the early side, and repeat in twenty-four hours.

PLANNING INSEMINATIONS WITH A FRESH SAMPLE THAT HAS BEEN SHIPPED OVERNIGHT

If you are having your known donor ship their sperm sample to you using an overnight preservation and shipping kit, time insemination the same as you would with a frozen sperm sample. The life span of sperm cells is reduced any time they leave the human body and are preserved, whether that is through refrigeration and shipping or cryopreservation at a clinic or sperm bank.

The tricky thing about getting the timing right with a shipped sample is that you need to have the sample shipped the day before you think you will need it. If you don't get your OPK positive at least twenty-four hours before ovulation, you will need to be aware of other preemptive signs that appear for you. This is most commonly based on the appearance of fertile fluid, or on knowing the number of days you typically get fertile fluid and shipping accordingly. For some, there is a pattern to how the lines on the OPK start to darken before turning positive, so this may be a useful signal for you. You may also opt to do more than one shipment if the first sample ended up being shipped too early, so make sure your donor has an extra kit on hand. Keep a close eye when your fertile signs appear on a Friday—overnight shipping is not typically available on Sundays, so you will need to give your donor an opportunity to collect their sample and ship it to you before the shipping office closes on Friday for delivery on Saturday.

TIPS FOR PROVIDING A FRESH SPERM SAMPLE

1. Abstain from ejaculating for one to three days prior to donation.

2. Find a small, widemouthed jar to collect your sample, such as the smallest-size mason jar or a plastic specimen container. The jar must be clean and dry prior to collecting the sample.

3. Be sure to be well hydrated on the day you provide your sample.

4. When it is time to provide your sample, wash your hands before you begin.

5. Keep in mind:

   - The more aroused you are, the more sperm you will release.
   - Take your time—let your arousal build as much as possible.
   - Provide yourself with your favorite magazines, videos, etc.
   - If you have a lover who would like to be involved, that is fine too.
   - If you need to use a lubricant, choose a sperm-friendly brand such as Pre-Seed.
   - Keep lubricants away from the tip of the penis.
   - The greatest number of sperm are in the first portion of ejaculate, so be sure to capture the sample as soon as you start to climax.

6. Once you have collected your sample, place the lid on the container. If the sample is spread thinly across the bottom of the container, you may need to tip it slightly so that the sample does not dry out.

7. If you are planning to draw up the sample into the syringe yourself, allow time for the sample to turn from a gel to a liquid. This typically takes five to fifteen minutes or up to half an hour.

8. Keep the sample at body temperature until it is time to inseminate. You can do this by placing the jar under your arm or between your legs while you are sitting or driving (do not turn on your seat heat).

9. A normal amount of ejaculate is two to four milliliters. If you notice that your sample is less than that amount, try drinking a lot of water next time so that you will be more hydrated. You can also try increasing your level of arousal while providing your sample, or allowing time for more buildup prior to ejaculation.

NAME:

MONTH: NOVEMBER **YEAR:** 2020

CYCLE DAY	1	2	3	4	5	6	7	8	9	10	11	12	13	14	15
DATE	3	4	5	6	7	8	9	10	11	12	13	14	15	16	17
DAY OF THE WEEK	T	W	R	F	S	S	M	T	W	R	F	S	S	M	T
CONCEPTION ATTEMPTS METHOD & TIME OF DAY												PM		PM	

AM FERTILE SIGNS

CERVIX high / med / low right / left soft / med / firm pink / red opening / +open / OPEN / closing / closed												firm	softening	medium	medium	softer
FLUID clear / white / yellow / brown dry / sticky / wet / slippery fertile / egg white (EW) Stretchy: How many inches/centimeters?											wet	stretchy	stretchy	^stretch	^stretch
OPK / FERTILITY MONITOR neg (-) / light line / darker / pos (+) Brand used:												neg	neg	neg	almost pos.
FERNING: none / partial / full															

PM FERTILE SIGNS

CERVIX high / med / low right / left soft / med / firm pink / red opening / +open / OPEN / closing / closed												"	"	softer	"
FLUID clear / white / yellow / brown dry / sticky / wet / slippery fertile / egg white (EW) Stretchy: How many inches/centimeters?												"	"	"	more
OPK / FERTILITY MONITOR neg (-) / light line / darker / pos (+) Brand used:												neg	neg	darker	+
FERNING: none / partial / full															
OVULATION SENSATION TODAY? What did you feel? (cramp, twinge, pressure, fullness, gas) Which side? When did it start/stop?													bloated	gas	crampy
FERTILITY MEDS / ULTRASOUND which medications / follicle size / L or R															

CYCLE NUMBER: 3   **CYCLE LENGTH:**   **DAYS OF INSEMINATION:**

16	17	18	19	20	21	22	23	24	25	26	27	28	29	30	31	32	33	34	35	36	37	38	39	40
18	19	20	21	22	23	24	25	26	27	28	29	30	1											
W	R	F	S	S	M	T	W	R	F	S	S	M	T											
AM																								
soft/open	less soft	firm/closed																						
LOTS	less	sticky																						
soft/open	firmer																							
LOTS	=																							
=																								

CYCLE DAY	1	2	3	4	5	6	7	8	9	10	11	12	13	14	15
DAY OF THE WEEK	T	W	R	F	S	S	M	T	W	R	F	S	S	M	T
Bleeding x = light day / X = heavy day / • = spotting															
Menstrual Cramps															

Basal Body Temperature: Mark your temperature on the graph each day, then connect the dots to make a line.

What time did you take your temp?	1	2	3	4	5	6	7	8	9	10	11	12	13	14	15
98.9	9	9	9	9	9	9	9	9	9	9	9	9	9	9	9
98.8	8	8	8	8	8	8	8	8	8	8	8	8	8	8	8
98.7	7	7	7	7	7	7	7	7	7	7	7	7	7	7	7
98.6	6	6	6	6	6	6	6	6	6	6	6	6	6	6	6
98.5	5	5	5	5	5	5	5	5	5	5	5	5	5	5	5
98.4	4	4	4	4	4	4	4	4	4	4	4	4	4	4	4
98.3	3	3	3	3	3	3	3	3	3	3	3	3	3	3	3
98.2	2	2	2	2	2	2	2	2	2	2	2	2	2	2	2
98.1	1	1	1	1	1	1	1	1	1	1	1	1	1	1	1
98.0	0	0	0	0	0	0	0	0	0	0	0	0	0	0	0
97.9	9	9	9	9	9	9	9	9	9	9	9	9	9	9	9
97.8	8	8	8	8	8	8	8	8	8	8	8	8	8	8	8
97.7	7	7	7	7	7	7	7	7	7	7	7	7	7	7	7
97.6	6	6	6	6	6	6	6	6	6	6	6	6	6	6	6
97.5	5	5	5	5	5	5	5	5	5	5	5	5	5	5	5
97.4	4	4	4	4	4	4	4	4	4	4	4	4	4	4	4
97.3	3	3	3	3	3	3	3	3	3	(3)	3	3	3	3	3
97.2	2	2	2	2	2	2	(2)	2	2	2	2	(2)	2	2	2
97.1	1	1	1	1	1	1	1	(1)	1	1	1	1	1	1	(1)
97.0	0	0	0	0	(0)	(0)	0	0	(0)	0	0	0	0	(0)	0
96.9	9	9	9	9	9	9	9	9	9	9	9	9	9	9	9
96.8	8	8	8	8	8	8	8	8	8	8	8	8	8	8	8
96.7	7	7	7	7	7	7	7	7	7	7	7	7	7	7	7
96.6	6	6	6	6	6	6	6	6	6	6	6	6	6	6	6
96.5	5	5	5	5	5	5	5	5	5	5	5	5	5	5	5
96.4	4	4	4	4	4	4	4	4	4	4	4	4	4	4	4
96.3	3	3	3	3	3	3	3	3	3	3	3	3	3	3	3
96.2	2	2	2	2	2	2	2	2	2	2	2	2	2	2	2

	1	2	3	4	5	6	7	8	9	10	11	12	13	14	15
Mood Changes anxious, depressed, content, creative, ecstatic, happy, irritable, "on," voluptuous, or anything else notable around ovulation														*sad*	*happy*
Sex Drive increase or decrease in libido														↑	♥
Breast / Chest Changes tender, full, areola darkening, nipples more erect or sensitive															
Increased Appetite / Food Cravings															
Sleep Changes / Dreams waking up in the night, vivid dreams													*dreams*	*dreams*	*dreams*
Intuition internal sense that ovulation is happening															+
Herbs / Supplements															
Exercise															
Stress / Alcohol / Travel / Illness															

16	17	18	19	20	21	22	23	24	25	26	27	28	29	30	31	32	33	34	35	36	37	38	39	40
W	R	F	S	S	M	T	W	R	F	S	S	M	T	W	R	F	S	S	M					

Pregnant!!

Mark your temperature on the graph each day, then connect the dots to make a line.

great!

-)

sore " " " " " " " full " " "

wakeful

+

What to Know about Self-Insemination

Self-insemination is easy. You don't need any special tools other than a syringe (without a needle) or medicine dropper. Fresh samples are less than a teaspoon, and frozen samples are only about one-fifth of a teaspoon. If you are using fresh sperm, use a 5 cc syringe—for frozen sperm, a 1 cc syringe is good. Please do not use a turkey baster—it's way too big! You also don't need an overpriced $100 plastic syringe with a curved tip, such as the Mosie. To make sure none of the sample is left in the tip of your syringe after inseminating, simply draw up your sample, and *do not* invert the syringe and flick it to remove the bubble of air that appears behind the sample. Instead, keep that air bubble where it is, so that as you press the syringe, the entirety of the sample will flow out, and the air bubble will end up at the tip of the syringe after the last bit of sample is pressed out.

All you need to do is elevate your hips on a couple of pillows, insert the syringe as far as it will go, and slowly press the plunger to place the sample in the genital canal. Please do not use a speculum! If you do, the sample will pool in the bills of the speculum, which means you will pull it back out again when you remove the speculum. You don't have to try to get the sample close to the cervix—inserting the syringe completely and elevating your hips will allow gravity to do that for you. You can put your legs up the wall, but this doesn't gain anything over simply elevating your hips on some pillows.

Once the sample is placed internally, the motile sperm cells enter your fertile fluid and swim upstream into the cervix, through the uterus, and into the fallopian tubes. Please do not insert egg whites or Pre-Seed lubricant! This is not at all necessary and will only confuse and disperse the sperm cells—all they need is your fertile fluid to guide them where they need to go.

The fastest swimmers will arrive in the fallopian tubes within two to ten minutes. You don't need to orgasm to help the sperm get into the cervix, although if you want this to be part of your insemination experience, you are welcome to. It is more helpful to be aroused and/or to climax before you inseminate because this shifts your internal pH to match the pH of the sperm sample, creating the optimal chemical environment.

Regardless of how you spend your time after inserting the sample, please remain lying down with your hips elevated for an hour or so. The viable sperm will continue moving into the upper reproductive tract until those that are left start to die off. If you remain lying down, there is absolutely no need to use a device such as a soft cup to hold the sample inside. Your cervical mucus filters out the duds from the strong swimmers, and your internal reproductive tract has everything the best sperm cells need to keep them alive and swimming—from macroproteins within crypts along the cervical canal to the cilia that provide safe harbor within the fallopian tubes.

The only reason to use a soft cup or other device that holds the samples close to the cervix is when you must inseminate on the go or you simply cannot lie down for an hour after inseminating. Seminal fluid only protects sperm cells for about an hour. After that, it starts to inhibit the function of the cells. Any sperm cells that have not left the seminal fluid by swimming into your cervical crypts or up into the fallopian tubes will be destroyed, so wearing a soft cup or insemination device for more than an hour is futile.

What to Know about the IUI Procedure

Intrauterine insemination is a simple, straightforward procedure that can easily be done by a pelvic health care provider in a clinic or in the comfort of your own home. A midwife, nurse practitioner, or physician has the skills to maintain sterility and to place the catheter successfully within the uterine cavity. This is done by inserting a speculum, bringing the cervix into view, passing a catheter through the cervix and into the uterus, and placing the sample by pressing the plunger on a syringe that is attached to the other end of the catheter. Some providers are even comfortable allowing a partner or loved one to press the syringe and inject the sample. Once the sample is placed, the catheter and speculum are removed. In a clinic, you can usually stay on the table for ten to fifteen minutes after the procedure. (If this is not offered, I encourage you to insist on this because research shows it results in higher success rates!) At home, clients are often encouraged to remain lying down for thirty to sixty minutes. Some people have some cramping after IUI, especially if it's the first time you have had sperm in your body. The procedure itself usually takes five minutes or less.

Your experience of IUI will depend on the skill and approach of the provider performing the procedure, as well as the accuracy of your timing and, to a certain extent, your anatomy. Some people experience cramping during IUI, and others don't feel anything at all. There are no two bodies alike. Some cervixes are wide open for days surrounding the time of ovulation, and others appear open but remain closed at the inner margin of the cervical os, except for just a few hours each month. Some uteruses are centered in the pelvic cavity, while others tilt frontward, backward, or to the side, making some procedures quick and easy while others may take more patience and skill.

Some things you can do to ensure a comfortable IUI experience:

- Make sure your timing is spot on—this will ensure your cervical os is as open as possible.

- Have an orgasm within an hour before the IUI procedure—this tends to open the cervix.

- Choose a care provider who is gentle and not rushed, and who uses a trauma-informed approach. Experience matters—if your IUI provider is newly in practice and your IUIs are uncomfortable, seek care with a provider who has more experience and finesse.

TRAUMA-INFORMED IUI—EVERY PERSON DESERVES GENTLE, RESPECTFUL CARE

The following information is for ensuring that your IUI is as comfortable as it can possibly be. Many of us have not had positive experiences with pelvic exams, but there are many things that can be done to make them more tolerable and even empowering. If you are receiving IUI, use the column on the left to guide your communications with your provider. Providers can use the column on the right for guiding trauma-informed pelvic care and IUI.

Trauma-Informed IUI Guide

Self-Advocacy for Receiving IUI	Guidelines for Care Providers
Does your provider welcome open communication about your care? Do you feel that they respect you and your personal boundaries? If not, find a different provider.	Establish open communication, respect client/patient boundaries, be clear about your own boundaries or expectations, and provide shared decision-making.
Let your provider know if there are specific words you prefer in reference to your gender, your family, or your reproductive anatomy. Body parts don't have a gender—people do. You deserve to have your gender affirmed no matter the situation.	Invite communication about the words a client/patient uses, from pronouns to familial nomenclature to the words they use to refer to their reproductive anatomy. Use these words consistently.
Let your provider know if you have a trauma history or if there are triggers that make exams difficult for you. Give specific information about words to avoid or what not to do, as well as what would make the exam more tolerable for you.	Ask if there is anything you should know that might make the procedure feel more comfortable or safe for the recipient. Listen carefully and be prepared to get creative in order to avoid re-traumatization and to keep the recipient in control.
Ask any questions you have. Get the information you need to feel comfortable and assured. Ask to see equipment and supplies that are used in the procedure—or not to see anything if that increases anxiety for you.	Explain the procedure before it begins. Give the client/patient an opportunity to see the catheter, and to participate in selecting the size of the speculum.
Wear your own clothing during the procedure if desired, and be sure to bring warm socks! Use the drape or don't use the drape—whatever makes you feel most comfortable.	Allow the client/patient to choose whether or not they use a gown or drape during the procedure.
Let your provider know if you prefer to be talked through the procedure, or if you would rather not know the specifics of what is happening. You can change your mind at any time.	Offer to inform the client/patient about what is happening at each step of the process, and allow them to determine how much they want to know.
Speak up if you need the provider to stop for any reason. You may need to take a break or use your breath to relax. You are in control and can ask for what you need.	Let the client/patient know they are in charge of when a procedure starts and stops, or when a break is needed. Be prepared to end the procedure upon request.

Self-Advocacy for Receiving IUI	Guidelines for Care Providers
Let your provider know that you prefer to give permission before being touched, and again at every step of the procedure. You can ask for things to go as slowly as you need them to.	Always ask permission before touching a client/patient. Get permission before advancing to each step of the procedure (touch, speculum insertion, advancing the speculum, placing the catheter).
If footrests are unsettling for you, request that you place your feet flat on the exam table instead. You can use a towel or bolster to elevate your hips instead of moving to the end of the table. Keep in mind that sometimes using footrests makes the internal exam more comfortable. See what works best for you.	Allow the client/patient to avoid using exam table footrests if this creates anxiety for them. Use a folded blanket or towel to elevate the hips and make room for the handle of the speculum. Cooperate to find a position that will allow for a comfortable internal exam while ensuring you will be able to perform the procedure effectively.
Be sure to let your provider know if they touch you in a way that feels uncomfortable. You can simply say, "Stop," and then figure out how to express more clearly what you need.	Verbally ask the client/patient to adjust their position—never move any part of their body for them. For example, you may place your hand outside and away from the knee without touching it while asking them to "please allow your knee to fall outward toward my hand, as much as is comfortable for you."
If speculum insertion is triggering for you, ask to insert the speculum yourself, and then the provider can adjust it as needed.	Allow the client to self-insert the speculum if desired, and adjust as needed. A light that fits into the speculum handle is helpful for this.
If anything feels like it is pinching or pulling as the speculum is placed, ask the provider to stop. Let them know where you feel the sensation so they can adjust as needed.	Ensure that no skin, hair, or external genitalia are being pulled or pinched by the speculum. Make adjustments with consent.
You can help ensure that your cervix is as open as possible by having an orgasm within an hour prior to your IUI procedure. If your cervix tends to be too high for the speculum to reach, jump up and down for thirty seconds before getting on the table. If your provider routinely needs to use a tenaculum to get through your cervix, reassess your timing and make sure you are inseminating when your cervix is most open (and consider changing to a provider who does not use instruments to force through your cervix).	Make sure you are using the appropriate-size speculum. It should reach securely around the cervix to hold it in place. A retroverted uterus can be accessed by tilting the pelvis forward with a bolster or the recipient's fists under their hips, and an anteverted uterus can be accessed by applying suprapubic pressure to bring the fundus into alignment with the cervical canal. Invite the client's participation in positioning. There is no need to use a tenaculum. If the internal os is tight, utilize patience and finesse, and be sure you are inseminating at the right time for the individual.

Self-Advocacy for Receiving IUI	Guidelines for Care Providers
If you have a partner who would like to push the syringe plunger to inject the sample once the catheter is in place, please be sure to ask about this. Trust your provider's judgment about whether the placement will be easy or if they recommend doing the sample placement themselves.	If there is a partner in attendance, offer to have them place the sample once the catheter has been inserted and you have ensured the sample will flow freely into the uterus. Brace the catheter against the speculum handle so it cannot be moved, and watch for any backflow. Instruct them to press the plunger very slowly so you can instruct them to stop if needed.
Afterward, let your provider know if there was anything that was especially helpful for you, or anything you would like to request they do differently next time. If you think of something later, make a note for yourself so you can be sure to talk about it at your next appointment.	Debrief the procedure once the client/patient is dressed. Ask if there is anything they would like you to do differently or to remember for next time. Keep an open mind and be receptive. Let them know you are open to feedback at any time, and reiterate that your goal is for the IUI procedure to be as comfortable, affirming, and empowering as possible.

GUIDANCE FOR CARE PROVIDERS

You don't have to be a midwife to assist people in timing their inseminations using an individualized, physiological approach. However, trusting people to gather accurate information about their bodies, and being willing to utilize that information to create individualized care plans, is a departure from the medical model in which we are taught to rely on labs, ultrasounds, medications, and standardized procedures. Keep in mind that an individualized approach to insemination timing does not contradict what is known about how the body ovulates. It simply keeps in mind that frozen sperm has a limited life span, and that while standardized timing protocols may work for some, they do not work for all. Your ability to use your own best clinical judgment in the service of each individual makes you a more proficient IUI provider.

That being said, for most people, charting takes considerable effort at the outset, and your skills in providing affirmation and nonjudgmental feedback will be put to good use here. Many people will not get a full set of data the first month they track, and it can be validating to normalize this experience for the people you serve. You will also find that you spend a fair amount of time debunking the erroneous information that circulates on the internet and social media about what OPKs mean, mostly because the same level of accuracy is not needed for conceiving via intercourse, and the information out there is primarily by, for, and about heterosexual couples having sex to conceive. You will find that people either stop charting after the positive OPK, thinking that the OPK itself has identified the day of ovulation, or they keep charting the rise and fall of LH, thinking that ovulation occurs at the peak of urinary LH secretion. Be prepared to gently reeducate your clients, explaining the pitfalls in these methods and presenting the more reliable approach of charting peak estrogen symptoms.

One of the best things you can do to support the families in your care is to give them feedback and encouragement every month as they begin charting. This will allow you to point out the helpful information they gathered, as well as to provide timely education and feedback so they don't lose time as they go on to chart the following cycle. It can be so disappointing for a client to faithfully track their fertile signs for three months or more, only to bring their charts to you all at once in preparation for insemination the following month . . . and then find out they are missing the data that is needed to time insemination accurately. Ask that your clients schedule a follow-up visit each month to review their cycle chart with you. This will help them keep on track with accurately identifying ovulation so that when they are ready to start inseminating, they have the information they need to get started right away and feel confident in their timing.

And finally, please take the time to incorporate trauma-informed techniques into your practice. The chart on pages 181–183 provides a step-by-step guide for comfortable, trauma-informed pelvic exams and IUI.

Resources

MAIA Cycle Chart and ovulation tracking supplies: MAIAMidwifery.com

The Beautiful Cervix Project*: BeautifulCervix.com

*Go to the Cervix Photo Galleries and click on "Entire Cycle" to view various cervixes as they change throughout the month. The language on the site is female gendered; however, there is no need to read the small print—just look through the photos and try to guess when ovulation occurred!

TROUBLESHOOTING AND COMPLICATED CONCEPTIONS

If you are trying but not conceiving, start with the basics as you investigate possible reasons why. Ask yourself the following questions—if the answer is no, go to previous chapters to get the information you need:

Is your sperm source viable?

- I/my partner/coparent/known donor has had a normal semen analysis in the past six months (Chapter 3).

- I'm having my donor ship to me, and I've had their shipped sample tested with normal results (Chapter 4).

- I'm using a sperm bank, and my vials have at least 20 million motile cells per cc—not bargain or "ART" vials (Chapter 4).

Are you having regular cycles, and ovulating each month?

- My periods come every twenty-two to thirty-five days. (If not, it's time to see a fertility specialist.)

- I have tracked my basal body temperature, noting a temperature rise after ovulation that continues through the luteal phase—or I've confirmed ovulation with a serum progesterone test (Chapter 3).

Is your timing spot on?

- I'm using frozen sperm, testing LH twice daily as ovulation approaches, and continuing to track high estrogen symptoms as they peak and go away. The interval between my LH surge and best fluid plus softest, most open cervix is consistent, and I have inseminated at the peak of those symptoms in at least three cycles (Chapter 6).

- I'm using fresh sperm and attempting conception on my fertile fluid days, including one to two inseminations within twenty-four to forty-eight hours prior to the release of my egg, in at least three to six cycles (Chapter 6).

Are you living a fertile lifestyle?

- I'm eating whole foods and focusing on anti-inflammatory proteins to keep my blood sugar stable (Chapter 2).

- I get moderate exercise three to four times a week (Chapter 2).

- I sleep eight hours each night (Chapter 2).

- My stress level is below a five out of ten (Chapter 2).

- I am avoiding toxins and endocrine disruptors (Chapter 2).

Have you completed all recommended lab tests and fertility evaluations?

- All recommended lab work has been completed within the past year, and my results are in the ideal range for pregnancy (Chapter 3).

- I have addressed any abnormal results and followed up with my practitioner to make sure everything is now in the normal range (Chapter 3).

Is It Time to Visit a Fertility Clinic?

If you answered in the affirmative to all of the aforementioned questions, and you have inseminated three to six cycles without success, it may be time to be assessed by a fertility doctor. Going in for an assessment simply gives you more information—the plan you choose going forward ultimately lies in your hands. Many people are trepidatious about going to a fertility clinic because there is a sense of losing agency while undergoing painful, costly treatments. But in an ideal world, your fertility doctor will provide you with their assessment and recommendations, allow time for your questions, and then support you in making the decision that is best for you. For some, putting the process into the hands of a fertility doctor feels like a relief from decision-making fatigue, so letting go of being the one in charge may support you in that regard. In any case, remember that the initial assessment is just that—an assessment. It's information about your body that you can use to help inform your next steps. The decisions you make about your care are ultimately up to you.

"IF I GO TO A FERTILITY CLINIC, THEY ARE JUST GOING TO TELL ME TO LOSE WEIGHT."

Just like homophobia, transphobia, and racism, anti-fat bias is everywhere, and it is rampant in our health care system. However, just like you may need to look past the rampant cis/heterosexism in fertility medicine in order to access care, you may need to reframe the bias against fatness too. Start by affirming your own lived experience. Having a large body intersects with multiple psychological factors that have a direct effect on overall health and well-being. Trauma and abuse from forced exercise and dieting during childhood, being socially ostracized and bullied by peers during school-age years, and continuing to navigate a world that values people according to their body size as an adult takes a toll. This lived experience contributes to disordered eating at any age, and if you have spent years recovering from an eating disorder and tuning out all the noise so you can truly love your body, being told you have to lose weight can feel defeating and put you at risk for landing right back into patterns you have worked hard to overcome.

The reality is that everything you have ever done to cultivate your own resiliency and self-love will serve you now. Pregnancy is a deeply embodied experience, so if there is a trauma history affecting how you navigate this time, make sure you have a good therapist to support you. Choose how to care for your body in the way that works best for you. If your BMI (body mass index) is above 25, your doctor is likely to tell you to lose 10 percent of your body weight, because the data says that improves success rates. If it works for you to focus on the numbers, get on a scale, and do what it takes to lose the weight, then do that. But this sort of approach is not required, especially if it makes you hate yourself. From a long-term health perspective, it is certainly not the best approach. Dieting may bring short-term weight loss, but studies show that without long-term changes in how you eat and how you move your body, the weight comes back.

A "health at every size" approach means focusing on building health rather than losing weight. Healthy eating, ample sleep, and consistent exercise are the goal, not a number on a scale. This is what will support you through pregnancy and into parenthood as you feed your kids. You are not just trying to get pregnant, you are trying to have a baby. Once you conceive, there is an entire pregnancy to navigate. Focus on nurturing your body, mind, and soul. Let the haters hate. Love yourself as well as you already love this child. Make sure your self-talk is as loving as the way you would speak to your child. Feed yourself as well as you would feed your baby, and encourage yourself to get out and move your body in ways that you enjoy, just like you would for your kiddo.

WHAT IS COVERED IN A FERTILITY ASSESSMENT

The following section assumes that you have already completed the basic lab work outlined in Chapter 3, which can uncover issues such as anemia, deficiency in vitamins D and B_{12}, thyroid problems, sickle cell anemia, thalassemia, diabetes or prediabetes, and STIs that can damage the reproductive system. If you have not already completed these health tests, make sure your fertility doctor orders them as part of your assessment. Additional components of the infertility workup are described in Chapter 3 as well.

COMPONENTS OF THE INFERTILITY WORKUP

- Health history and physical exam
- Blood work to uncover causes of infertility and assess markers of "ovarian reserve"
- Ultrasound for antral follicle count and assessment of the uterine lining
- Hysterosalpingogram or saline infusion sonogram
- Laparoscopy may be performed if you have symptoms of endometriosis or to assess for structural issues, scar tissue, or fibroids

Common Causes of Infertility and How They Can Be Addressed

The rest of this chapter covers the most common causes of infertility. For each condition, you will find the definition, symptoms, how it is diagnosed, and a care plan including nutrition, exercise, supplements, herbs, and complementary or conventional medical treatments.

PCOS

Polycystic ovary syndrome, or PCOS, is not just about having cysts on the ovaries—in fact, sometimes the ovaries are not polycystic at all! PCOS is the most common endocrine issue affecting those with ovaries who are of reproductive age. It affects anywhere from 8 to 13 percent of people with ovaries. What we call PCOS is actually a complex condition that involves ovulatory dysfunction, hyperandrogenism (high testosterone), and/or polycystic ovaries.

DIAGNOSIS

PCOS is diagnosed when at least two of three factors are present:

1. Ovulatory dysfunction
   - Cycles that are fewer than twenty-one days or more than thirty-five days in length, or

- Anovulatory cycles as diagnosed by serum progesterone less than 4 ng/mL at mid-luteal phase

2. Hyperandrogenism

- Hirsutism (hair growth on the face, lower abdomen, back, or chest) that occurs without taking exogenous testosterone, alopecia (hair loss), and/or acne

- Elevated lab values for free testosterone, free androgen index, or bioavailable testosterone

3. Polycystic ovaries

- More than twenty follicles on either ovary

- Ovarian volume over 10 milliliters

ACCESSING CARE FOR PCOS

You may or may not need to see a doctor to know that you have PCOS based on these guidelines. If you have very short or very long cycles and physical symptoms such as facial hair, you meet the criteria for diagnosis of PCOS. However, an ultrasound and lab work can be useful in identifying the type of PCOS you have.

All forms of PCOS benefit from the same lifestyle adjustments, which you can start implementing on your own right now. That being said, there are a number of factors that affect emotional well-being for those with PCOS, so making use of health care providers to support you can make a huge difference, especially if you experience depression or anxiety; low sex drive, inability to orgasm, or genital dryness; anorexia, bulimia, or disordered eating; or negative body image. You don't have to do this alone, especially if there are multiple factors at play in your lived experience addressing PCOS. Many clinics have their own mind/body medicine program, nutritionists, or counselors, and if not, they should have referrals available in your community.

PCOS is associated with other conditions that should receive follow-up from a physician for your overall health as well as your health during pregnancy. PCOS is a condition of insulin resistance, and half of all people with PCOS develop metabolic syndrome, which leads to cardiovascular disease as well as type 2 diabetes. Cardiovascular disease is an important concern, especially if you have clinical risk factors such as high cholesterol, hypertension (high blood pressure), large body size, or high blood sugar, or if you have life-style factors such as smoking or minimal exercise. During pregnancy and the days after birth, you might be more likely to experience preeclampsia, which is a life-threatening situation. If you have sleep issues such as snoring, fatigue, or waking unrefreshed after a full night of sleep, especially if these factors may be contributing to anxiety or depression, you may benefit from screening and a referral for obstructive sleep apnea. There is a high prevalence of anxiety, depression, and eating disorders in those with PCOS, which means that caring for your mental health is a vital aspect of your care plan. And while the overall risk is still low, those with PCOS are at increased risk for endometrial cancer, so be sure to reach out to your doctor if you start having cycles that are even longer than usual, excess spotting or bleeding during or between periods, or unexplained weight gain.

THE PCOS CARE PLAN

While there are medications and supplements that can be helpful for conceiving with PCOS, they will only be minimally effective without addressing insulin resistance through nutrition and exercise. Not only will these lifestyle adjustments make other treatments more effective, they are things you can start doing on your own right now, even before you are seen by a physician.

Nutrition

Nutrition is a vital aspect of any care plan for PCOS, and the good news is you can use the same guidelines as in Chapter 2. In the medical community, weight loss is a primary approach to treatment, as measured by BMI and waist circumference. If this approach is not helpful for you, then skip it and focus instead on the foods you are eating, portion sizes, and frequency of meals and snacks instead of pounds on a scale or body measurements. Keeping your blood sugar in check is essentially what matters.

During pregnancy, gestational diabetes is common for those with PCOS. Because of the risks presented by gestational diabetes during pregnancy, if you have PCOS, you may be offered a glucose tolerance test early in pregnancy before the routine screen that is offered at the end of the second trimester. This is all the more reason to work on your blood sugar before becoming pregnant. As with PCOS, the first-line approach to treatment for gestational diabetes is also nutrition and exercise, which means you are going to need to implement these changes sooner or later anyway. However, waiting until pregnancy and then dealing with a gestational diabetes diagnosis has implications for your care, including limiting your choices of care providers and place of birth, an increased likelihood of induction of labor, and a higher chance of cesarean delivery. The risks of gestational diabetes are very real, but if your blood sugar stays in the normal range, the risks can be mitigated. Essentially, you can avoid a problem-based approach to your entire pregnancy if you are able to get your blood sugar under control before becoming pregnant.

Whether or not you do this with support from a midwife, nutritionist, and/or a therapist, implement a plan of action geared toward moving your body and keeping your blood sugar stable and in range. Make goals that are SMART (specific, measurable, achievable, realistic, and timely) and ask for support from your loved ones in achieving them. If you decide to focus on losing weight, do this by limiting portion sizes and increasing physical activity instead of following nutritionally unbalanced diets or starving yourself. What you eat is still important, but do what you can and take it step by step. Often the changes we make to support our health build upon one another. Incremental shifts lead to new habits and long-term lifestyle choices, so make sure you aren't rushing it. Unless you are over forty, there is time (and if you are over forty, get help in all the ways, without delay). Ideally, the changes you make should not result in more than 10 percent weight loss over six months. (You can use an app that calculates weight loss over time based on caloric intake and exercise to help check yourself.)

Exercise

The guidelines for exercise include a combination of focused physical activity, as well as time spent walking, cycling, or other activities that are part of your daily life, such as commuting to work or physical exertion that is part of your job (including taking care of your home and caring for children). Perhaps the most important aspect of exercise is doing something you love. If you haven't been exercising at all, especially if you work at a desk or another sedentary occupation, start small and work your way up. It is better to exercise for ten minutes a day and add one to five minutes per week than to start at a level that is so extreme you injure yourself and can't workout anymore. The goal per week is 150 minutes of moderate exercise or 75 minutes of vigorous exercise, or an equivalent combination of both, including at least two nonconsecutive workouts that include weight-bearing or muscle-strengthening activities. If you have a larger-than-average body size, the benefits will be enhanced by reaching a weekly total of 250 minutes of moderate exercise or 150 minutes of vigorous exercise, with the same guidelines for two muscle-strengthening workouts per week.

Moderate-intensity activities include brisk walking, easy jogging, using an elliptical trainer, riding a bike with minimal hills, dancing, rollerblading or skating, gardening or heavy housework like vacuuming, leisurely swimming, water aerobics, softball, volleyball, or doubles tennis.

Vigorous-intensity activities include running; racewalking; hiking or biking uphill; lap swimming; step aerobics; spin classes; heavy gardening or shoveling snow; running sports like basketball, hockey, or soccer; singles tennis or other court sports such as racquetball or squash.

Muscle-building activities can be anything that utilizes your body weight or activates large muscle groups, such as circuit training, HIIT (high-intensity interval training), weight lifting, resistance bands, stair climbing, hill walking, push-ups, sit-ups, squats, martial arts, or yoga.

Supplements

Omega-3 improves the LH/FSH ratio (important for ovulation) and helps address lipid ratios (high cholesterol), which are so common in PCOS. When taken with vitamin D, it has been found to reduce elevated testosterone levels, improve depression, and reduce inflammatory markers. For therapeutic benefit, take 2,000 to 4,000 milligrams daily with meals (adjust dosage based on your body size and dietary intake of fish).

Vitamin D levels are often found to be low in those with PCOS, which makes supplementation that much more important. Some of the data on vitamin D and PCOS shows improved glucose and lipid metabolism, especially when combined with **calcium**, **magnesium**, and **zinc**. In IVF cycles, people with PCOS have been shown to increase rates of egg retrieval and fertilization by ensuring their vitamin D levels are ample—as many as one more fertilized egg per 3 ng/mL of vitamin D. Another study showed that people with PCOS and vitamin D deficiency were less likely to ovulate, more likely to experience pregnancy loss, and had a 40 percent lower chance of live birth.

Inositol is a plant-based antioxidant supplement that increases insulin sensitivity. It is often used as an alternative or adjunct treatment to metformin (see medical treatments on page 194). It is better tolerated than metformin with fewer gastrointestinal side effects. Although it is safe and effective, the use of inositol is currently considered experimental. There is evidence showing lower testosterone levels and improved insulin sensitivity. Inositol has also been shown to improve mental health parameters so common in those with PCOS, and it can be used during pregnancy to prevent gestational diabetes. The myoinositol form is specific to ovarian tissues, while the D-chiro-inositol form is active on non-ovarian tissues. Studies are still being done, but if you choose to add this supplement, go for myoinositol or a combination of the two that is higher in myoinositol (one study suggests a forty-to-one ratio). The dosage indicated by the available evidence is 1,000 to 4,000 milligrams daily.

Coenzyme Q10 is an antioxidant supplement that supports the mitochondria (energy-producing organelles) in cells. CoQ10 lowers testosterone and LH levels and increases insulin sensitivity in those with PCOS. When given with **vitamin E**, it has an even more pronounced effect on the production of sex hormone binding globulin (SBGH), which is part of how insulin resistance occurs in PCOS. In a 2014 study, 180 milligrams daily of CoQ10 combined with clomiphene citrate increased the ovulation rate so significantly (65.9 percent versus 15.5 percent) and with such a higher pregnancy rate (37.3 percent versus 6.0 percent) that the author of the study recommended it as an effective and safe option before considering gonadotropins or laparoscopic ovarian drilling. Look for the active ubiquinol form for best absorption.

Cinnamon and black cohosh have been shown to be beneficial in treating PCOS without any negative side effects. Cinnamon helps with lipid profiles and insulin sensitivity, especially alongside lifestyle interventions. Black cohosh improved hormonal markers better than Clomid in one small study, with fewer side effects, at a dose of 40 milligrams daily for ten days during the follicular phase.

Complementary Treatments for PCOS

Acupuncture can be helpful for regulating menstrual cycles, reducing testosterone, and improving symptoms of depression in PCOS. Treatments must be done weekly for three months or more in order to be fully effective.

Mental health care is just as important as care for your physical health, especially when you are having a baby. People with PCOS are up to four times more likely to experience depression and five and a half times more likely to experience anxiety than the general population. Eating disorders range from 12 to 36 percent, depending on the study. During pregnancy, depressive symptoms are 25 percent more likely, and during the weeks and months after birth, postpartum depression is 50 percent more likely. This means that taking care of your mental health is important for the entirety of your transition to parenthood. Nutrition, exercise, and quality sleep are imperative for supporting your mental health at every stage of the process. There are medications for mood regulation that are well studied and safe for use during pregnancy and lactation, so there is no need to go without pharmacological support during this time. It's important to have a prescribing provider who is well versed in perinatal mental health, just as it is important to have a talk therapist who fully understands all of the phases of the transition to parenthood.

Medical Treatments for PCOS

Metformin is a medication that increases insulin sensitivity, which can cause the ovaries to start ovulating more regularly again. However, since nutrition and exercise also increase insulin sensitivity, it is considered a secondary treatment if lifestyle adjustments do not bring your glucose levels into range. Some people have digestive side effects on metformin, and while it can be used safely long term and through pregnancy, it is associated with low vitamin B_{12}, so be sure to have this checked. The use of metformin is considered off-label in the United States (meaning that the FDA has not approved its use for this specific indication); however, it is commonly used in fertility medicine.

Letrozole (Femara) is also used off-label in fertility medicine in the United States; however, it is the recommended first-line pharmacological treatment for ovulation induction in those with PCOS who are not ovulating on their own. Letrozole is a pill that is taken for five days early in the cycle, stimulating the ovaries to develop more robust follicles with enhanced function such as timely ovulation and ample progesterone production. Letrozole improves rates of ovulation, pregnancy, and live birth; however, it also comes with an increased likelihood of twins (around 10 percent).

Clomiphene citrate (Clomid) is also a pill taken for five days early in the cycle for ovulation induction; however, the way it works presents potential drawbacks such as decreased fertile fluid and thinner uterine lining. Clomiphene citrate also presents a 10 percent chance of twins.

Gonadotropins are used if the oral medications above have not been successful in inducing ovulation. These medications are given by injection, and they are more expensive than the oral meds. The risk of conceiving twins is 25 percent and triplets is 5 percent when gonadotropins are used for ovulation induction. Careful ultrasound monitoring must be done to assess for ovarian hyperstimulation as well as monitoring follicular growth, which also increases the cost of using these medications.

Laparoscopic ovarian drilling involves creating small holes on the surface of the ovaries, which reduces testosterone production, increases ovulatory function, and makes the ovaries more sensitive to stimulation medications. This procedure has similar success rates to gonadotropins without the increased risk of twins. While 80 percent of recipients will begin ovulating again, there are risks including scarring and damage to the ovaries that could inhibit their function.

ENDOMETRIOSIS

Endometriosis is a condition of inflammation and oxidative stress that occurs when cells that normally make up the interior lining of the uterus grow outside the uterus, invading the tissues they are attached to. This can happen anywhere within the abdomen, but most commonly, it happens on the ovaries, in the areas just behind or in front of the uterus, on the ligaments that hold the uterus in place, on the outside of the uterus itself, on and within the fallopian tubes, or on the colon, bladder, or appendix. Endometriosis lesions can more rarely be found almost anywhere in the trunk of the body, including on the major organs and on the lungs.

Pelvic pain is the most prominent feature of living with endometriosis. Because endometrial cells proliferate in response to estrogen, the pain often increases during your period. The pain can be incapacitating, affecting overall quality of life throughout the reproductive years, and sometimes extending into menopause.

Endometriosis doesn't always cause infertility, but it can when the endometriosis cells block the fallopian tubes or they grow on the ovaries, limiting their function. When it grows on the peritoneum, the inflammation causes chemical changes that affect the function of the reproductive system, including the health of the eggs. Endometriosis can also affect the uterine lining in such a way that implantation cannot occur.

Endometriosis can have effects on pregnancy, including increased likelihood of miscarriage, ectopic pregnancy, placenta previa, bleeding during pregnancy, preeclampsia, preterm birth, postpartum hemorrhage, and cesarean delivery. It's also possible for endometriosis on the abdominal organs to become exacerbated during pregnancy, so be sure to contact your prenatal care provider immediately if you have abdominal pain or bleeding during pregnancy.

Risk factors for endometriosis include alcohol use and smoking, as well as having a smaller-than-average body size. Other associated factors include early onset of menses (before age eleven to thirteen), shorter menstrual cycles (fewer than twenty-seven days), heavy periods, anatomic differences of the reproductive system that inhibit the outward flow of menstrual blood, exposure to severe physical or sexual abuse during childhood or adolescence, and a high consumption of trans unsaturated fats. Your risk of endometriosis is double if you were fed soy formula during infancy.

DIAGNOSIS

Diagnosis of endometriosis can be based on symptoms or laparoscopic evaluation. Laparoscopy allows lesions to be visualized clearly; however, if there is no pelvic pain, then laparoscopy is not typically recommended because, without pain, endometriosis is likely minimal to mild, and outcomes are the same whether those lesions are removed or left alone. On the other hand, if there is pain, then it is more likely that the endometriosis is moderate to severe, which increases the chances that it is affecting your ability to conceive. Laparoscopy allows for simultaneous identification and surgical removal, because the endometrial lesions can be both identified and excised or cauterized during laparoscopy.

Pain is an important indicator of where endometrial lesions are occurring. While the pain is often chronic, it typically worsens during the menstrual period. This happens because endometrial cells are affected by rising levels of estrogen that occur in the first half of each cycle, no matter where they are located in the body.

Pelvic pain: If endometriosis occurs within the pelvic cavity, there is usually pelvic pain that worsens during or after sex.

Bladder pain or UTI symptoms: With endometriosis on the bladder, there may be symptoms similar to a UTI such as urinary frequency or urgency, or pain with urination, often worsening during menses.

Bowel pain or digestive symptoms: If endometriosis is on the bowel, it can cause digestive problems such as constipation, diarrhea, cramping, or pain and/or straining with bowel movements.

Abdominal pain: If there is endometriosis on the abdominal wall, there can be a palpable mass as well as pain that is either chronic or happens during menses.

Chest, neck, or shoulder pain: Endometriosis that is in the chest cavity can cause chest pain, shortness of breath, coughing up blood, and/or neck or shoulder pain, all typically occurring during menses.

ACCESSING CARE FOR ENDOMETRIOSIS

If you have had difficulty conceiving and you experience chronic or cyclic pain as described previously, a fertility specialist can help with laparoscopic evaluation and surgery, followed by medications to help you get pregnant quickly before the growth returns. However, this approach does not treat the underlying cause of endometriosis, so while it may help you conceive, it does nothing to address the ongoing implications of endometriosis during pregnancy and into the future. This is why the endometriosis care plan presented in this chapter is focused on a nutritional approach, which is not only evidence based but can also support you over the long term.

For the sake of your overall health, it is important to follow up with your primary care physician if you think you may have symptoms of endometriosis occurring outside the reproductive system. Additionally, while the overall risk is low, there is a slightly increased risk of ovarian cancer with endometriosis on the ovaries, so be sure to have your pelvic exams and Pap tests on time, and don't skip the internal exam that allows the provider to palpate the ovaries for masses.

THE ENDOMETRIOSIS CARE PLAN

Endometriosis is a condition of inflammation and oxidative stress, so it is imperative to follow the recommendations in Chapter 2, specifically the guidelines for nutrition, supplements, and avoiding endocrine disruptors. Remember that the goal is not just to get pregnant, it is also to carry a healthy pregnancy to full term with good outcomes and long-term health and well-being. The following section highlights evidence-based nutritional guidance specific to endometriosis, as well as supplements and herbs, and options for medical support.

Nutrition

Anti-inflammatory proteins: Eliminate beef, lamb, and pork. Instead, get your protein from fish, poultry, eggs, nuts, dairy, soy, legumes, lentils, and whole grains. Make sure that your dairy is full fat and hormone free, and limit intake to one serving daily. If you are vegan, make sure most of your protein comes from legumes, lentils, whole grains, nuts, and seeds, with no more than one serving of soy daily.

Healthy fats: Eliminate trans fats. Focus on healthy fats, going for a high ratio of omega-3 to omega-6 fatty acids. One study showed that for every 1 percent of nutritional intake from omega-3 versus omega-6, the risk of endometriosis decreased by 50 percent! Use lots of olive oil and limit your intake of butter, but complete elimination of butter is not necessary.

Fruits and vegetables: Maintain a high intake of these antioxidant powerhouse foods, including choices from a range of colors. Vitamins A, C, E, and folic acid, along with the mineral zinc, work together to reduce inflammation, and taking a supplement has not been shown to be as useful as getting these nutrients through foods. Intake of these nutrients has been shown to reduce pelvic pain as well as markers of inflammation and oxidative stress in those with endometriosis. Organics are important in order to avoid endocrine disruptors such as PCBs and pesticides, as well as avoiding cooking and storing foods in plastic.

Whole grains: Unprocessed whole grains contain fiber and B vitamins, namely B_6, which are important for hormone regulation. Some people with endometriosis experience a decrease in pelvic pain after going gluten free, so if you suspect you might be sensitive to wheat and other glutenous grains, it is worthwhile to eliminate them altogether and see if your symptoms improve. Gluten-free grains include: quinoa, brown rice, wild rice, buckwheat, sorghum, tapioca, millet, amaranth, teff, and oats.

Low-FODMAP diet for bowel endometriosis: If you have endometriosis on your bowels, whether that diagnosis is based on laparoscopy or symptoms, reducing inflammation is an important part of your overall health during the entirety of your reproductive years, and especially during pregnancy. You can greatly reduce pain and IBS symptoms before you conceive by following a low-FODMAP diet for a few weeks and then reintroducing foods slowly in order to identify foods that exacerbate your symptoms.

The low-FODMAP diet consists of three stages. The elimination stage should be followed for three to eight weeks, but not longer than that because of the long-term need for a balanced diet. Consult a nutritionist or naturopath, or look for lists of high- and low-FODMAP foods online or use an app.

Stage 1: Eliminate all foods high in "fermentable oligo-, di-, monosaccharides, and polyols," including wheat, garlic, onion, some fruits and vegetables, legumes and pulses, some sweeteners, and some forms of dairy. You can eat gluten-free grains (except amaranth), low-FODMAP fruits and vegetables, tofu, eggs, nuts, seeds, some sweeteners, and some forms of dairy.

Stage 2: Reintroduce high-FODMAP foods systematically to see how your body reacts. While maintaining a low-FODMAP diet, test each new food, one at a time, for one to three days. You can also track the amount of that food you eat to see if small versus large amounts are OK for you.

Stage 3: Maintain your health by following a modified low-FODMAP diet that includes the foods you have tested to make sure they are not a problem for you. It is important to follow this throughout conception and pregnancy in order to avoid the issues returning.

Supplements

Vitamin D: As with many fertility issues, low vitamin D is associated with endometriosis. Vitamin D helps regulate the immune system, decreasing the inflammatory process that happens in endometriosis.

Omega-3: Taking an omega-3 supplement helps reach the ideal balance of essential fatty acids, which some sources claim is most therapeutic at a two-to-one or even a four-to-one ratio of omega-3 to omega-6, which is only possible with supplementation. Take 2,000 to 4,000 milligrams daily with meals (adjust dosage based on your body size and dietary intake of fish).

Probiotics: Beneficial bacteria are present throughout the reproductive tract, and studies have found a reduction in pain associated with endometriosis when there is a proper balance of microflora.

Magnesium: Magnesium helps relaxation of smooth muscles and may influence the appropriate flow of menstrual blood out of the body through the cervix, rather than the retrograde flow that carries it through the fallopian tubes and into the pelvic cavity in endometriosis. Adjust your dose of magnesium to bowel tolerance (diarrhea will occur above your maximum dose) starting with 100 milligrams daily.

N-acetyl cysteine (NAC): NAC is a potent antioxidant that helps the body rid itself of reactive oxygen species (oxidative stress), which limits the proliferation and growth of displaced endometrial cells. Various studies have been done to demonstrate this effect, along with reducing pain and the need for NSAID medications, without any negative side effects. One study showed decreased growth and proliferation of endometriosis cells when subjects took 600 milligrams three times a day for three consecutive days, followed by a rest period of four days, over a period of three months. The rest period allows for levels of NAC to stabilize in the plasma rather than being excreted. Another study used NAC along with the antioxidants alpha-lipoic acid and bromelain.

Resveratrol: An anti-inflammatory substance found in the skin of red grapes, berries, and peanuts, resveratrol limits oxidative stress and insulin-like growth factor, which contributes to the growth and proliferation of endometriosis. Research shows the greatest benefit without any negative side effects with supplementation of 2.5 grams daily, although some people have some digestive upset, so split or adjust your dose as needed.

Curcumin: The active component of turmeric root, curcumin contains potent antioxidant and anti-inflammatory properties. It is widely used in Ayurvedic and Chinese medicine for treating endometriosis as well as a variety of other inflammatory conditions and cancer. Daily doses up to 2,000 milligrams have been shown to be safe and without side effects.

Milk thistle: This herb's active component silibinin is a bioactive flavolingan that has been used to treat liver conditions, inflammation, diabetes, and cancer, even enhancing the effects of chemotherapy treatments. It is currently being studied in the treatment of endometriosis and is being found effective in limiting a number of cellular processes in the disease. In addition to its anti-inflammatory properties, it helps the liver excrete excess estrogen, which is an important aspect of limiting the growth and proliferation of endometriosis tissue.

Medical Treatments for Endometriosis

Most of the conventional treatments for endometriosis involve inhibiting the menstrual cycle, which is not compatible with fertility. The only conventional treatments available for endometriosis while trying to conceive are medications to limit pain and inflammation, such as NSAIDs (ibuprofen, acetaminophen, etc.). Because endometriosis can vary in terms of severity and location, the treatment plan will be different from person to person. In the absence of pelvic pain, even in cases of suspected minimal to mild endometriosis, the treatment is the same as in cases of unexplained fertility: stimulate the ovaries and do intrauterine insemination, and/or proceed to IVF. If endometriosis lesions are surgically removed, ovarian stimulation and IUI or IVF is recommended expeditiously before the lesions have a chance to grow back.

UTERINE FIBROIDS

Uterine fibroids, or leiomyoma, are benign tumors of the uterus that may or may not affect fertility. Lots of people have them (35 to 77 percent of all people with a uterus), although they are much more common in Black people than white or Asian people. Because they occur over time, they are more likely in those who are over age thirty-five. If you have a first-degree relative (parent or sibling) with fibroids, you are two and a half times more likely to have them yourself. Most of the time fibroids do not interfere with fertility; however, when they do, it is because they are blocking the passage of sperm through the cervix, uterus, or fallopian tubes, or they are affecting uterine blood flow and/or the receptivity of the uterine lining, which impedes implantation and/or embryonic development. Overall, only 5 to 10 percent of people evaluated for infertility have fibroids.

Fibroids can interfere with pregnancy if they are large to begin with (over 3 centimeters), or if they grow during the time you are pregnant. On the other hand, even those with fibroids over 10 centimeters can have a normal physiological birth 70 percent of the time. A quickly growing fibroid can cause pain during pregnancy, so be sure to contact your care provider for assessment if you have new-onset or increased pain. A primary concern is miscarriage, although preterm labor is also more common, especially if a fibroid is large, there are multiple fibroids, or the placenta attaches next to or on top of a fibroid. A fibroid can also affect the baby's ability to assume a head-down position for birth and/or affect the baby's ability to descend into the pelvis, both of which are indications for cesarean birth. On the other hand, when a fibroid is significant enough in size that it must be removed via abdominal surgery, the risk of uterine rupture during pregnancy or birth is higher, so cesarean birth may be recommended (although you can often find a provider who is comfortable with VBAC and other prior uterine surgeries if this is your preference). There are also concerns for postpartum hemorrhage if the presence of a fibroid interferes with the delivery of the placenta or uterine involution after birth. Fibroids that grow during pregnancy usually get smaller in size (about 50 percent reduction) within six months after birth.

DIAGNOSIS

There are three types of fibroids, categorized according to their location.

Intramural fibroids grow within the muscular fibers of the uterine wall. This is the most common type of fibroid, and it can cause heavy menstrual flow, urinary frequency, and low back or pelvic pain, as well as an increased rate of miscarriage.

Submucosal fibroids grow within the uterine lining and may protrude into the uterine cavity, and they are sometimes pedunculated (growing on a stalk).

This is the least common type. This type of fibroid can also cause heavy menstrual bleeding, and it is most closely associated with infertility and pregnancy loss.

Subserosal fibroids grow on the outside of the uterus and can also be pedunculated. This type of fibroid doesn't cause heavy periods, but it can cause pelvic pressure, and if it gets twisted or starts breaking down, it can cause pelvic pain.

Symptoms associated with fibroids depend on where they are located. Very long, heavy periods can be indicative of fibroids in the uterine cavity or in the uterine muscle. A fibroid that presses on the bladder can cause urinary incontinence or frequent urination. A fibroid that presses on the colon can cause rectal pressure or constipation. Other symptoms include pelvic pain or pressure, leg or back pain, or pain with penetrative sex. Sometimes fibroids can grow pretty significantly, so if you are experiencing increased weight gain in the lower abdomen, especially with any of these symptoms, be sure to get it checked out. Fibroids can sometimes be palpated by an internal pelvic exam during routine gynecological care. Fibroids can be diagnosed by ultrasound, MRI, saline infusion sonogram (SIS), or hysteroscopy.

ACCESSING CARE FOR FIBROIDS

If you have had difficulty conceiving, recurrent miscarriage, or you experience any of the aforementioned symptoms, a fertility specialist can help with evaluation and treatment for fibroids. It's important to see a provider who is experienced in fertility-preserving surgical options for uterine fibroids, because some treatments (for example, uterine artery embolization) are not recommended when there is a desire for future fertility, and the recommended care plan will be informed by the expertise of the surgeon.

Surgery is not the end of the story, however. Not only can fibroids grow back, they are associated with other health concerns such as insulin resistance, PCOS, and diabetes, as well as hypertension and metabolic syndrome. Like so many causes of infertility, fibroids may signal the alarm to pay closer attention to your health.

THE FIBROID CARE PLAN

Fibroids are associated with insulin resistance, which means the guidelines on nutrition and exercise in the previous PCOS section also apply to those with fibroids. They are also associated with inflammation and oxidative stress, which means the guidelines on nutrition in the endometriosis section apply as well. Review these sections, as well as Chapter 2, to gain a thorough understanding of how to manage blood sugar, inflammation, and oxidative stress through nutrition and exercise.

Specifically, those with a history of fibroids should avoid red meat, trans fats, milk, soy products, and alcohol. Vitamins A, B3, C, D, E, and K are known to be beneficial for those with fibroids, so eat lots of fruits and vegetables from a range of colors, as well as nuts, whole grains, and legumes. For fertility, it's ideal to eat vegetarian whole foods and limit soy. It's especially important to eat cruciferous vegetables such as broccoli, brussels sprouts, cabbage, cauliflower, collard greens, and kale for their tumor-limiting effects. Focus on lower glycemic foods and avoid sugar. Eat more berries, which are low-glycemic antioxidant power foods that have anti-fibroid properties. Quit coffee and switch to green tea. Get regular exercise—ideally an hour each day.

Take special care to avoid PCBs in fish, which you can do in a number of ways. One is to limit your intake of fish to those with known low PCB content (see Chapter 2). In general, go for wild Pacific salmon instead of farmed Atlantic salmon. Limit intake of canned Pacific salmon to twice a week, fresh or frozen wild Pacific salmon up to twice a month, and fresh or frozen farmed Atlantic salmon once every two months. Take special care to find out the PCB level in local areas that provide you with fresh-caught fish, especially large bottom-feeders such as striped bass, bluefish, American eel, and sea trout, and predator species such as bass, lake trout, and walleye. When you cook fish, remove the skin, fat, and dark meat portions of the fish before cooking, and prepare it in ways that allow the fat to drip off, such as grilling, baking, or broiling. Do not fry fish, as this seals in the fat, which also seals in PCBs.

Supplements

Omega-3: Get your supplemental omega-3 from fish oil rather than flax oil, and always choose an omega-3 supplement that is well regulated and guarantees no PCBs.

Vitamin D: The lower your vitamin D, the more likely you are to develop fibroids. It is thought that the relationship between vitamin D and fibroids may explain the increased incidence of fibroids in those of African descent, given that serum vitamin D levels are low in 80 percent of this population. Keep your levels up with ample supplementation. In those who have had fibroids removed, maintaining adequate vitamin D levels (above 38.6 ng/mL) can prevent a recurrence. The ideal target is about 50 ng/mL. Vitamin D can be safely administered up to 50,000 IU per week in those with uterine fibroids.

Green tea extract: Green tea, and its active polyphenol component EGCG (epigallocatechin gallate), has been shown to significantly reduce the volume of uterine fibroids as well as associated symptoms including anemia when taken over a four-month period, with no adverse effects. Take 800 milligrams with 45 percent EGCG.

Curcumin: Curcumin is a potent anti-inflammatory that is used to treat tumorous growths. In a study on cancerous ovarian tumors, it was shown to be effective in suppressing tumor growth when taken with EGCG, which helped with the absorption of curcumin. It has been shown in various studies to limit the growth of benign uterine fibroids, although absorption is a concern, so either take it with EGCG or choose a highly absorbable form.

Medical Treatments for Fibroids

Sometimes hormonal medications can be used for a few months to shrink a fibroid in preparation for surgery, or to stop menstrual periods temporarily in order to allow treatment for anemia from heavy menstrual flow. While there are many medications being investigated for the long-term treatment of uterine fibroids, to date, there is no medication that both reduces the size of fibroids while also reducing heavy uterine bleeding without undesirable side effects. Most medications currently in use only provide a temporary reduction of symptoms.

If you have intramural or submucosal fibroids and you have had difficulty getting pregnant, surgical removal (myomectomy) is usually recommended to increase fertility and reduce complications during pregnancy and birth. If you are planning to do IVF and you have submucosal fibroids or intramural fibroids greater than 5 centimeters in size, myomectomy can double your chances of pregnancy and live birth. Minimally invasive techniques such as laparoscopy or hysteroscopy are the methods of choice; however, some fibroids are large enough to require abdominal surgery (laparotomy).

The benefits of myomectomy are not permanent. Fibroids can grow back again 15 to 51 percent of the time, so it's important to conceive expeditiously following recovery. Myomectomy comes with the same risks as any surgery, and it's possible for postsurgical adhesions to occur, which may impact future fertility.

POLYPS

Polyps are small growths that occur in the uterus and sometimes in or near the cervix. They are made of endometrial cells, which means they grow in response to estrogen and bleed during menses. Polyps may also bleed outside the normal menstrual period, so if you have very long or heavy periods, this is something to rule out. Polyps are typically identified by saline infusion sonogram or hysteroscopy. It is beneficial to remove polyps because their presence can disrupt endometrial receptivity, inhibiting implantation. They are especially disruptive if they are growing at the junction of the uterus and the fallopian tube. In one study, those who opted for polypectomy, regardless of size and location, were four times more likely to conceive than those who did not. As opposed to fibroids, which are completely benign, polyps can sometimes lead to cancerous growths, which is another reason to have them removed once identified.

AUTOIMMUNE CONDITIONS

There are a variety of autoimmune conditions that are associated with infertility and pregnancy loss. If you are having difficulty conceiving, and you experience symptoms such as fatigue, joint pain, skin problems, digestive issues, fevers, or swollen glands, be sure to check in with your doctor, and keep checking in until you get to the bottom of it. Many autoimmune conditions have similar symptoms, so you may need to see a rheumatologist or other specialists for an accurate diagnosis. Some of the more common autoimmune conditions that can be ruled out with simple blood work include:

- **Antiphospholipid syndrome**: a clotting disorder that causes repeat miscarriage

- **Autoimmune thyroiditis**: a thyroid problem that can cause miscarriage

- **Celiac disease**: a condition of gluten intolerance that can cause irregular cycles, miscarriage, and infertility

GUIDANCE FOR CARE PROVIDERS

Many people seek care after they have been trying on their own without success. Whether this is the case, or you are providing care from the very beginning of the conception process, it is important not to overlook the basics. The checklist at the beginning of this chapter can be used to guide the focus of any sort of investigation into why someone is not conceiving.

If you are supporting someone with a known issue such as PCOS, endometriosis, or fibroids, be sure to address the influence of nutrition and exercise. No supplement or complementary treatment can overcome the hour-to-hour, day-to-day effects of a constant state of inflammation and oxidative stress. Take the time to discuss the barriers people have to implementing these aspects of self-care, help with problem-solving, and provide perspective as parents-to-be reorganize their priorities during this time of transition. Be sure to remind folks that the changes they plan to make once they are pregnant may actually need to be made in order to become pregnant in the first place. Taking the time to prepare healthy food or to exercise, or even to chart fertile signs, can seem insurmountable until you compare the time spent doing these things with the amount of time it will take to care for a newborn. Ultimately, the personal growth that takes place during preconception and pregnancy helps us be better parents, if only to support us in filling our own cup, or putting our own mask on first, so that we can better care for our children.

Resources

Mindfulness-based food tracker: YouAte.com

Low-FODMAP diet guidelines and app: MonashFODMAP.com

IN VITRO FERTILIZATION AND EMBRYO TRANSFER

For many queer and trans parents-to-be, in vitro fertilization (IVF) represents hope, promise, and the possibility of becoming a parent through both love and high-tech reproductive science. Whether making use of gametes stored prior to gender transition, carrying a pregnancy with a partner's egg, or having a baby through surrogacy or embryo adoption, for our families, IVF can feel exciting, empowering, and celebratory.

On the other hand, many people in our community have complex emotional landscapes to navigate when the hope was to get pregnant without fertility medicine. The one thing we may have in common with straight people experiencing infertility or pregnancy loss are feelings of grief, hopelessness, or even desperation. However, that's where the commonalities end. Most of us never anticipated becoming pregnant without some sort of outside help. We bond with our communities over shared experiences of donor conception, creating a sense of pride and affirmation of queer capability, embodiment, and resiliency. But when insemination does not result in a pregnancy, or the process is complicated and prolonged by pregnancy loss, that sense of camaraderie is often forgone. Our friends and loved ones no longer understand what we are going through, and when we share our experiences, it's as if we are speaking a foreign language. This can bring about feelings of loss and even estrangement from others in the queer community who have no understanding of the complexities of seeking pregnancy through IVF.

However, one of the most overlooked aspects of successful parenting is the way we avail ourselves of resources when needed. Our human nature is to take note of shortcomings quite easily, while we are less likely to cultivate feelings of success and self-affirmation when we access the resources we need. If you are looking to harness the best of what modern medicine has to offer in pursuit of parenthood, good on you—this is a success! Keep reminding yourself of that. Utilizing reproductive science is about your ability to access support when you need it. Decode and let go of internalized messages about failure, and embrace your choices fully, regardless of the circumstances that brought you there.

Navigating Cis/Heteronormative Clinic Environments

That being said, navigating care at a fertility clinic that is designed by, for, and about cisgender, heterosexual people can feel deeply dysphoric, no matter if you are there by choice or by default. Holding space for the validity of our families and maintaining a celebratory spirit in our pursuit of parenthood is additional emotional work we must do every time we interact with forms, receptionists, and care providers who use words to describe our bodies and our relationships in ways that do not reflect our lived experience. Honor all the ways you choose to cope with this on any given day, whether you correct the person speaking to you aloud or silently in your own mind, and whether you ask the clinic to change their forms to better represent your family or you opt to keep your head down and ignore it. Just showing up for yourself, as yourself, is all you need to do, and as with all the ways queer and trans people show up in the world, our mere presence invites people to reconsider their cis/heterocentric perspective—what they choose to do with that is on them.

Centering Embodied Experience While Honoring Emotional Labor

You may be reading this chapter as an intended parent or as a surrogate; as a parent-to-be going through egg retrieval and/or embryo transfer; or as a partner, coparent, or loved one of someone going through IVF. No matter where you sit within the constellation of people involved in bringing this baby into the world, you will want to know what to expect and how to support one another. While this chapter provides information that is useful from any perspective, the language centers those who are going through IVF with their bodies, which is intentional. While everyone is navigating the process emotionally, embodying this experience means a great deal of physical and psychological vulnerability, and centering the most vulnerable is one of the ways we show up for one another in community. The role of nongestational parents is to hold space for ourselves and our own emotions while centering the experience of the person who is gestating and carrying the child through pregnancy. This parallels the experience of a pregnant person, who must simultaneously care for their own needs while considering the effect on the pregnancy with every decision made, big and small, every hour of every day. Becoming a parent means caring for another while caring for the self. Whether gestation occurs in your own body or not, this is how pregnancy grows us and ultimately prepares us for a lifetime of this practice, commonly known as parenthood.

Whether you step into a fertility clinic in full awareness of the complex emotions underlying the experience, or your coping mechanisms allow you to put those feelings aside in order to get what you need, either approach takes a lot of work. The simultaneous emotional labor we do while navigating our health care can make it difficult to process clinical information and to participate fully in the care we receive. The goal of this chapter is to provide you with a framework for understanding the process of IVF so you already have some of the basics down. From there, you can focus on relationship building with your doctor, asking questions, and taking in what they have to share with you about how their practice works and what protocols they recommend for you.

Decoding the Acronyms of ART

Broadly defined, assisted reproductive technology (ART) is any type of assisted reproduction, including insemination with or without the use of medications. However, it is more commonly associated with IVF. In IVF, medications are used to stimulate the development of as many egg follicles as possible, and then the eggs are taken out of the body and combined with sperm cells in a lab. The resulting embryos are incubated for a few days, and then they are either frozen or transferred to the uterus for pregnancy. The language of ART separates these two distinct aspects of the process:

In vitro fertilization (IVF) refers to the stimulation, retrieval, and fertilization of eggs.

Embryo transfer or frozen embryo transfer (FET) refers to the transfer of embryos into the uterus.

IVF and embryo transfer sometimes take place all in one cycle; however, it is increasingly common to do cycles of stimulation and retrieval until the desired number of healthy embryos are collected, freezing them after each retrieval, and then proceeding to FET in a later cycle.

Indications for ART

- Couples who have the anatomy for one partner to carry a pregnancy created with their partner's egg

- Parents-to-be via gestational surrogacy

- Families using a donor egg or donor embryo to conceive

- Those with a sperm count that is too low to conceive via insemination

- Parents-to-be with diminished ovarian reserve who have been unsuccessful with IUI or who are using a donor egg

- Those with blocked fallopian tubes, making it impossible for inseminated sperm to reach the egg

- People who want to prevent passing on known genetic disorders to their offspring by using donor eggs or testing their own embryos prior to transfer

- Those who saved eggs when they were younger and are now ready to carry a pregnancy themselves or have a partner carry a pregnancy with their eggs

- Families for whom insemination or intercourse has been unsuccessful

EXCITING NEW TECHNIQUES IN FERTILITY MEDICINE FOR QUEER AND TRANS PARENTS-TO-BE

- An embryo created via IVF can be harbored in a vaginal incubator called INVOCELL prior to being transferred to the uterus that will carry it to term. This means that a partner with a vagina has the opportunity to "carry" the pregnancy for a few days prior to implantation. At the time of this writing, it is unclear whether or not trans women can use INVOCELL—but here's hoping!

- For transmasculine people going off testosterone to retrieve eggs and/or conceive via ART, some clinics will monitor your testosterone level and start the stimulation protocol when your testosterone reaches the appropriate range, before you have a menstrual bleed, which avoids the dysphoric experience of having a period.

Understanding ART Success Rates

A good place to start gathering information about your chances for success is the Society for Assisted Reproductive Technology (SART), a US-based nonprofit professional organization that establishes and maintains standards for ART. They collect data on outcomes and set guidelines for best practice based on the evidence. The SART website has a patient predictor tool that allows you to put in some basic data and calculates your chance of live birth. You can also look up fertility clinics in your area to view and compare their success rates. One thing to keep in mind as you look at the success rates for each clinic is that there are aspects of success that may not be reflected in the raw numbers. For instance, some providers may be more willing than others to tailor treatment plans to your individual desires for or against certain treatments, taking into account your experience going through the process. If there is a provider in your community who has been highly recommended to you based on the patient experience but their success rates are slightly lower than other clinics, take some time to meet each of the providers and decide for yourself. Your experience matters, and you may personally find that you have indicators for what you feel is "success," such as the bedside manner of the physician and the ability to be involved in decision-making about your care, that are not reflected in the published stats.

Funding for ART

For the vast majority of us, the economic disparity we experience as queer and trans people may put ART out of reach, or only accomplishable at the expense of our long-term financial security, which only deepens the sense of vulnerability we carry with us as we navigate this process. The baseline cost for a single cycle of IVF in the United States is $10,000 to $15,000, with the average cost around $12,000. Costs vary based on the treatment protocol that is recommended for you. Medications can run an additional $1,500 to $3,000; ICSI (intracytoplasmic sperm injection, a method of inserting an individual sperm cell into each egg, rather than putting the cells in a petri dish and letting them combine on their own) can add $1,000 to $2,500; genetic testing of embryos is an additional $1,800 to $3,000 plus; and frozen embryo transfer adds $3,000 to $5,000. This adds up to a total range of about $10,000 using oral medications only, without additional testing or treatments, up to $30,000 for "the works." You may need to do more than one cycle in order to reach your ultimate goal of a live birth. This is why recommendations for ART treatment are always weighed against your likelihood of conceiving in other ways, and this probability is measured against cost. If you are more likely to end up with a baby in your arms after one IVF cycle than you are after a year's worth of IUI cycles, then IVF may be less expensive overall.

Choices in reproductive health care are all too often determined by privilege, and ART is no different in that regard. Systemic racism and the legacy of white privilege offers white people, on the whole, more connections to financial resources than families of color. Gender-based income inequality means that more cis men will be able to access IVF than cis women or trans people. The economic disparities experienced by trans people through employment discrimination, combined with lack of financial and emotional support from families of origin, as well as intersectional forms of oppression, make access to IVF exponentially difficult.

However, there is hope. Access to care is a hot topic in fertility medicine, and some US states and Canadian provinces have begun to mandate health care coverage for ART. At the time of this writing, more than one-third of US states require insurance companies to cover some level of assisted reproductive services, whether limited to fertility testing, partial coverage, or a limited number of cycles. However, only a few states cover ART benefits without a requisite number of unsuccessful attempts at unassisted conception, which is, of course, a cis/heterocentric model that completely overlooks the reality that many of us can have endless sex with our partners without any possibility of a pregnancy. There are a number of organizations that are doing legal advocacy and/or generating and distributing funds to queer and trans families pursuing IVF:

- RESOLVE is a nonprofit organization for families who experience infertility, and it is actively pursuing legislation to secure options for family building for LGBTQ+ people. Their website has a tool kit for requesting that your employer add infertility coverage to their employee health care plan. They also have a list of grants for funding ART, as well as a list of financial aid programs.

- Family Equality has a list of LGBTQ+ family-building grants.

- FertilityIQ also has an excellent rundown of IVF grants and charities.

- The organization Men Having Babies has created a Gay Parenting Assistance Program to offset the costs associated with surrogacy, including a list of discounted and free medical and legal services as well as cash grants funded through the organization.

- Some fertility clinics have funding resources. When selecting a fertility clinic, ask about cash pay discounts and grant programs. Compare pricing at different clinics in your area. You may be surprised to find a range of pricing strategies; however, be sure to find out what is included in the costs you are quoted, and take the time to add up costs for monitoring, storage, and procedures as well as medications.

- Other approaches include taking out a loan, using credit cards, creating an online funding request such as GoFundMe, asking friends and family members for help, getting a job with fertility benefits, or moving to a state that guarantees insurance benefits.

The Initial Assessment

The first step is to see a fertility doctor who will do ovarian reserve testing (see Chapter 3) in order to make recommendations for you and determine how your body is likely to respond to fertility medications. Keep in mind that regardless of the results of your ovarian reserve testing, it is commonly understood that age is the single most predictive factor for IVF success. You need good-quality eggs in order for IVF to work, and egg quality is directly impacted by age. This means that even if you have "diminished ovarian reserve" at a young age, you may have fewer eggs available, but those eggs are likely to be better quality than if you were older. And the older you are, the more your ovarian reserve matters, because you may need to have a greater number of eggs retrieved in order to end up with the one you need to create a healthy embryo.

Ovarian reserve is determined by the following:

AMH: This is a blood test that measures anti-Mullerian hormone, which is produced by the pool of dormant eggs in your ovaries.

AFC: The antral follicle count is the number of egg follicles your ovaries are developing in a given cycle, measured by transvaginal ultrasound.

FSH and estradiol: Follicle-stimulating hormone and estradiol levels inform the appropriate stimulation protocol to recommend for you.

The more eggs that can be retrieved, the greater the potential for ending up with healthy, usable embryos. If you have low ovarian reserve, it will take more cycles to get the number of eggs you need to result in the desired number of embryos (and the more it will cost). Most clinics recommend at least two euploid (genetically normal) embryos for each child you want to have in order to allow for an additional attempt if the first embryo transfer doesn't succeed.

How IVF Works

From here, things start to get a bit complicated . . . but this overview should break it down for you. If you already have a solid understanding of how conception happens physiologically (Chapter 6), you can use this to springboard your understanding of how science takes over the process in an IVF cycle. Here is a review:

- People with ovaries are born with all the eggs they will ever have. From the time of puberty, each month, the body recruits a few eggs that are nourished inside follicles within the ovary. That selection process starts a few days before your period begins.

- By the time your period ends, the follicles grow in response to rising levels of estrogen (from the ovaries) and FSH (from the pituitary gland in the brain).

- A few days before ovulation occurs, FSH production goes down and then rises again, causing the ovaries to select one dominant follicle while the others die off.

- Then FSH comes back on line, honing in on the development of what we call the dominant follicle, and estrogen keeps rising until it causes the pituitary gland to release LH (luteinizing hormone).

- The surge of LH tells the egg cell to prepare itself for fertilization and then burst free from the follicle to be swept up by the fallopian tube.

- If sperm are awaiting the arrival of the egg in the fallopian tube, they will swim quickly toward it and work together to break through its outer shell (the zona pellucida).

- Finally, one lucky sperm enters the egg and its tail falls away. Each of these gametes (sperm and egg) has a half set of chromosomes, so when they combine, a full set of chromosomes comes into being within this new single cell.

- That cell splits, and then those cells split, over and over again, following the instructional code within the DNA, eventually forming a new baby human.

In ART, the conception process is carefully controlled by medications:

- The ovaries are encouraged to produce as many eggs as possible in a process called controlled ovarian hyperstimulation. This relies on mediating the activity of the hypothalamus gland, which regulates the production of FSH and LH through the messenger hormone GnRH (gonadotropin-releasing hormone).

- Medications called GnRH agonists are used to stimulate FSH production so that the ovaries develop as many follicles as possible.

- Medications called GnRH antagonists are used to prevent the body from ovulating on its own so that a doctor can go in and retrieve the eggs into a test tube.

- Just before retrieval, the final step in egg cell maturation is induced by an injection of hCG (human chorionic gonadotropin), which takes over the role of LH in telling your eggs to ready themselves for fertilization. The retrieval is timed precisely according to the administration of hCG.

Different medication dosages and protocols are used based on your physician's best guess about what will be most effective for your body. If the desired results are not achieved, the protocol can be changed in subsequent cycles, in hopes of improving on retrieval rates. If you are thinking this sounds a lot like trial and error, you are right—it is. And this can be incredibly frustrating given how much money it takes to keep trying until it works.

Coping with the Unpredictability of ART

ART is a highly advanced science, but given the intricacies of the human endocrine system and the gametes it produces, applying that science to the individual is somewhat unpredictable. The doctor will use scientific evidence to inform the protocols they recommend, as well as to help guide you in the decision-making process. But statistics only provide probabilities, not guarantees. What this means is that as you navigate cycles of stimulation, retrieval, and embryo transfer, there are points at which things may go differently than expected. Whether you are a prospective parent, an egg donor, or a surrogate, I want you to be aware of the places where pitfalls may lie so that you feel informed and prepared if they happen to you. But even more than that, I want you to be able to reframe the notion that lack of success, or a less-than-anticipated response, equals failure. On the contrary, when the body does not have an ideal response to a certain medication protocol, this information is used to inform your treatment plan. It is not necessarily a loss but a potential gain in terms of getting to the protocol that will ultimately bring you success.

In fertility medicine, as in life, success may tell us what we are doing right, but lack of success tells us what we need to do differently. Of course, we want things to go smoothly, to be able to do A plus B and end up with C (and certainly where ART is concerned, the longer it takes, the more costly it becomes). But weathering the unexpected is part of the process—an experience not unlike parenting. The emotional skills and capacity for resilience you gain during this time will serve you well in the years to come.

Overall, an IVF cycle takes about four to six weeks. There is usually a two-week window of time when you know you will have lots of appointments, but how it all plays out is unpredictable. For prospective parents, this lack of predictability is excellent practice for what it is like to live with an infant, never knowing for sure how long they will nap (and therefore how much you can get done before they are awake again) or when they will get sick and you will need to take time off work to care for them. However, being plunged into the day in, day out uncertainty of an IVF cycle can put enormous strain on you emotionally, as well as on your responsibilities at work, not to mention how you are navigating this in your relationship. Added to this is the stress of sidesteps and adjustments to the plan based on how your body responds each step of the way.

To help you and your loved ones understand what the process can look like, the chart on the following pages describes IVF and embryo transfer alongside a parallel physiological conception cycle. The column on the right-hand side provides anticipatory guidance for other possible outcomes at each step of the way.

Step-by-Step Guide to the IVF Process

What Happens in a Physiological Conception Cycle	How Conception Is Managed in IVF and Embryo Transfer	Sidesteps That May Occur along the Way
About a week before your period starts, your body starts to recruit a pool of eggs to develop in the upcoming cycle.	You may be asked to take oral contraceptive pills before your IVF cycle begins. If you are planning a fresh embryo transfer with a partner's egg or donor egg, you and the egg provider will both take contraceptive pills in order to sync your cycles. In a "long protocol" IVF cycle, you are given injectable medication (Lupron) to keep FSH and LH from being released so that you will have a cohort of eggs that will grow at the same rate once stimulation medications begin. This "downregulation" causes a temporary menopausal state and may come with associated symptoms such as night sweats and hot flashes. This process takes about two weeks.	If you are young, or you have PCOS or other indications that put you at a higher risk for OHSS (ovarian hyperstimulation syndrome), you will skip this step and follow what is called a "short protocol."
Your period begins.	Your period begins.	Your period may not occur, or it may be too short to render your uterine lining thin enough to begin ovarian stimulation. In this case, you will be given progesterone for a few days, which will then cause your period to start once the progesterone is withdrawn.

Physiological Cycle	IVF & Embryo Transfer	Sidesteps
The uterus sheds its lining while your recruited egg follicles begin to respond to low levels of FSH and estrogen.	You go into the clinic on cycle day two or three for baseline blood work and ultrasound.	Your blood work may indicate that it's not an ideal time to go ahead with stimulation this cycle. Your ultrasound may reveal a cyst that was left over from your last cycle, which usually means the cycle has to be canceled.
In the days following your period, increasing levels of FSH are released from the pituitary gland to further develop the egg follicles.	This is the stimulation phase. If you have ample ovarian reserve, you will be given injectable medication (Follistim, Menopur, Gonal-F, Bravelle, or Repronex). If your ovarian reserve is low, you may be given a lower dose of FSH, or letrozole or Clomid—this is called a minimal stimulation cycle. If you are on the long protocol, you will continue the Lupron injections, although the dosage will be reduced. If you are on a short protocol, you will start Lupron now to prevent premature ovulation.	Aside from the emotional stress of injections, you may develop bruising, redness, or irritation at the injection sites. Sometimes stimulation medications can impede the growth of your uterine lining, in which case, it will be recommended that you freeze your embryos and delay the embryo transfer until a later cycle. Your follicles may not grow all at the same rate, in which case, the cycle may or may not continue based on the doctor's clinical judgment for how to get the greatest number of eggs.
Meanwhile, estrogen levels rise, causing the uterine lining to build up and eventually making the cervical fluid become clear and stretchy as ovulation approaches.	Meanwhile, you go into the doctor's office every few days for internal ultrasounds and blood draws. The ultrasounds look to see how the follicles are growing. The blood work tracks your estrogen levels, allowing your medication dosages to be changed as needed.	Medication dosages may be changed based on how your body is responding to ovarian stimulation.
Just before ovulation occurs, FSH decreases and then rises again, which helps the ovaries select one dominant follicle, while the others dissolve and go away.	As your pool of follicles grows, the doctor determines when looks to be the best time for retrieval based on the rate of growth.	If the rate of growth is slower than anticipated, your retrieval date may be pushed out by a few days to a week.

Physiological Cycle	IVF & Embryo Transfer	Sidesteps
When estrogen levels are at their peak, the pituitary gland responds by flooding the bloodstream with a surge of LH (luteinizing hormone). This causes the final maturation of the egg cell (meiosis 1), which makes it fertilizable.	Once your follicles are large enough, you are given an injection of HCG (the "trigger shot"), which does exactly what your own LH would do—it causes the final maturation of the egg cells (meiosis 1), which makes them able to be fertilized.	If the number of mature eggs is too low for a retrieval, you may be offered IUI instead.
The egg cell erupts from the follicle anywhere from a few hours to one or two days after the onset of the LH surge.	Mature eggs are retrieved about thirty-six hours after the HCG shot. Retrieval is performed under IV anesthesia (fentanyl and propofol), and the eggs are aspirated using a needle that enters the pelvic cavity through the vaginal wall. When you wake up, the doctor will be able to tell you how many eggs were retrieved.	It is important for the doctor to avoid damage to surrounding structures such as the bowel and bladder. For this reason, some of the eggs that were seen on the ultrasound may not be able to be retrieved. Risks associated with egg retrieval are higher in those with larger bodies, which means you may need to have your retrieval done in a hospital setting rather than in the clinic.
The egg cell is swept into the fallopian tube where it may find sperm cells awaiting its arrival for fertilization.	Egg cells are taken to the lab for (in vitro) fertilization. If you are using fresh sperm, the sample may be collected the same day, or a day or two before. If you are using a frozen sperm sample, it will be thawed and prepared in the clinic. The egg cells will either be combined with sperm cells to let them fertilize on their own, or each egg may be injected with a sperm cell by the embryologist in a procedure known as ICSI (intracytoplasmic sperm injection).	Some of the egg cells that were retrieved may not be able to be fertilized. If you are conceiving with a partner, donor, or coparent who has a very low sperm count, especially in cases where testicular extraction is being used to collect sperm cells, there is a chance of not having enough healthy sperm cells to adequately fertilize the egg cells that have been retrieved. Those egg cells can be frozen at this point; however, the survival rate of cryopreserved eggs is not as high as cryopreserved embryos.

Physiological Cycle	IVF & Embryo Transfer	Sidesteps
The empty egg follicle, now called the corpus luteum, produces progesterone, which thickens and sustains the uterine lining.	If your embryos are being transferred in the same cycle, you (or the person carrying) will start supplemental progesterone following egg retrieval. Progesterone will be continued for the first nine to ten weeks of pregnancy.	If you are not receiving a transfer in this cycle, you will continue your cycle as usual—although you will be eagerly awaiting news of how many of your embryos survived. The sudden discontinuation of hormonal medications can be jarring and may affect your mood.
The sperm and egg cell each have a half set of chromosomes. Once they combine, a single cell with a complete set of chromosomes is formed. That cell replicates itself and splits, and the same happens over and over again as the action of the fallopian tube carries what is now called a zygote along toward the uterus.	Your embryos will be kept in a culture medium inside an incubator in the lab until they reach the cleavage stage (day three) or blastocyst stage (day five). Another option is to incubate the embryos in an INVOCELL vaginal incubator, although this option only allows for day-three embryos.	Some of the embryos will naturally die off before reaching the blastocyst stage. Growing to day five provides increased confidence that the remaining embryos are healthy and increases your chance of successful implantation.
By the time it is ready to implant in the uterine wall, the embryo has around one to two hundred cells and is called a blastocyst.	Embryos that reach the day-five blastocyst stage are more likely to implant successfully and result in a live birth, so this is becoming the gold standard method.	If you have extra embryos, they can be cryopreserved for later use—either for another transfer cycle if this one doesn't take, or for future children.
Implantation	**Embryo Transfer**	
About six days after fertilization, the embryo implants into the uterine lining.	The embryo transfer procedure is a lot like IUI. A catheter is passed through the cervix, and the embryo is placed inside the uterus. Some people experience pain or cramping, and for others, it's no more than the sensation of a Pap test. You may be given Valium if you anticipate this will be difficult for you.	You may transfer an embryo in the same cycle, or your embryos may be frozen for transfer in a later cycle. These two options are presented on page 221.

Physiological Cycle	IVF & Embryo Transfer	Sidesteps
Fresh Embryo Transfer		
You may opt for embryo transfer in the same cycle as your IVF process if: - You aren't doing genetic testing. - You or your partner are incubating your embryos vaginally using INVOCELL. - You have used a minimal stimulation protocol (usually if you are older). - You are trying to keep costs down.		You may not be able to opt for a fresh embryo transfer if you are at risk for ovarian hyperstimulation syndrome (OHSS).
In a physiological cycle, you wait and see if pregnancy has occurred. If it has, the corpus luteum will continue to produce progesterone until nine to ten weeks of pregnancy, when the placenta has grown enough to take over this function.	Fresh embryo transfers are scheduled based on the day of retrieval and the stage at which you plan to do the transfer, day three or day five. In a fresh embryo transfer, supplemental progesterone is given, but you will also be making your own progesterone, so the doses are not as high as in a frozen embryo transfer (FET).	If your embryos are growing a little slower than expected, your transfer might be pushed out to day six or seven. If there are a small number of embryos, a day-three transfer may be recommended instead of day five. Some embryos don't do well in the culture medium and can be seen degrading from day three to day five. If this happens, a day-three transfer will be recommended in subsequent cycles.
Frozen Embryo Transfer		
Frozen embryo transfer offers the advantage of allowing the IVF protocol to focus on egg development without simultaneous concern for the development of the uterine lining. It is also the way conception will occur if you are using donor embryo. There are two ways to do an FET cycle: "controlled" or "natural," each of which is addressed on pages 223–224. FET also allows for genetic testing of the embryos.		FET is preferred if you are at risk for OHSS—usually those who are young, or in cases of polycystic ovary syndrome (PCOS).

Physiological Cycle	IVF & Embryo Transfer	Sidesteps
The most common cause of miscarriage is chromosomal error. Around 30 to 50 percent of zygotes do not make it to the blastocyst stage, and at least 40 percent of blastocysts do not successfully make it to implantation. It is believed that up to 50 percent of conceptions never make it to a missed period. In this case, your cycle begins again.	Genetic testing can be performed at the blastocyst stage; however, it takes seven to ten days to get results, so the embryos will need to be frozen for transfer in a future cycle. Genetic testing allows you to only transfer one genetically normal (euploid) embryo, increasing your odds for a live birth while reducing your chance of complications associated with a multiple pregnancy. Genetic testing is especially important if you need to screen for heritable conditions, or if you have had multiple miscarriages or unsuccessful embryo transfers. It is also recommended over age forty to offset the high miscarriage rate in this age group due to the high rate of chromosomal abnormality as we approach the end of our fertile life span.	Genetic testing results are the ultimate moment of truth. The numbers go down from the number of eggs retrieved to the number that successfully fertilize to the number than make it to day five. But you really don't know how many viable embryos you have until the genetic testing results are in. On the other hand, your confidence in a successful transfer goes up and your chances of miscarriage go down when you know the embryo being transferred is genetically normal.

IVF & Embryo Transfer	Sidesteps
Controlled FET Cycle	
In a controlled FET cycle, you are given two weeks of supplemental estrogen (usually a pill, sometimes along with a patch or vaginal suppository, and less commonly by injection) from the start of your period to the time of the transfer.	
You will have a baseline ultrasound at the beginning of your transfer cycle, and another one before the transfer to make sure your uterine lining is thick enough and has a uniform three-layer or "trilaminar" appearance.	Your transfer may be delayed for a week to give the lining more time to develop. If not, your cycle may be canceled. In subsequent cycles, your doctor may try other options to support the uterine lining, from different modes of delivery of synthetic estrogen to using other medications such as Viagra. However, some people don't respond to synthetic estrogen and will build a better uterine lining on their own estrogen. If this turns out to be the case for you, it will be recommended that you try a "natural" cycle instead.
High-dose estrogen should keep you from growing a follicle or ovulating, but you may also be given contraceptive pills or Lupron to prevent breakthrough ovulation.	If you develop a large follicle or ovulate during a FET cycle, it will cause progesterone to release, throwing off the timing of the transfer and canceling your cycle.
Progesterone will be administered once your uterine lining has reached optimal conditions. Progesterone administration starts the clock on your transfer, because the transfer must happen precisely on the appropriate day for the age of your embryo. Progesterone is an oil-based formulation that is given in daily injections or a combination of daily vaginal suppositories plus injections every three days. The embryo will be thawed and transferred on the sixth day of progesterone administration.	If you forget to start your progesterone, or if something happens that keeps you from taking your progesterone on time, your transfer cycle may be canceled. Out of all the injections given during ART, progesterone shots are the worst. However, the high-dose estrogen used to prepare your lining in a controlled cycle prevents you from making any progesterone at all, so it's worth it to do what you need to do to hold on to that lining and support a successful implantation. You can apply heat or ice for pain relief, and it may help to rub the area of injection in order to disperse the medication.

IVF & Embryo Transfer	Sidesteps
Natural FET Cycle	
Rather than doing a controlled embryo transfer cycle, you can do a natural (unmedicated) or modified natural (letrozole or low-dose gonadotropins) cycle. This is only an option if you regularly ovulate on your own and you typically develop a robust uterine lining.	
Even in a natural cycle, once your follicles are large enough, a trigger shot will be given, followed by supplemental progesterone (usually vaginal suppositories). This is necessary to time the FET appropriately.	Natural embryo transfer cycles require frequent monitoring because your body will be dictating the timing of the transfer. This presents a higher level of stress and unpredictability than a controlled cycle.
Whether you do a controlled or natural FET cycle, supplemental progesterone is continued through nine to ten weeks of pregnancy.	

Multiple Pregnancy and ART

Historically, IVF was known for high rates of multiple pregnancy because the only way to increase the odds of pregnancy was to transfer multiple embryos. However, now, with genetic testing and frozen embryo transfer, an equally successful live birth rate can be achieved by transferring only one genetically normal embryo. Multiple pregnancy is the single most important risk of ART, but keep in mind that this is a risk that can be mostly avoided by only transferring one embryo. Although the overall rate of multiples is low, there is still a higher chance of multiple pregnancy with embryo transfer due to splitting, where the embryo splits on its own after transfer, creating identical twins (2 percent versus 0.5 percent in the general population).

While having twins may seem super cute—and if you desire two children, it could mean achieving your family-building goals with a single pregnancy— carrying multiples puts the entire pregnancy at risk. A healthy, full-term pregnancy and live birth are more likely with a singleton pregnancy. If you are in your late thirties or early forties and you do not do genetic testing, it may be recommended to transfer more than one embryo to account for the rate of miscarriage. However, because this puts the overall health of your pregnancy at risk, genetic testing and single embryo transfer is the gold standard of care.

In multiple pregnancy, there is an increased chance of gestational hypertension, gestational diabetes, postpartum hemorrhage, and cesarean birth. The chance of premature birth is increased sixfold. When babies are born early, mortality rates are higher. Preemies can spend weeks to months in the hospital NICU, and they are at risk for lung problems, intestinal infections, cerebral palsy, learning disabilities, language delays, and behavioral issues. Preterm birth is a traumatic event for parents due to prolonged experiences of uncertainty, feeling helpless in the situation, and shattered expectations of what new parenthood would look like. These experiences can be mitigated by family-centered NICU practices such as kangaroo care and supporting lactation and chest/breastfeeding; however, the experience of having a baby in the NICU is unavoidably traumatic.

Side Effects of ART

If you lead into your cycle with suppression medication, you are likely to experience menopausal symptoms such as night sweats and hot flashes. Medications that stimulate follicular growth can cause nausea (and sometimes vomiting), chest/breast tenderness, increased genital discharge, mood swings, and fatigue. These are all common symptoms of pregnancy, so you are going to get a swift preview of what is to come. Additionally, there will be pelvic pressure and bloating as estrogen levels rise and the ovaries become heavy. You will be advised to limit your exercise in order to prevent ovarian torsion. (The ovarian ligaments can stretch and twist from increased weight of the ovaries.)

During egg retrieval, there is a risk of damaging surrounding structures (bladder, bowel, blood vessels), and this risk is higher for those with larger-than-average bodies. If this is the case for you, it might be recommended to do the retrieval in a hospital rather than your doctor's office so that acute care can be immediately available if needed. Your anesthesia is an important part of the procedure, so there may be recommendations made by the anesthesiologist on the team about what type of anesthesia will be most effective for you—and anesthesia always comes with risks, which will be discussed with you ahead of the procedure. Most retrievals cause some pelvic and abdominal pain for one to two days, but this can usually be managed with over-the-counter pain medications. There is a risk for infection, but this is mitigated by taking antibiotics at the time of retrieval. Be sure to follow up with a high-quality probiotic supplement to replace beneficial microflora after antibiotic treatment.

After a stimulation and retrieval without immediate embryo transfer, you can have a pretty big hormone crash once the hormonal medications are discontinued. However, the frozen embryo transfer cycle is easier, and at that point, the painful progesterone shots are the worst of it.

When an ART Cycle Is Not Successful

The reason you will ideally have two healthy embryos for each desired child is that it often takes two transfer cycles for a successful pregnancy. If at first you don't succeed, try again—but not without investigating why it may not have worked the first time. You may have tests to look for problems with the uterine lining, or you may be tested for autoimmune factors. But given that there is not an unlimited supply of embryos, and you can't do an endless number of ART cycles, at a certain point, you may need to look at adoption or opt for child-free living.

In the meantime, while you are still trying, do everything you can to increase your chances for success. If you have issues such as PCOS or endometriosis, review Chapter 7. Be sure to follow the guidelines in Chapter 2—everything you need to know to support the development of healthy egg cells is there. Reproductive technology can't correct for the health of your eggs, it can only build upon the potential for success you already have.

GUIDANCE FOR CARE PROVIDERS

Unless you are a specialist in reproductive endocrinology and infertility (REI), you will be providing referrals to clinics in your area for ART. It is imperative to know which doctors and clinics are welcoming and affirming to queer and trans patients. Most fertility clinics market themselves to the LGBTQ+ community, given that for most of us, building a family via pregnancy requires assisted conception. However, a sticker on a website does not always accurately reflect the attitudes, language, and experiences people have inside the clinic. Get to know the REIs in your community: join the local reproductive medicine society, take a colleague out to lunch, attend local conferences, and invite fertility doctors to speak at educational events you organize for your clients—and require them to use inclusive language when they do so. Solicit feedback from your clients after you have made referrals, and listen to the experiences of pregnant people and new parents as they describe their encounters in the local health care system.

Another important aspect of referring prospective parents to ART is providing education and anticipatory guidance (such as the information provided in this chapter), as well as allowing ample time for counseling. Make sure your clients feel listened to and heard. Affirm the validity of the emotions that come up. Reframe the option for medical support as a positive intervention that can bring them closer to holding their baby in their arms. Name that reproductive science has come a long way over the years—success rates are higher and the risks are lower than they have ever been. The financial implications can be immobilizing, so make sure people know about options for funding and insurance mandates in your state or province. This can be an excellent time to make a referral to a therapist who specializes in infertility and perinatal mental health. It's also important to remind people that everything they are doing to support their body still counts and will enhance their chances of success.

If you are reading this as an REI or someone who works in a fertility clinic, please do everything you can to make your clinic more welcoming and appropriate for queer and trans families. Engage in a formal gender-inclusivity process that addresses queer and trans sensitivity at all levels of your practice, from the website, to forms and electronic health records systems, to the language used by employees at every level of the organization, to policies that present barriers to care or make us feel marginalized at best. I look forward to hearing from clinics that have been able to successfully remedy the broad and repeated instances of cis/heteronormativity, transphobia, and/or homophobia so uniformly reported by LGBTQ+ families using fertility clinics, but until then, please, do better.

Resources

Society for Assisted Reproductive Technology

Patient predictor tool: w3.abdn.ac.uk/clsm/SARTIVF

Fertility clinic directory and success rates:
www.sartcorsonline.com/members/Search

Resources for Funding ART

RESOLVE: www.resolve.org/what-are-my-options/lgbtq-family-building-options

Family Equality: www.familyequality.org/resources/lgbtq-family-building-grants

FertilityIQ: www.fertilityiq.com/topics/fertilityiq-data-and-notes/free-ivf-grants
-and-charities

Men Having Babies: www.menhavingbabies.org/assistance

Video Resource for Improving Queer/Trans Sensitivity in Fertility Clinics

LGBTQ Parenting Network's "Scenes from a Fertility Clinic":
https://vimeo.com/129461617

COPING WITH CYCLE ATTEMPTS

At the first sign of blood, your cycle begins, again. Or perhaps your partner comes out of the bathroom in tears and tells you it didn't work, again. Or you get a call from the clinic letting you know that there were no viable embryos, or that your surrogate is not pregnant. Whether you are the one conceiving or your partner, coparent, or surrogate is, even one unsuccessful cycle attempt can feel disheartening. If this is not your first go-round, or your second, or even your third, you might be feeling disappointment, sadness, or anger—or you might simply feel numb. Not far behind these emotions is knowing that your expenses in this process are mounting, accompanied by escalating stress and worry. If you are planning to try again right away, disappointment may fade as feelings of anticipation and hope start to arise, tempered by the self-protective voice in your head that may be warning you not to get your hopes up too high. If you decide to take a break, your disappointment may be tempered by relief—but at the same time, having time and space to fully process the emotions of not having conceived is also not easy.

After a couple of days, if you are trying again this month, you take a deep breath and start making calls. You let your midwife, doctor, or clinic know your cycle has started. You call the sperm bank, or give your known donor a heads-up, or inform the intended parents. You may feel a sense of defeat as you settle into the feeling that this unwished-for situation is becoming all too familiar. As the tasks involved with the coming cycle start to take over your headspace again, your feelings of excitement and anxiety grow. You take note of the changes your body goes through as midcycle approaches, and you start to feel hopeful again. Even if you are trying not to get your hopes up, you may have a feeling that this could be the one.

Finally, the day arrives. You make the necessary arrangements. Doubts continue to crop up, but it's not time for that now. You muster all the hope you can, even if it's no more than blind faith—but what other choice do you have? You go through the motions, welcoming this pregnancy to take hold in your body, or the body of the person carrying. Afterward, you settle into a brief post-attempt calm. However, just like the eye of a hurricane, the sense of calm does not last long, especially in the conceiving body. Your mind keeps asking questions: Did it work? When will I know? Is that a cramp? Am I peeing a lot? Was I tired today because I'm pregnant? Is that implantation spotting? Is my temperature going up again? When can I test? Should I test or should I wait?

How can I stay focused at work when this is all I think about? What will pregnancy be like for me? Will I be a good parent? Do I deserve this? Will I have enough money to keep going if this one doesn't take? Should I go for a run today or should I take it easy? If I have sex, will that disrupt the pregnancy? Should I start making plans for the next cycle, or will that jinx it? I really want to know, but can I handle it if I get a negative test today? I'm sure I'm pregnant. I'm sure I'm not pregnant. This is the longest two weeks of my life!

No matter how you go about coping, cycle attempts can start to take over your very existence. There are a million things to worry about and fixate on, and an internet full of advice about what you should or shouldn't do when trying to conceive. Thoughts and emotions spin out of control, including how we feel about our bodies, about becoming a parent or having another child, financial pressures, relationship dynamics, decision-making . . . it is just a lot. With each cycle that ends in yet another period, those feelings come up again and again, sometimes compounding one another and hitting harder and harder each time. The emotional roller-coaster ride is no joke.

Dealing with an unsuccessful conception attempt is often compounded by physical pain from cramps, the constant reminder of menstrual blood, and the dysphoria many of us feel around having periods at all. Be gentle with yourself. You don't have to figure it all out today.

That thing you are not supposed to do because it's not good for your fertility? Do it now, just once, during your period. You get a free pass for one day. Give yourself space to cope in the best way you know how. You can make a new plan tomorrow.

What not to do? Think that it's going to be possible to not let this get to you. In other words, allow yourself to feel your feelings. If you are disappointed and upset, let yourself feel that. Don't participate in gaslighting yourself. Have a good cry, go for a run, make some art, talk it through, or dance it out. Process the feelings so that they don't get stuck in your body.

Managing the Stress of Trying to Conceive

Luckily, there are various ways to cope with stress. The hard part is actually doing them. This will not be the last time you must force yourself to engage in a practice of self-preservation for the sake of this child. Consider it more preparation for pregnancy and/or parenting.

Move your body: Science has shown us time and again that the number-one way to move stress out of the body is through physical activity. Get out of your head and into your body. Let the endorphins flow. According to authors Emily and Amelia Nagoski in their research-based book, *Burnout: The Secret to Unlocking the Stress Cycle*, moving your body is the single most effective way to complete the cycle of a stress response. Because stress is always happening, they recommend twenty to sixty minutes of physical activity every day. In fact, the Nagoskis' book talks a lot about the stresses of motherhood, so if you are trying to conceive while already parenting and you identify as a mother, their book is definitely for you.

Be in your body without movement: If you need to let go of stress you hold in your body and exercise is simply not on the table for you, take a hot bath, go to the spa or get a massage, get some acupuncture, have sex or masturbate. You can even release stress lying down by tensing and releasing parts of your body from head to toe.

Breathing practices: One common technique is slow, deep breathing that is stronger on the exhale (similar to taking a big sigh), or some type of measured breathing such as equal counts of in breath and out breath while pausing after each. Look for pranayama classes at your local yoga studio.

Be with people you love: Positive social interactions can go a long way toward helping us feel connected and less alone. Try a twenty-second hug, or keep hugging until both you and your hugging partner become relaxed. Affection with pets counts too.

Laughter is the best medicine: Deep belly laughter changes your brain chemistry in a way that reduces stress and supports well-being.

Cry: Sometimes it helps to just have a good cry. Letting your feelings flow can feel scary at first, especially if you've been keeping things bottled up. But your tears are there for a reason. Let them come, and they will carry worry, stress, fear, and frustration out of your body. Having a big cry can ultimately help you feel a bit lighter, even if it's just the relief that comes from not resisting your feelings for a while.

Creative expression: Drawing, painting, singing, playing an instrument, knitting, coloring, or even preparing a beautiful meal help get you into parts of your brain that don't harbor anxiety and stress about conceiving.

Have a daily self-care practice: If you don't have a solid self-care plan, make one now. What do you typically do to mediate stress in your life? Are you doing that now? The stress of trying to conceive is happening daily, so your stress mediation plan needs to happen daily too. If your typical methods of blowing off steam are not available to you because they negatively affect your fertility (alcohol is a common example), make sure you've got an alternate plan. If you normally like to have a drink when you get home at the end of the day, make a delicious mocktail or circumvent the drinking thing altogether by having a planned wind-down activity you will do instead.

Meditation: While meditations that include visualizations of conception can be helpful during or after procedures, the rest of the time it is more helpful to clear your mind. A technique called mindfulness-based stress reduction (do an internet search for classes in your area) has been shown to reduce anxiety, depression, stress, anger, and to increase feelings of well-being in those experiencing infertility. The reduction in physiological stress improves the quality of sleep, regulates cortisol levels, and supports the HPA (hypothalamic-pituitary-adrenal) axis and the immune system, all of which support fertility.

Get support from a professional: Whether you see a therapist or you opt for a fertility doula to support you through this time, having someone who is not a friend or family member to witness your experience and help you process your emotions can be extremely helpful.

Rearrange your priorities: The fact remains that trying to conceive is inherently stressful. The trick is to make getting pregnant a top priority without letting it take over your life completely. You may need to reduce other stressors in your life (change to a less stressful job, take a break from leadership roles, or say no more often) while at the same time building in more time and space to blow off steam and truly let go.

Create opportunities for joy: Do what it takes to make time for things you enjoy. The goal is not necessarily to make the stress and worry go away but to set things up for even momentary reprieves. The more you can incorporate positive experiences into your daily life, the more balance you will have in the range of emotions you are experiencing.

Complete tasks: Completing tasks can help you feel more in control. Ordering your sperm samples, going to appointments, filling in the cycle chart—this might hit the spot more for one person in a partnership than the other, so make sure you divvy up the work so that everyone gets to participate in a way that helps them thrive and feel connected to the process.

Put the Process into Context

It can be immensely helpful to locate yourself in time, intentionally (and often repeatedly) acknowledging where you are at in your self-determined process. Specifically, having a solid sense of exactly what your next step will be if the current cycle or procedure doesn't work can keep a "landing pad" in sight, so to speak. The following suggestions can help guide you as you navigate this aspect of coping.

Have an overall plan: Think of trying to conceive in sets of three cycles, rather than one cycle at a time. The physiological reality is that you could do everything right, and still conception may not happen in a given cycle. Depending on age or circumstances (see Chapter 1), you may already have an overall plan about how many cycles to try with one method before trying something else. Regroup at three-month intervals, and in the meantime, stick to the plan rather than constantly trying to figure it all out. This measured approach can bring about a sense of containment and reassurance.

Remember your ultimate goal: It may feel like your ultimate goal is to be pregnant, but given that pregnancy is a very short chapter in a lifetime of parenthood, you most likely have a larger goal in mind. Is your ultimate goal a life of fulfillment, and is having a kid just one way to attain that? Is your ultimate goal to be a parent, and is pregnancy just one way to accomplish that? Trying to conceive can create a state of tunnel vision, so when you notice this happening, step back and bring your ultimate goals into focus. This can help keep the day-to-day, cycle-to-cycle ups and downs in check.

Keep the cost-benefit in mind: Let's face it, there are aspects of this process you could do without. For some, it's having to deal with the clinic, or even the fact that you have to go to a clinic at all. For others, it's dietary restrictions, needing to exercise, going to acupuncture, or taking supplements or medications—or not taking medications that you can't take while trying to conceive, including gender-affirming hormones. And for still others, it's charting, checking fluid, looking at your cervix with a speculum, peeing on a stick for days at a time. Often, it's the things that just suck, yet they come with the territory and there's not much we can do about them—the trying, the waiting, dealing with unexpected hitches in the plan, disappointment, frustration. I'm here to tell you that I've never heard a parent holding their baby in their arms say it wasn't worth it. Everything you do gets you one step closer to your goal, and every experience you weather is for a greater purpose. Everything you learn about yourself, about dealing with hard things, about coping when you ultimately have no real control, will serve you as a parent. After the conception process, you will have a pregnancy to navigate, and a birth, and recovery, and caring for a newborn around the clock with very little sleep. . . . This is just the beginning of the ways this process will grow you.

Take a break when you need to: Sometimes taking a cycle off from trying is the best way to find your ground again and regroup. If you are considering taking a cycle off, consider if you need to be completely freed of everything to do with trying to get pregnant, or if you can take some time to boost your fertility or do some cycle charting. Consider carefully what you really need. Taking some time off can help you find yourself again outside of the all-consuming mental energy of conception cycles. Stress reduction is an excellent way to support your fertility, so why not take a breather from trying and effortlessly boost your efforts to conceive in the process?

Even if you feel you are racing against time because of your age, if the stress is too overwhelming or your mental health is suffering, taking a month off could be the best thing for you—it may even support the healthy maturation of the egg you will release in the following cycle. Below age forty (unless you have lab work or imaging that indicates you are closer to menopause than the average person your age), you can take a month off and let the negativity and fear about "advanced maternal age" go. Your body does not know the difference between being thirty-nine years and three months old and being thirty-nine years and four months old—I promise.

If you are age forty or over, you might decide to take time off from inseminating, but during that time, focus on other things that move you forward in the process of achieving pregnancy. There is no time to lose, so even if there isn't an attempt happening, make sure you are continuing with fertility support, tracking your fertile signs to make sure your next insemination is timed appropriately, or setting things up for yourself so that when you start trying again, you can do so with less stress and more support.

Take time to troubleshoot: Whether you are taking time off or diving right back in to try again in your next cycle, most people start to wonder what they can do to increase the chances of success. It's hard to just "try" when doing so is costing you hundreds or thousands of dollars, and it has to be done with a great deal of intention, not to mention logistical coordination and an emotional roller-coaster ride that dominates every waking thought. (See Chapter 7: Troubleshooting and Complicated Conceptions.)

Should I Stop Trying, or Am I Just Burned Out?

It can be hard to know if you are really done trying or if you are just done feeling so much stress. One way of sorting out your feelings is to make a list of pros and cons. It sounds simplistic, but going through the exercise can be enlightening. Be sure to include the short-term and long-term effects of stopping versus the short-term and long-term effects of continuing. No matter how you decide to move forward, going through a process of self-investigation will help put you back in the driver's seat, and the sense of empowerment and self-determination you gain will make all the difference in how it feels to approach the next phase.

Keep in mind that it can be hard to make big decisions when we are exhausted, or when we feel isolated, or when we are overcome with feelings of shame or inadequacy. The Nagoskis point to three critical elements of managing stress:

1. Connection

2. Rest/sleep

3. Tempering your internal critic and toxic perfectionism with self-compassion, healing, and gratitude

This last point is similar to what Sonya Renee Taylor calls radical self-love. In her book *The Body Is Not an Apology*, Taylor guides readers through the process of radical self-love as the foundation of making peace with our bodies. If you are feeling bad about yourself or having difficulty staying embodied through this process, you have been given a golden opportunity for healing. Take a deep dive into transforming feelings of shame and inadequacy and unlocking the ways that systems of oppression undermine the self-love that is and has always been your birthright.

What to Do If You and Your Partner Are at Odds with How to Best Cope

It is rare that both/all partners in a relationship have similar ways of coping with the stress and uncertainty of trying to conceive. As in everyday life, there may be one of you who tends to be optimistic, while another prefers to hold all possibilities with equal weight, and still others gravitate toward negative expectations. Because achieving pregnancy is ultimately beyond our control, it is a leap of faith every time we put the process in motion and then wait to see what happens. We are left only with hope—and hopes can be either dashed or fulfilled. Some feel more grounded by holding on to hope, while others attempt to keep disappointment at bay by not allowing themselves to feel hopeful. This makes staying emotionally connected really complicated.

Understanding how the brain responds to stress can help us navigate our own emotions as well as help us support our partners as they navigate theirs. Because our brains are always working to protect us, they go into reaction mode even faster than we can think our own thoughts. This means that we can be swept away by overwhelming emotions, or shuttered into emotional withdrawal, before we even have a chance to understand what is happening—let alone communicate with our partners about what we are feeling and experiencing.

Work on Your Psyche as Preparation for Parenting

If you are experiencing internal conflict or conflict with a partner during the process of conceiving, it might be an indication that you are being called to strengthen your relationship with yourself and/or with your partner. Here is an opportunity to go deep, because having a baby is not something you add to your life, it's something that completely transforms your life. The experience of bringing a new life into the world brings up memories of what our own childhood was like, and it triggers all the ways we have learned to love, to connect, and to protect our hearts. Even though your baby is not here yet, everything you are learning in the process of getting your baby into your arms is teaching you about parenting. In fact, the most commonly chosen discussion topics in our Queer/Trans Early Parenting Support group at MAIA are "nurturing self-esteem in our babies and ourselves," "dealing with anger, frustration, and grief as a new parent," and "tending your relationship after becoming a parent." The work you do now will only serve you in the future. Honor this time for what it has to offer.

Even if you are already a parent, this is a great time for individual as well as couples therapy. Attachment-based approaches can be particularly helpful as we live our lives as parents. Every one of us has a foundation for attachment, laid down in early childhood and evolving over the course of a lifetime, informed by each one of our primary relationships. Our brains respond in times of stress based on the ways we learned to survive emotionally in relation to our parents or caregivers, our closest friends, and our romantic partners. Having a solid understanding of your attachment style, as well as the attachment style of your partner(s), is critical for cultivating compassion and understanding during times of stress.

Author and social scientist Brené Brown conveys in her book *Daring Greatly: How the Courage to Be Vulnerable Transforms the Way We Live, Love, Parent, and Lead* that our sense of self-worth is formed during childhood and continues to affect the ways in which we interact in our relationships as adults. Secure attachment and attentive parenting provide us with a lifetime of resiliency, and lack of it requires a continued struggle to reclaim our rightful place in the world and a sense of being "enough." The science clearly reveals that the way to foster true connection, heal underlying hurts that sabotage our ability to connect, and maintain healthy relationships is by engaging in deep conversation with our own hearts and the hearts of our loved ones. When we become parents, we are in the role of primary attachment figure for our children. Your own healing, especially those parts of you that need healing in relationship to others, is a foundational part of learning how to foster secure attachment in your child.

The process of trying to conceive is going to bring up a whole lot of feels, reaching deep into your psyche and the ways you have acquired and exhibited resiliency since your own infancy. Whether for the purpose of coping with stress, or healing so that you can be the best parent you can be, your therapist will be a valuable resource during this time. So many in our community are coping with post-traumatic stress, estrangement from our families of origin, and lack of validation within cultural institutions. This major life transition requires just as much care for our mental health as it does for our physical health and the health of our partnerships. We are not at fault for the wounds we carry, but if you are standing at the precipice of welcoming a new life into your heart and your home, the time to heal is now.

GUIDANCE FOR CARE PROVIDERS

Trying to conceive is one of the most stressful aspects of becoming a parent. Learning how to cope when you ultimately have no control may be central to what parenting has to teach us, but this lesson is received prematurely when conception does not come easily. Your involvement as a provider in the conception process means coming forth with affirmations of hope and understanding as families navigate the emotional ups and downs of cycle attempts. Remind people to create balance in their lives so that seeking pregnancy does not take over completely. Preservation of self is necessary for navigating the major life transition of welcoming a child. You can guide parents-to-be in the dance of caring for their own needs while also caring for the needs of a baby—even before the baby is conceived. This ultimately represents an advantage for queer and trans families. Our introduction to these central aspects of what it takes to be a parent comes early in the process, which makes us well prepared once our babies arrive. This sort of reflection can be extremely comforting to those who are frustrated with all the extra steps it takes for us to conceive.

Resources

Radical Self-Love for Everybody and Every Body

The Body Is Not an Apology: TheBodyIsNotanApology.com

The Body Is Not an Apology: The Power of Radical Self-Love
by Sonya Renee Taylor

Navigating Vulnerability, Shame, Courage, and Connection

Research professor and author Brené Brown: BreneBrown.com

Queer and Trans Pregnancy Program and Early Parenting Support Groups

MAIA Midwifery & Fertility Services: MAIAMidwifery.com

TEN

MISCARRIAGE

As much as no one wants it to happen, miscarriage is one of the most natural things a body can do. It is believed that up to 50 percent of all conceptions end before being confirmed with a positive pregnancy test. The rate of loss in confirmed pregnancies increases with age, from 10 to 11 percent at age twenty to thirty-four, 17 percent at age thirty-five to thirty-nine, 33 percent at age forty to forty-four, and 53 percent at age forty-five and over. Most pregnancy losses occur in the first trimester—once you are in the second trimester, the risk drops to 2 to 3 percent overall.

Causes and Risk Factors

The most common cause of miscarriage is chromosomal abnormality—in losses that occur at six to ten weeks of pregnancy, 70 percent are genetically abnormal, and at ten to twenty weeks, genetic abnormalities are present 30 percent of the time. Other direct causes include some uterine anomalies and trauma (typically from chorionic villi sampling or amniocentesis, but also from intimate partner violence). Risk factors for pregnancy loss include diabetes, untreated thyroid disease, infection, chronic stress from systemic inequities such as racism, high BMI, clotting disorders, teratogenic medications or substance use, and toxic environmental exposures. Ultimately, what this means is that there are a variety of risk factors, most of which are completely outside of our control. It also means that the approaches in this book to supporting fertility and ensuring optimal preconception health, such as screening for thyroid disorders and keeping blood sugar in check, also serve the purpose of preventing miscarriage.

Symptoms of Pregnancy Loss

The most common symptoms of pregnancy loss are bleeding and cramping, although sometimes there is a decrease in pregnancy symptoms such as nausea and vomiting as well. On the other hand, first trimester bleeding can also be completely normal—it occurs in 20 to 30 percent of all pregnancies, but only 12 percent of those who bleed in the first trimester actually miscarry. The time of greatest risk is when bleeding occurs at six to eight weeks of pregnancy. It is very important to get an ultrasound if you have bleeding or cramping in early pregnancy, because ectopic pregnancy (when implantation occurs outside the uterus) and molar pregnancy (when the cells form a mass with or without an embryo present) may also present this way, and these conditions warrant follow-up in order to protect your future fertility and ongoing health.

Chemical Pregnancy versus First Trimester Pregnancy Loss

In a chemical pregnancy (also called blighted ovum), conception occurs but no embryo forms. This can result in a positive urine or serum pregnancy test that is ultimately followed by a menstrual period that comes more or less on time. In first-trimester pregnancy loss, the pregnancy starts to form but stops growing at a certain point. If you are following your hCG levels and they are not doubling as they should, this may be an indication of early pregnancy loss, which can be further evaluated by ultrasound.

Ectopic Pregnancy

If there is any question about the location of your pregnancy, such as a slow rise in hCG, vaginal spotting or bleeding, or abdominal pain, ultrasound can be used to confirm that the pregnancy has implanted within the uterus or to detect an ectopic pregnancy. While the overall rate of ectopic pregnancy is low in the general population (around 2 percent), there are many conditions that present increased risk, including prior ectopic pregnancy; IVF pregnancy; previous pelvic infection, tubal pathology, or abdominal surgery; past or current smoking; conceiving while under contraception or IUD use; vaginal douching; previous miscarriage or medically induced abortion; history of infertility; or being over age forty. Ectopic pregnancy is a dangerous situation, because if the pregnancy is allowed to grow, it can damage the organs it is attached to, causing life-threatening internal bleeding. Most commonly, an ectopic pregnancy attaches to the fallopian tube, which can rupture as the pregnancy grows. An undiagnosed ectopic pregnancy typically presents with bleeding and severe abdominal pain, and it requires immediate medical attention.

Experiencing Pregnancy Loss

If you find out that your pregnancy is no longer viable, the news can be devastating. Anyone who goes through a pregnancy loss, even if the pregnancy was not in your body, experiences a range of emotions, from numbness or shock to sadness, anger, and feelings of immense loss. The emotions surrounding a miscarriage can feel enormous and out of control, and because this experience is not commonly talked about in our society, it can be incredibly lonely. Underlying mental health concerns can be exacerbated or triggered by the experience, making symptoms of anxiety or depression even more intense. All of these things are true for anyone experiencing a pregnancy loss; however, for queer families, there are additional concerns that make miscarriage even more emotionally complex.

For queer and trans families, the conception process requires so much: a deep and lengthy decision-making process around who will carry and who will provide the necessary gametes; major financial investment in accessing donor gametes and reproductive health services; confronting internalized homophobia and/or transphobia in pursuit of your dream of becoming a parent; navigating cis/heterosexism in clinical settings; fielding obtrusive questions from family members, coworkers, and friends; and various instances of vulnerability and erasure experienced by nonbiological and nongestational parents within medical and legal systems. In addition, transgender parents may have discontinued or delayed gender-affirming hormones in order to achieve pregnancy. We work so hard to get a baby, which means that the trauma, loss, and grief we experience when we lose a pregnancy is amplified. Research on queer women, specifically, indicates that anxiety symptoms following a pregnancy loss typically continue for four months, and grief lessens in intensity by six months. However, the overall sense of loss often has a long-lasting impact, continuing for up to eighteen months and, for some, never completely going away.

All of this means that if you are struggling with the loss of a pregnancy, you are not alone. It means that you are experiencing something that many people go through, and the depth of your grief is shared by every other queer family who has ever lost a pregnancy. Be gentle with yourself. Take the time you need to grieve, to be numb, and to process this experience in whatever way it is unfolding for you. Advocate for yourself, whether you were the pregnant person or not, to get the support you need. Find out who in your community is offering support groups or other resources around pregnancy loss, and see if they can connect you with other families like yours who have gone through it. You can also find solace in the book *Reproductive Losses: Challenges to LGBTQ Family-Making* by Christa Craven, and the companion website (see page 246) that provides commemorations as well as advice for parents and support people.

Guidance for Miscarriage

The loss of a pregnancy is often diagnosed by ultrasound, whether you were already suspecting it due to spotting or cramping, or whether it comes as a complete surprise on a day you were simply hoping to see a heartbeat for the first time. Sometimes the information you receive is not conclusive, such as indicators of fetal age that do not correspond to the date of insemination or your LMP (last menstrual period). You may be in limbo for another week or more before a definitive diagnosis can be made with a follow-up ultrasound.

If it is confirmed that your pregnancy is not viable, you will be offered information so that you can make a decision about how to proceed. You can allow time for your body to release the pregnancy on its own, you can take medication to induce the miscarriage, or you can opt for surgical management, which involves removing the contents of the uterus through the cervix. Sometimes one option is preferred over another due to clinical risks such as uterine fibroids, bleeding disorders, or the age of the pregnancy, but often, the decision will be up to you.

EXPECTANT MANAGEMENT

Waiting for the body to do its thing is called "expectant management," which is only recommended in the first trimester. Most of the time, miscarriage happens on its own within two weeks, but it can sometimes take longer for the process to begin. Most providers will want to conduct a follow-up visit if the miscarriage has not occurred within four weeks. Living with the knowledge that there is an unviable pregnancy in your body is very difficult emotionally, which can be intensified by not knowing when the body is going to actually miscarry. However, you may prefer a natural approach, or you may have fears about medical or surgical procedures. Some people opt to wait for a while, and if the miscarriage doesn't happen within an emotionally manageable period of time, another method of resolving the pregnancy can be pursued.

MEDICATION MANAGEMENT

Medication management consists of one or two medications: an oral medication called mifepristone followed by misoprostol, or misoprostol alone. Misoprostol is dissolved under the tongue or inserted vaginally to avoid digestive side effects, although the dosages are different so make sure you follow your care provider's instructions for the dose you received. You can also take some ibuprofen for pain management. Cramping typically begins within two to four hours, but sometimes it takes longer, especially if you have not yet experienced any spotting or bleeding. If miscarriage has not occurred by twenty-four hours after the initial dose of medication, it may need to be repeated.

THE MISCARRIAGE PROCESS

Whether miscarriage occurs on its own or is medically induced, you will experience a mini labor. Uterine cramping can be intense, coming and going in waves until the tissue is passed. This typically takes about two hours in the acute phase, although generalized cramping usually continues for about twenty-four hours. Make sure you have someone with you during this time for emotional support and physical comfort measures such as providing heat or counterpressure to the low back area. While miscarriage is a normal physiological process, if the uterus is having difficulty passing the tissue, you may experience very heavy bleeding. If you are filling more than two large pads in an hour, or if you start to feel faint or have an increased heart rate with heavy bleeding, seek emergency medical care. Once the tissue passes, you may opt to catch it in a basin so that you can examine it or submit it to a lab for evaluation using a test kit provided by your midwife or physician.

SURGICAL MANAGEMENT

You may choose surgical management at the outset, or this may be the option you are left with if expectant or medication management does not successfully expel all of the tissue from the uterus. Surgical management is highly effective and offers the most rapid resolution of the miscarriage. If you have anemia or a bleeding disorder, or if you are experiencing repeat pregnancy loss and you want to make sure the pregnancy tissue can be collected for testing, surgical management will be recommended. Pain medication or sedation is administered ahead of time. The procedure takes about fifteen minutes and consists of dilating the cervix to aspirate the contents of the uterus with a vacuum, and you can go home within about half an hour afterward. If you lost your pregnancy in the second trimester, you may need cervical preparation, which is administered the day before your procedure. While the technique for surgical management is the same as that for elective termination of pregnancy, loss of a wanted pregnancy is a very different scenario. Double-check with your provider to make sure that you are not being sent to a facility that is providing elective termination on the same day you are going in for surgical management of pregnancy loss. Miscarriage is hard enough without being subjected to a situation that could be very confusing emotionally.

FOLLOW-UP AFTER MISCARRIAGE

After miscarriage, you will continue to have period-type bleeding for one to two weeks. If at any time you have fever or chills, foul-smelling discharge, or increased bleeding that soaks more than two pads in an hour, call your care provider. If you have an Rh-negative blood type, you will need to receive Rh immune globulin within three days of having a miscarriage, or it may be provided at the time of medication or surgical management.

Even if you feel that everything went as expected, please be in touch with your care provider to make sure you are getting the follow-up you need. Your hCG levels will be monitored to make sure they are going down. If not, this could indicate that there is still pregnancy tissue in the uterus, which can cause infection if not removed. You may also want to know when your hCG level is low enough to try to conceive again.

Additionally, you may be screened for mood disorders, which can occur more frequently with any pregnancy, and even more so after a pregnancy loss. If you experience increased anxiety, depression, or post-traumatic stress, please do not hesitate to be seen by a mental health provider. The hormones of pregnancy can trigger changes in brain chemistry that may require medication management, and even if you are still processing emotions from this specific experience, you deserve to be well.

Going through Miscarriage as a Nongestational Parent

Nongestational parents may also suffer deep grief with pregnancy loss; however, it can be difficult to access support in a world that is designed for heterosexual people and doesn't expect partners experiencing pregnancy loss to express emotions due to cultural expectations of masculinity. If you find yourself in this situation, be sure to let people close to you know what you are experiencing. You may find the best support comes from other queer nongestational parents who have gone through this experience themselves, or from a mental health provider who is also a part of the queer community and has experience with family building and pregnancy. You are not alone, and your feelings are valid.

Telling People about the Loss

If you have already told people about the pregnancy, you will at some point be faced with telling them about the loss. This can sometimes feel like reliving the experience every time you have to talk about it, which may not be the best way to support your mental health. On the other hand, telling people who are close to you may be a way to ensure you have the support you need. Sometimes you learn about other people's experiences with pregnancy loss that they did not disclose previously, and you may end up finding connection and support in ways you did not expect. Keep in mind that who you tell, when you tell, and how much detail you choose to share is completely up to you. If someone who doesn't know asks how the pregnancy is going, you can simply say, "I/we lost the pregnancy, and I'm not ready to talk about it." If your miscarriage occurred after a widespread pregnancy announcement, you can ask a friend to circulate notification of the pregnancy loss, along with resources for how to support you.

What to Say When Someone Miscarries

"I'm so sorry for your loss."
"You are not alone."
"Be gentle with yourself."
"Take the time you need."
"I'm thinking of you."
"Sending love."
"I'm here for you."

GUIDANCE FOR CARE PROVIDERS

Because the majority of miscarriages occur before routine prenatal care begins, you are likely to care for pregnancy loss as an extension of your preconception practice. Be aware that pregnancy loss is much more impactful for families who must conceive via assisted conception, and the resources for pregnancy loss in your greater community are likely to overlook the needs of queer and trans people completely. This means you may be providing additional counseling and support to families who experience loss, and you will need to have resources readily available. Christa Craven's book *Reproductive Losses: Challenges to LGBTQ Family-Making* is an excellent resource for providers, and you can guide clients to the accompanying website as well. Approach those in your community who provide support groups for pregnancy loss and see if their offerings might be appropriate to some or all of the families you serve, and consider collaborating with them and/or providing support groups in your practice to fill this need.

Resources

LGBTQ+ reproductive loss: LGBTQReproductiveLoss.org

ELEVEN

EARLY PREGNANCY AND LACTATION INDUCTION

In addition to queering pregnancy, this chapter covers what you need to know in the early weeks, from taking pregnancy tests to coping with nausea to choosing a care provider. If you are a nongestational parent of any gender and you want to induce lactation, the process takes three to six months, so you will want to get a jump on this during the first half of pregnancy. Here you will find lactation induction protocols, options for chestfeeding after top surgery, and guidelines for infant latch, all within an inclusive, nonjudgmental approach to infant feeding.

Am I Pregnant?

When have you *not* been asking yourself this question over the past two weeks? With every cramp, twinge, need to pee, wave of nausea, and feeling of heaviness or sensitivity in your chest, you have probably wondered if this could be it. As the expected date of your next period grows closer, you are most likely grappling with the choice of whether or not to take a pregnancy test, and if so, when. Can you handle seeing a negative result, or would you rather have forewarning if your period is just going to show up anyway? Should you just wait and see if you miss your period and then test for confirmation? How accurate are pregnancy tests anyway?

URINE PREGNANCY TESTS

A urine pregnancy test is a reagent strip that indicates the presence of the pregnancy hormone hCG in your urine. Some tests give two lines, and others give a plus sign, a "yes" or a "pregnant" to indicate a positive result. While most tests promise 99 percent accuracy, this isn't true until the date your period is expected, and only with concentrated urine when you first wake up in the morning. The biggest risk with a urine pregnancy test is a false negative, which can happen if your urine is too diluted, if you test too early, or if the test is not sensitive enough for an early result. A false positive can occur if you induced ovulation with an hCG trigger shot, especially if you take the test sooner than two weeks later. (Although rare, some tumors can produce hCG, so if you always get a positive on a pregnancy test, be sure to see your physician.) An early detection kit such as First Response can turn positive with a lower level of hCG (6.5 mIU/mL), while other kits turn positive at 10 to 20 mIU/mL.

SERUM PREGNANCY TESTS

A serum pregnancy test requires a blood draw. A qualitative serum test gives you a yes or no answer, but a quantitative serum test actually measures the amount of hCG in your blood. If you are going to the trouble of getting a blood draw, you may as well know the actual level of hCG. The production of hCG can vary from pregnancy to pregnancy, so the range of normal is very wide. For this reason, serum pregnancy tests are typically repeated every two to three days so that the rate of increase can be monitored. This is often called beta hCG testing. The production of hCG begins with implantation, and levels double every two to three days for the first six weeks of pregnancy. Some clinics recommend skipping the urine pregnancy test and getting a serum test instead because hCG can be detected earlier in the serum. If you opt for this method of testing, you can get your blood drawn as soon as ten days after ovulation. The test can be repeated every two to three days over the next week or two to ensure the levels are doubling appropriately.

ULTRASOUND

Dated from the first day of your last menstrual period, or LMP, a gestational sac can be visualized with an internal (transvaginal) ultrasound by five weeks. By six weeks, the yolk sac appears, followed shortly after by the presence of a fetal pole with observable cardiac activity. If you prefer abdominal ultrasound, wait until eight weeks of pregnancy (from the first day of your LMP). Ultrasound evaluation can confirm that the pregnancy is viable, inside the uterus, and the appropriate size for dates. If you do not know when you conceived and you don't have the date of your last period, an early ultrasound can help determine the age of the pregnancy and assign an accurate due date.

DOPPLER

A fetal heartbeat can be heard as early as ten weeks with a high-frequency medical doppler. If your body is a larger-than-average size, you may need to wait until eleven to twelve weeks to hear the heartbeat with a medical doppler due to adipose tissue over the lower abdomen. While there are many home dopplers on the market, these are typically low-frequency dopplers that won't reliably detect a fetal heartbeat until the second trimester of pregnancy. It also takes some skill to find the heartbeat of a fetus who is the size of a strawberry and is tucked deep in the pelvic cavity behind your pubic bone!

Who to Tell

Once you have confirmed your pregnancy, you may be so excited that you want to share your news with the whole world—or at least a few dozen of your closest friends! While it is always a good thing to cultivate shared joy, you might want to be selective about who you come out to in the beginning. Aside from the buzzkill of fielding intrusive, uninformed, and cis/heterocentric questions from people who have no context for queer or trans pregnancy, there is a vital reason to hold back on making a widespread announcement in the first trimester. Whoever you tell about your pregnancy, you will also have to tell if you have a miscarriage. Until you pass age forty-five, the odds are in your favor (see Chapter 10). But because there is a chance of this no matter your age, I encourage you to only share your news with people you would want to have supporting you if a miscarriage were to occur. If you are partnered, make sure you are on the same page about who to share the news with. When you do share, make sure the person you are telling understands that you are maintaining privacy until you feel confident that the pregnancy will continue. Typically this is around the end of the first trimester when the miscarriage rate goes down significantly and testing for chromosomal anomalies is complete (if you opt for it).

Symptoms

Many people experience symptoms of pregnancy even before being able to take a pregnancy test. You might feel chest heaviness and nipple sensitivity, cramping in the lower abdomen, fatigue, and the need to pee more frequently in the first couple of weeks after conception. In addition to those symptoms, nausea, sensitivity to smells, and sometimes vomiting can start within a week or two after a positive pregnancy test. You will start to notice your pants getting snug much earlier than anticipated as your body grows to make room for the baby, expanding the nest your babe will grow into. Soon, your emotions will start to be all over the place, and you may catch yourself crying at TV commercials.

The experience of being pregnant is all-consuming. No matter how intentionally you invited this life to take hold in your body, you may be overwhelmed by how it actually feels to be pregnant. You may feel pride in what your body has accomplished while at the same time feeling betrayed by waves of nausea and daily vomiting sessions. The physical expansion and enhanced sensation in your chest may feel exciting and erotic, or unwanted and deeply dysphoric, or both, depending on the day. You may not want to be touched, or you may experience a surprisingly ravenous libido. You may worry about your ability to keep up with your responsibilities at work and at home as you pass out the moment you get home at the end of the day, and you still feel tired after nine, ten, eleven hours of sleep or more.

How can such a tiny bean make you feel so . . . inhabited? It's because your body is completely renovating itself for the sake of growing another human. It's important to remember this when it feels like you are doing "nothing"—during pregnancy, there is no such thing as doing nothing. Every minute of every day, you are making a human being with your body. Everything else is extra.

Understanding the Pregnant Body

Physiological Changes of Pregnancy	You may experience symptoms like . . .
Progesterone increases by 50 percent by the end of the first trimester.	dizziness, heartburn, reflux, nausea, vomiting, belching, gas, constipation, decreased blood pressure, and/or increased capacity for sleep.
Estrogens increase exponentially over the course of pregnancy (estrone by a hundred times and estriol by a thousand times by the end).	glowing skin, increased appetite, nausea, spider veins, nose bleeds, and/or dental problems (bleeding gums, gingivitis, periodontal disease, and cavities).
Human chorionic gonadotropin (hCG) maxes out at ninety days, then falls to an elevated baseline throughout pregnancy.	nausea, vomiting, increased appetite, increased thirst, changes in taste and smell, bloating and weight gain, and/or rapid changes in blood sugar.
Relaxin levels increase by ten times in the first trimester and sustain throughout pregnancy.	loose connective tissue, contributing to shoulder, knee, hip, and ankle pain, as well as pain and inflammation in the low back and increased clumsiness.
Adrenal and pituitary hormones increase.	frequent urination; increased cardiac output; and/or increased skin pigmentation on nipples/areola, face (the so-called mask of pregnancy), freckles, scars, and navel to pubis (linea nigra).

Thyroid hormone production increases.	dizziness, heartburn, reflux, nausea, vomiting, belching, gas, constipation, decreased blood pressure, and/or increased capacity for sleep.
Uterine muscle changes in size, shape, and contractile activity, eventually becoming the largest muscle in the human body.	rapid enlargement of the lower abdomen as the neck of the uterus lengthens from 7 to 25 millimeters and the top of the uterus extends above the pubic bone by twelve weeks, putting pressure on the bladder which causes increased frequency of urination.
Blood flow to the sexual organs increases.	internal tissues becoming more stretchy and accommodating, increased lubrication and discharge, and possibly increased libido.
Vascularization of chest tissue increases.	superficial veins becoming more prominent, resulting in a marbled appearance, while chest tissue becomes heavy and sensitive or achy.
Total blood volume as well as cardiac output increases by up to 50 percent by midpregnancy.	easily running out of breath, heart palpitations, and swelling of hands and feet.
The diaphragm is displaced upward by 4 centimeters in the first trimester, and the rib cage widens and expands. Respiratory effort increases so that by the end of pregnancy, 16 to 20 percent more oxygen is consumed.	labored breathing, even in early pregnancy.
Changes occur in the upper respiratory system such as engorgement of nasal capillaries and swelling of the vocal cords.	difficulty breathing through the nose, hoarseness and deepening of the voice, increased severity of respiratory infections, sleep apnea, and/or snoring.
Kidneys enlarge, ureters distend, and bladder tone decreases to accommodate greater excretion of waste as metabolism increases.	frequent and copious urination, increased susceptibility to urinary tract infections, and/or stress incontinence.
Sensitivity to glucose and insulin increases in the first half of pregnancy for enhanced nutrient absorption.	rapid drops in blood sugar between meals and overnight, contributing to nausea, vomiting, fatigue, and emotional ups and downs.
Insulin resistance occurs in late pregnancy to enhance protein synthesis for the fetus. Insulin levels double by the third trimester.	gestational diabetes as the pancreas struggles to produce enough insulin to process excess glucose from a high carbohydrate diet, ultimately shunting excess sugar to the baby and increasing the risk of birth complications and neonatal hypoglycemia.

Caring for Your Body
During Pregnancy

First of all, understand that being pregnant is a lot of work. If you can't exercise like you used to, you are not weak or out of shape—you're pregnant. If you want to sleep all the time, you are not lazy—you're pregnant. If you want to have sex all the time, or you don't want to have sex at all, there's nothing wrong with you—you're pregnant. Do not underestimate the work your body is doing. The chart on pages 250–251 provides perspective on a wide array of pregnancy symptoms and why they occur. Because so many of them are due to hormonal and physiological changes of pregnancy, they may be somewhat beyond your control. However, you can diminish the severity of some of the discomforts of pregnancy by ensuring your body has the nutrients, movement, and rest it needs to function to the best of its ability.

EXERCISE

Exercise regularly but be ready to pull back or stop if you tire easily. Aim for thirty to sixty minutes of moderate physical activity every day (walking, dancing, swimming, stationary cycling, aerobic workouts, resistance bands or weights, yoga), including warm-up, cooldown, and stretching. Use the "talk test" to make sure your heart and respiratory rate are not too high to carry on a conversation during exercise. If you are an athlete or regularly did vigorous workouts prior to pregnancy, you can continue as long as you consult with your care provider and you don't overheat, you stay hydrated, and you get enough nutrition to support the increased caloric needs of a very active pregnancy. Avoid activities that are prone to physical impact or falling. Be aware that your connective tissue can easily overextend due to increased relaxin and joint mobility, so pay attention to body mechanics and core strength, especially during yoga. Benefits of exercise during pregnancy include reduced risk of gestational diabetes, gestational hypertension, preterm birth, low birth weight, and cesarean delivery. You will also find your digestion is improved, decreasing constipation and hemorrhoids.

SLEEP

Sleep when you need to. Nap often. Sleep in the position that is most comfortable for you. Current evidence debunks earlier studies that promoted specific positions for sleep during pregnancy, although most people are most comfortable sleeping on their side. As your belly (and your chest) grows, use lots and lots of pillows—one between your knees, one under your top arm, and one under your abdomen—or invest in a body pillow. Allow extra time to get the rest you need in late pregnancy when your bladder is unlikely to let you sleep through the night. Nutrient deficiencies can disrupt your sleep, such as restless leg syndrome brought on by iron or folate deficiency, and leg cramps, which can be mediated by calcium/magnesium and vitamin B complex (B_1 and B_6, specifically).

NUTRITION

Nutritional recommendations in pregnancy are essentially the same as preconception (see Chapter 2), although you will need to increase caloric intake by about five hundred calories per day. Many obstetricians and even some midwives perpetuate strict guidelines around weight gain in pregnancy, which are intertwined with societal bias against fat bodies. As long as you are eating nutrient-dense foods, avoiding excess sugar and junk food, exercising regularly, and getting enough rest, you can trust the pattern at which your physical body adjusts to pregnancy. Some people with large bodies don't gain at all or even lose weight in early pregnancy. Some people with small bodies gain weight quickly and feel alarmed by the changes. Keep in mind that obstetric guidelines for weight gain in pregnancy merely reflect the weight of the uterus, fetus, amniotic fluid, placenta, expanded blood volume, and growth of milk-producing anatomy. They do not account for the ways a human being changes when going through a major life transition, and all the ways our emotions, our relationships, and our social lives intersect with food. Healthy practices, and getting the support you need to maintain them, are worthy of your time and attention. Body shaming is not.

BLOOD SUGAR IN PREGNANCY

In terms of healthy eating practices, one of the primary things to focus on during pregnancy is your blood sugar. Because of the ways that carbohydrate metabolism changes in pregnancy, maintaining glucose levels can make a huge difference in how you feel as well as in avoiding major complications of pregnancy.

Starting in the early weeks of pregnancy, the body is primed by hCG to absorb glucose quickly and efficiently. This means that you may need to eat something before getting out of bed in the morning. It also means that you will need to eat more frequently in order to keep your glucose levels stable. Changes in blood sugar can happen so rapidly that by the time you feel hungry and then make something to eat, you might feel too nauseous to eat the food you have prepared for yourself. Keep an eye on how much time lapses after a meal or snack before you feel hungry or nauseous again, and use that as your guide for when to eat. If you tend to feel hungry or nauseous again after two hours, make sure there is food available for you to put into your mouth at two hours. Don't wait for the two-hour mark and then rummage around in the kitchen, and end up finally eating (or not being able to because you feel awful) at two and a half or three hours.

It is not uncommon for pregnant people to need to eat every two hours, or even every hour, in order to keep nausea at bay in the first trimester. It is also not uncommon for pregnant people to only be able to eat bland, white foods, which typically are high in carbohydrates. Your best bet is to eat frequently enough that nausea doesn't prevent you from eating. And eat what you can, when you can. If you can get ahead of your blood sugar curve, you may be more successful in being able to stomach protein, fruits, and vegetables. Try to find some protein sources that you can eat on a regular basis (blanched almonds are also white!) so that you can work toward mitigating the blood sugar ups and downs of eating too many carbohydrates. If you can only do cooked veggies, or you can only do fresh veggies, or you can only do certain veggies but not others, so be it. However, if you aren't feeding yourself frequently enough, the nausea will inhibit you from getting the nutrition you need. In the same way you will need to be available to feed your baby frequently in the first weeks of life, you must feed your body frequently now as you grow your baby inside.

As your nausea (hopefully) subsides in the second trimester of pregnancy, and even if it doesn't, be sure to start shifting to a more focused attempt at maintaining your blood sugar with protein rather than high-carb foods. This is because your body will be shifting from an insulin-sensitive state to an insulin-resistant one, and if you eat too many carbohydrates, your pancreas might not be able to keep up. This results in a condition called gestational diabetes, which is a complication of pregnancy. Screening for gestational diabetes doesn't happen until twenty-four to twenty-eight weeks, but prevention of gestational diabetes starts much earlier—even before you are pregnant. There are significant risks associated with gestational diabetes (gestational hypertension, preeclampsia, large-for-gestational-age infant, birth trauma and operative delivery, and neonatal hypoglycemia and jaundice). However, just because you are diagnosed with this condition does not mean these risks will come to pass. As long as you are able to maintain normal glucose levels, the risks can be mitigated (this is called "diet-controlled" gestational diabetes). In addition to exercising daily and taking medication or supplements to help with insulin sensitivity (metformin or inositol), you will monitor your glucose levels using a home glucometer, which provides in-the-moment feedback to guide you in your food choices. Ultimately, there is no escaping the need to pay attention to your blood sugar. In most cases, the prevention of gestational diabetes is also the cure: keeping blood sugar stable with consistent doses of protein and regular exercise.

UNRESOLVED NAUSEA

If eating something every hour or two does not resolve your nausea or if you are vomiting more than once per day, you need and deserve more help. If your supplements are making you nauseous, try taking them at night, or skip them all together until your nausea improves. Drink fluids at least half an hour away from foods. Non-pharmacological remedies for nausea in pregnancy include crystallized ginger or ginger candy, lemon or peppermint tea or ice cubes, ginger ale, lemonade or bubble water, acupressure wrist bands designed for motion sickness (Sea-Bands), acupuncture, or homeopathic remedies as indicated. Vitamin B6 can be used alone in doses of 25 milligrams three times daily, or check with your care provider about taking it in combination with doxylamine (Unisom). If you are having a lot of vomiting, there are a variety of other medications available, so keep reaching out to your care provider if the situation is not resolving. If you can't keep food or fluids down for twelve hours, you will need to be evaluated to rule out other causes of the vomiting, assess for electrolyte imbalance, and receive IV fluid therapy. Hyperemesis gravidarum is a horrible and dangerous condition that occurs in 0.3 to 2 percent of pregnancies, in which vomiting is persistent and severe and does not resolve on its own, requiring hospitalization to prevent adverse effects on the fetus and the pregnant person. If you are vomiting a lot, you feel faint when you stand up, or your urine is scant or dark, please contact your care provider or go to the nearest emergency room.

CARING FOR YOUR MENTAL HEALTH DURING PREGNANCY

If you have a history of depression, anxiety, or another mood disorder, the hormones of pregnancy and/or the transition after birth may bring back or exacerbate your mental health concerns. The same is true for nongestational parents, who can also experience increased depression and anxiety after the arrival of a new baby. During pregnancy, it is important to establish care with a therapist who specializes in perinatal mental health, as well as a prescriptive provider who can manage medications appropriately for pregnancy and lactation. Referrals can be found through Postpartum Support International. You can also set things up well for yourself by doing everything you can to access a trauma-informed provider for your birth and hiring a doula to assist you and your family during labor and postpartum recovery.

PROTECTING YOUR PREGNANCY

- To prevent contracting listeria, avoid the following: unpasteurized juice and dairy products such as raw milk and soft cheeses; raw, smoked, or undercooked meats, fish, and eggs, including raw cookie dough; and meat or seafood products from the deli counter. Always reheat precooked hot dogs or sausages.

- To prevent contracting toxoplasmosis, wash fruits and vegetables before eating, avoid raw sprouts, and wash cutting boards and food preparation surfaces thoroughly. Avoid contact with cat feces by wearing a mask while cleaning the litter box and washing your hands thoroughly after handling cats or gardening.

- Avoid consumption of high-mercury fish (see Chapter 2).

- Wear your seat belt low across your lap instead of across your abdomen.

- Avoid hot tubs and saunas during pregnancy, or limit duration of use to avoid elevating core temperature (fewer than ten minutes at 102 degrees).

- Get your flu vaccine as soon as it is available each year, and get the COVID-19 vaccine as currently recommended. The Tdap vaccine will be offered in the third trimester of pregnancy to provide temporary immunity to your newborn.

- To avoid contracting childhood infections such as CMV, varicella, rubella, and parvovirus during pregnancy, wash your hands thoroughly after contact with diapers or oral/nasal secretions of children, and avoid sharing food, drinks, or utensils or kissing young children on the mouth or cheek.

Thoroughly clean toys, countertops, and surfaces that may come into contact with young children.

- Be sure to protect yourself from STI transmission during pregnancy.

- Do not travel to Zika areas, and use barriers for sexual activity with any partners who have traveled to a Zika area for the duration of your pregnancy. If you live in a Zika area, prevent mosquito bites by wearing long pants and sleeves, maintain screens on your home, sleep under a mosquito net, and use mosquito repellent that is safe for pregnancy.

- Intimate partner violence may escalate during pregnancy. Talk to a trusted friend, therapist, or pregnancy care provider. Have an escape plan, including a safe place to go; memorized phone numbers; and a bag with important documents, ID and passport, cash, clothes, and valuables in case you need to leave with little notice. You and your baby deserve a home that is filled with love, safety, and respect.

Choosing a Prenatal Care Provider

You need not decide on your place of birth at the outset of your prenatal care. In fact, many people find that their ideas about where they would feel most comfortable giving birth change as they learn more about the available options and do more soul-searching about what feels right. You can change care providers and alter plans for your birth at any point in time. Your prenatal care lasts seven to eight months, while your labor and birth will only last a matter of hours or days. For all of these reasons, start your search for a care provider based on what you want out of your prenatal care, and hold off on the final decision about place of birth until you can make a more informed decision.

MIDWIFERY CARE

If you appreciate the ways that this book approaches you as a whole person, teaches you how your body works, respects your agency to make decisions for yourself and your family, provides a preventive approach to health, normalizes conception and pregnancy, and takes a critical approach to evaluating and applying available scientific evidence, congratulations! You are experiencing the midwifery model of care. Midwives are independent health care providers who serve pregnant people and families throughout the childbearing process. People who choose midwifery care for their pregnancies:

- Want to take an active role in supporting their health.
- Desire a relationship with their care provider built on mutual trust.
- Value shared decision-making as a vital aspect of care.
- Prefer a model of care that upholds bodily autonomy.
- View pregnancy and birth as normal, physiological events.

Some people worry that being in care with a midwife means that you don't have access to medical care, but nothing could be further from the truth. Midwives provide the same clinical prenatal care as physicians do, we just approach it as an opportunity to help you understand and build trust in your body's abilities and stay connected to your pregnancy. Receiving care from a midwife doesn't mean you don't have access to a physician or a hospital if you need it. Independent midwives who are not part of a hospital system generally have a positive outlook on physician consultation and referral and a solid plan for transfer of care when indicated.

Just as with any health care provider, some midwives are queer and trans inclusive, and some are not. This is ironic when you consider that trans people opt for midwifery care at much higher rates than cis/hetero populations. Some midwives seem to be queer inclusive or are queer identified themselves, but their consideration only extends to cisgender women. This may seem acceptable if this is how both you and your partner identify, but be aware that this approach can still marginalize the nongestational mother-to-be, especially when the word "mother" is used exclusively in reference to the pregnant parent. Pay attention to red flags on provider websites such as language that is exclusive to cisgender women and images that only include heterosexual couples. Inclusivity is such a breath of fresh air that you will know it when you see it. No matter how a practice appears on the surface, if you find that you are put in the position of having to educate your provider, if you are misgendered or repeatedly have the wrong name or pronouns used to refer to you, or you find yourself fielding intrusive questions that are unrelated to your care, pay attention and give credence to how these interactions make you feel. It's never too late to change care providers. Ask around in your community or on social media, or contact the Queer and Transgender Midwives Association for referrals in your area.

Certified Professional Midwives (a.k.a. Licensed Midwives, Direct-Entry Midwives, Certified Midwives, Registered Midwives) typically spend thirty to sixty minutes with you at every prenatal visit. Visits are held once a month until the third trimester, then every two weeks, and weekly during the final month of pregnancy. Postpartum care is frequent and attentive, often consisting of two to three home visits in the first week after birth, plus additional visits at three and six weeks postpartum. CPMs typically work solo or in small two- to three-person midwife teams and attend births in homes or birth freestanding birth centers, but in Canada, registered midwives also attend births in hospitals.

Certified Nurse-Midwives typically spend fifteen to thirty minutes at each prenatal visit, sometimes less. The schedule of prenatal visits varies, and part of the care may be provided in a group model. Postpartum visits are conducted in the clinic, and there may be only one to three postpartum visits in total. CNMs typically provide care in a clinic setting as part of a larger group practice and attend births in hospitals; however, there are a few who practice independently, in a practice model similar to CPMs, including attending out-of-hospital births.

OB CARE

Obstetricians typically spend five to ten minutes performing a brief exam at each visit, and the remainder of assessments such as vital signs and blood draws are performed by adjunct staff. Prenatal visits are the least frequent in this model, every four to six weeks until the third trimester, then every two to three weeks, then weekly in the final month of pregnancy. There is typically only one postpartum visit, which is conducted at six weeks after birth. OBs provide care in clinics or as part of hospital systems. OBs care for normal pregnancies as well as complicated pregnancies, although some, called perinatologists or maternal-fetal medicine specialists, focus on high-risk pregnancies. OBs typically espouse an authoritative approach to care rather than the participatory, shared-decision-making model used by midwives. There is little participation on the part of the pregnant person other than showing up for appointments and completing tests as directed. On the other hand, if your pregnancy is complicated, you will need an OB or perinatologist, and finding a caring and affirming one can really make a difference in your experience.

Options for Place of Birth

As long as your pregnancy is healthy and uncomplicated, you can safely choose to give birth at home, in a freestanding birth center, or at a hospital. Many people feel torn between a desire for a more holistic experience and the cultural messaging about hospitals being the safest place to give birth, but the science proves otherwise. Large studies show that home birth is at least as safe as birth in the hospital—often safer—and always with lower rates of intervention. If you choose to give birth in a hospital, know that you will reduce your chance of interventions, including cesarean birth, by going with a hospital-based midwife team, as well as having a doula present during labor.

Queering Pregnancy

The experience of pregnancy puts us face-to-face with rampant cultural stereotypes based on binary understandings of gender. Heterosexual norms permeate social constructs at every level. Your queerness means that you will run into experiences of otherness over and over again as you walk through the world as an expectant parent. If you are nonbinary or transgender, your sense of marginalization and dysphoria may be so heightened that navigating care during pregnancy pits your needs as an expectant parent against your needs for affirmation, embodiment, and safety.

Meanwhile, you are undertaking one of the most significant life changes you will ever experience. Becoming a parent changes everything. Every aspect of identity we have affects how we walk through the world, and the identity of "parent" intersects with all of them. Going through such a transition in isolation can be completely disorienting, but seeing ourselves reflected in community offers affirming points of contact and a deep level of camaraderie as everything about who we are shifts into who we are as parents.

This is why community is so vital to well-being during the formation of family. The sense of resonance we feel when we are with others who have shared experience means shared vulnerability, which is the pathway to heart-centered connection. Alone, you might wonder if you are doing it right, if there is something wrong with you for feeling how you feel, if you are good enough. In connection with others, we see that there are many valid ways of being, that all new parents cope with a surprising range of heightened emotions, and that, of course, we are all good enough—in fact, we are amazing!

When there is a history of being questioned, invalidated, and even hated for our queerness and/or our gender, this core aspect of identity needs to be affirmed in any circle we seek for support. You may find you have more in common with straight people than you ever have as you enter parenthood, but you may ultimately find a deeper level of kinship with other queer and trans parents, especially if you also share intersectional identities such as race, socioeconomic class, or disability. It stands to reason that the more aspects of identity we share with another person, the less we have to explain ourselves. Being in queer community can provide a sense of openness that happens when we are free from monitoring whether or not we need to have our guard up. It can be extremely powerful to see ourselves reflected and feel that we truly belong.

On the other hand, trans people who are excluded from queer spaces, as well as BIPOC people trying to access queer community in a sea of whiteness, often find the lack of inclusivity heartbreaking. When queer communities do not hold themselves accountable for undoing an internalized sense of cis and white superiority, there is no safe harbor for those of us who need it most. Considering the added implications of racism and transphobia for a person's physical and emotional safety during pregnancy, it stands to reason that many trans and BIPOC people must gravitate toward spaces that offer the greatest sense of refuge, and unfortunately, queer spaces often fall way too short. Consider that Black and Indigenous people are two to three times more likely to die from complications of pregnancy than white people (four to five times higher when over age thirty), and Black babies die at more than twice the rate of white babies in the first year of life. Because of this, BIPOC parents-to-be often feel a greater sense of safety and connection with BIPOC communities specifically, even if they are predominantly straight. For words of solidarity and healing, including queer, trans, and nonbinary voices, check out *You Are Your Best Thing: Vulnerability, Shame Resilience, and the Black Experience*, edited by Tarana Burke and Brené Brown.

If you walk through the world with white and/or cisgender privilege, it is your responsibility to find ways to utilize that privilege in a way that restores justice to our community as a whole. Read *So You Want to Talk About Race* by Ijeoma Oluo. View the documentary *I Am Not Your Negro*, inspired by the work of James Baldwin. Flip through *Gender: A Graphic Guide* by Meg-John Barker and Jules Scheele, check out the tips for allies of transgender people on the GLAAD website, and watch *Disclosure: Trans Lives on Screen*, directed by Sam Feder and produced by Laverne Cox. Be quiet and listen when those from marginalized communities speak. Step aside and make space for trans and BIPOC leadership in your organizations. Our task as a community is to circle around to welcome and protect those of us who are most vulnerable. Participate in creating community that is by us, for us, and about us—and that includes all of us.

Being able to share the ways in which we are confronted with our otherness as queer and trans parents is powerful. The more we can create spaces for sharing our stories and truly being heard, the more we can cultivate a sense of connection and belonging. It is vital to have a safe space to talk about day-to-day interactions in a cis/heterocentric world, from coming out at work in order to access family medical leave, to navigating medical forms and a health care system based on the gender binary, to dealing with family of origin, to how to find gender-appropriate pregnancy clothing, to the ways in which childbearing is affecting the dynamics of our relationships. We become each other's role models as we actively navigate our changing identity. These moments of shared experience not only provide support, they build our sense of pride in ourselves, our relationships, and our families.

The experience of parenting in community has the potential to bring us together in deeper, more heartfelt ways than bar culture ever did. So many of us came out and were able to access community through the gay bar scene, which presented valuable opportunities for self-expression within a celebratory atmosphere. Whether your queer enculturation was built around the consumption of drugs and alcohol, or you found yourself using substances to help you cope in a homophobic, transphobic world, accessing queer parenting community has the potential to provide validation and affirmation without the need for liquid courage. It is worth acknowledging that many members of our community are in recovery, and we can do a great service toward inclusivity and mutual support by keeping alcohol and recreational drugs out of our gatherings of queer and trans parents.

Even if you are not typically someone who gravitates toward being social or participating in groups, this is a unique time of life when you truly do need your community. Soon, you will be cultivating your child's self-esteem and sense of belonging in the world, which means that being in connection with other queer families with broad representations of gender and racial identities is even more important. If you are not already connected with a community of queer families, make this a priority during your pregnancy. Once your baby arrives, you will benefit deeply from the social nest you have created for yourself as you launch into parenthood. In fact, once your baby is here, it will not only be difficult to muster the energy for forging new relationships, but the level of vulnerability all new parents feel can inhibit your capacity for reaching out (although you will soon find that your reluctance is unfounded, because everyone is struggling, and I promise, you are not the only one).

Use social media not as the container for accessing community but as the launching point for bringing real relationships into your life. Connect with local families through queer pregnancy groups and classes. Ask your midwife, doctor, doula, therapist, or childbirth educator if they know other families like yours they can connect you with. Take the initiative to reach out and meet up at a park, even if you have to do it masked and six feet apart. Offer a time to meet up on Zoom or FaceTime, even if it's just a short twenty-minute chat over coffee on a Saturday morning. Yes, you are cruising for queer and trans friends! Reach out and make it happen. You have everything to gain by building the community that will hold, nurture, and support you and your family through the transition to parenthood and the years of raising a child.

Planning for Lactation and Infant Feeding

It is true that there are real benefits to human milk; however, if human milk is not available, then formula is the next best thing. The decisions we make about feeding our babies affect how we feel about ourselves, how we feel in our bodies, and the level of stress we experience in the early weeks of parenting. How we feed our babies is but one aspect of parenting. There is truly no place for anyone else's opinion in how you choose to use your body, and that includes the decision about whether or not to use your body to feed your baby.

OPTIONS FOR FEEDING YOUR BABY

- Babies can be fed human milk or formula, or a combination of the two.

- They can be fed through a bottle, a feeding tube, a milk-producing chest, or a combination of these methods.

- Anyone can use a supplemental nursing system to feed their baby with their body, whether or not their body makes milk.

- Human milk can be accessed by producing it yourself, direct donation from another lactating person, or through a milk bank, and various types of infant formula can be purchased in stores or online.

- Transmasculine and nonbinary people who have had top surgery may still be able to produce milk following pregnancy, and it's possible to do so while on gender-affirming hormones.

- Anyone who has the glandular framework to make milk can induce lactation, including trans women and people with ovaries who have not carried a pregnancy.

PHYSIOLOGY OF HUMAN LACTATION

Regardless of other aspects of our reproductive biology, we are all born with the same basic anatomy capable of producing milk. This means that anyone can potentially produce milk to feed their baby! The chart on the opposite page provides an overview of how lactation occurs in the human body. The column on the left describes the hormonal events that cause the body to lactate. The following columns outline how each step occurs in different bodies.

LACTATION INDUCTION

For the past twenty-plus years, people have been inducing lactation based on a protocol developed by Jack Newman, MD, in collaboration with his patient Lenore Goldfarb, PhD, who wanted to induce lactation to feed her baby arriving via surrogacy. Very little has changed because the protocol they designed works relatively well based on anecdotal and clinical evidence; however, no large-scale studies have been conducted. In 2018, Reisman and Goldstein published a case study of a trans woman who successfully induced lactation by following a modified Newman-Goldfarb protocol, but there is no research yet to inform the ideal protocol for transfeminine lactation induction.

Meanwhile, people who wish to make milk to feed their babies have been using the protocols, although outcomes vary from person to person. Some people are not able to utilize some of the medications in the protocol due to health considerations, and still many are able to make some amount of milk. Some people follow every part of the protocol and still don't achieve a full milk supply. However, a range of outcomes can still be considered "success" because success is defined by no one else but you. What you term success may also change over time as the reality of what it takes to induce lactation sets in. Many reflect that it is like a part-time job. And, making milk and/or feeding a baby with your body does not happen in a vacuum. It requires constant interaction with your chest. It often happens in the midst of learning to care for a newborn, on very little sleep, while trying to support a partner who is recovering from birth and possibly establishing lactation themselves. Medications and supplements are costly and may have side effects. Pumping equipment must be rented or purchased, and attachments must be cleaned and disinfected on a regular basis. You will definitely want a queer or trans-sensitive IBCLC (International Board Certified Lactation Consultant) to support you—ask your care provider or others in your community for a referral. Lactation induction is no small undertaking, but for many, it's worth it to try.

Physiology of Human Lactation

How Lactation Occurs . . .	in Bodies with Ovaries and Pregnancy	in Bodies with Ovaries without Pregnancy	in Bodies without Ovaries or Pregnancy
Chest development with onset of estrogen and progesterone	Natal puberty	Natal puberty	Feminizing hormone therapy
More chest development with an increase in estrogen and progesterone	Pregnancy	Oral contraceptive pills	Increase estrogen dose and consider adding progesterone, continue antiandrogen if needed
Production of prolactin, the hormone that makes milk	Pregnancy, plus further enhancement via hand expression of colostrum in late pregnancy	Domperidone/herbs plus pumping, hand expression, or feeding	Domperidone/herbs plus pumping, hand expression, or feeding
Rapid drop in estrogen and progesterone	Childbirth	Stopping oral contraceptive pills	Decrease estrogen and progesterone dose, continue antiandrogen if needed
Prolactin receptors multiply in response to the release of milk	Feeding, pumping, or hand expressing	Feeding, pumping, or hand expressing	Feeding, pumping, or hand expressing

MEDICATIONS, HERBS, AND PUMPS
FOR LACTATION INDUCTION

Estrogen/progesterone: For people with ovaries, oral contraceptive pills (OCPs) can be used. Recommended formulations are Yasmin (drospirenone, 3 milligrams, and ethinyl estradiol, 0.03 milligrams) or Microgestin (norethindrone, 1 milligram, and ethinyl estradiol, 20 micrograms). A $\frac{1}{35}$ combination formula can also be used, although if chest changes don't occur within two weeks, add 1 milligram oral progesterone, or switch to Yasmin or Microgestin. At minimum, OCPs must contain at least 1 milligram oral progesterone, ideally 2 to 3 milligrams, and no more than 0.035 milligrams estrogen. The pills must be taken continuously (no break for menses—remember, you are mimicking pregnancy). Contraindications are the same as for anyone using OCPs (cardiac conditions, clotting disorders, hypertension, smoking). Alternatively, an estrogen patch can be used along with oral progesterone. If you experience depression while taking oral contraceptives, consider an SSRI that is compatible with human milk feeding, such as sertraline (Zoloft).

For people who already utilize exogenous estrogen and progesterone due to lack of ovarian production (such as trans women), case studies show estrogen can be gradually increased to 12 milligrams a day or triple the baseline dose, and oral progesterone can be increased to 400 milligrams or double the baseline dose. If you are unable to find a health care provider to write these prescriptions for you, know that some people have been able to save up estrogen by ordering refills ahead of time, and some are able to get the changes they need with topical progesterone, which is available over the counter. Once lactation is established, estrogen can be reduced to a 0.025 milligrams daily patch and oral progesterone to 100 milligrams daily.

As with so many aspects of queer and trans health, finding a provider to support you in lactation induction can be difficult. However limited, evidence does exist to demonstrate the safety and nutritional adequacy of human milk after lactation induction. Start the conversation early and provide your doctor or nurse practitioner with the information in this book, or find a more affirming provider so that you have the care you need when you need it.

Domperidone is a dopamine antagonist used for nausea and vomiting, indigestion, and reflux, and it is used off-label in many countries for increasing prolactin levels and stimulating lactation. The most common side effects are GI upset, chest engorgement, weight gain, headache, dizziness, irritability, and fatigue. Domperidone is contraindicated in those who have a history of cardiac arrhythmias, or in those who experience abnormal heart rate or rhythm while taking the medication. People in the United States must import domperidone from Canada or other countries due to FDA restrictions, although sometimes it can be made available at a compounding pharmacy. When importing medications to the United States, no more than a three-month supply can be shipped at one time. There is always a risk that your order will be confiscated at customs, but a large shipment is almost guaranteed to be confiscated.

The Newman-Goldfarb protocol recommends starting domperidone at a dose of 10 milligrams four times a day for the first week, followed by 20 milligrams four times a day, although if you are short on time, you can start with the 20-milligram dose. (Be prepared for strong side effects if you don't have time to ramp up.)

Many people continue domperidone for the duration of lactation, but you may be able to stop taking it once lactation is well established. However, it's important to wean off very slowly to avoid psychiatric side effects such as anxiety and insomnia, while keeping a close eye on your milk production to ensure you are maintaining your supply.

A typical schedule for weaning off domperidone looks like:

- Drop one daily dose for two weeks (20 milligrams, three times a day).

- Drop dosage to 10 milligrams for two weeks (10 milligrams, four times a day).

Then, every two weeks:

- Drop to 10 milligrams, three times a day.

- Drop to 10 milligrams, two times a day.

- Drop to 10 milligrams, one time a day.

Herbal galactagogues used in the Newman-Goldfarb protocol include fenugreek (1,500 to 1,800 milligrams) and blessed thistle (1,000 milligrams) three times daily with food. Fenugreek makes your sweat and urine smell like maple syrup, and it may be contraindicated for those who have diabetes or asthma. The protocol also mentions that eating oatmeal three times a week can be helpful. Other herbs commonly used to support lactation include goat's rue, which is used to enhance the development of milk-producing framework in the last trimester of pregnancy, and alfalfa, milk thistle, shatavari, and moringa, which are used to boost the supply of milk. Herbal medicine is most potent in tincture or capsule form, although infusions of whole herbs steeped overnight can also provide a medicinal potency. While there is no reason not to use commercial herbal tea bags for lactation support, if your desire is to use herbs medicinally, the dose from a tea bag steeped for ten minutes is very small in comparison to an infusion.

Fluids such as water and herbal teas are very important to support the production of human milk. Drink at least eight glasses per day, and avoid anything dehydrating, including high amounts of caffeine.

A hospital-grade, double electric pump is preferable for initiating lactation. The most widely available model is the Medela Symphony, which can be rented from a lactation consultant, hospital, or other business that serves families with newborns in your area. Once lactation is established, you can switch to a pump of your choosing. Many people enjoy the convenience and efficiency of a double electric, variable-speed model such as the Medela Pump In Style, which is an easy switch if you were previously using the Symphony, because all the tubes and flanges are compatible with both.

It is imperative to ensure that you are using the proper-size flange. Select your size by measuring the diameter of your nipple (nipple only—not the areola). When applied, there should not be areola tissue inside the tunnel of the flange, only the nipple, which should have enough space to move freely. If pumping hurts your nipple or you see any blanching around the base or tip of your nipple, the flange is too small.

LACTATION INDUCTION PROTOCOL

The Canadian Breastfeeding Foundation has outlined the Newman-Goldfarb protocols (see page 279) based on the amount of time available before baby's arrival as well as adjusted protocols for those who cannot use oral contraceptive pills. A summary of the basic protocol is presented here with integration of the case study protocol for trans women.

1. Start OCP or increase estrogen/progesterone, and/or

2. Start domperidone, 20 milligrams, four times a day

This phase of the protocol takes at least thirty days, until significant chest changes occur, including fullness, heaviness and soreness, and an increase in cup size. This protocol can be started as soon as six to nine months prior to baby's arrival. If you have more than two months until baby arrives, ramp up slowly with 10 milligrams domperidone for the first week to make it easier for your digestive system to adjust. If you are postmenopausal, allow sixty days for initial changes to occur. If you are unable to use OCP, just start with domperidone alone, but add herbal galactagogues after one week on the full dose of domperidone.

Then, during the final six weeks of the protocol, which could be before or after your baby arrives, do the following:

3. Discontinue OCP or decrease estrogen/progesterone.

4. Continue domperidone, 20 milligrams, four times a day.

5. Add herbal galactagogues if you haven't already.

6. Start pumping every three hours and ideally once at night. Pump for five to seven minutes, then massage, stroke, shake, then pump five to seven minutes more. Frequency is more important than duration—pumping for a longer time at each session will not help and may increase discomfort. Start with a low setting until you get used to the sensation.

Feed Your Baby

Once you start feeding, continue domperidone 20 milligrams, four times a day, for the duration of lactation. You can continue using herbal galactagogues as well. For a full supply, feed baby or pump at least eight to twelve times a day. You can follow feeding sessions with ten minutes of pumping to further ensure supply. If co-nursing, pump when your partner feeds, and your partner should pump when you feed. If you (or your partner) do not desire a full milk supply, you can do fewer pumping or feeding sessions. If you decide to decrease the number of pumping sessions, do this gradually so you don't become engorged, and watch for pain or redness that could indicate a plugged duct or infection.

Adjust the Protocol Based on Your Needs

How you go about lactation induction depends on your goals. If you want the greatest assurance of a full milk supply, all steps must be followed, and ideally, you will start the protocol six months before baby arrives. If you are going to be sharing feeding with a lactating partner or you just want to produce a partial supply, you can skip the birth control pills, or the domperidone, or pump less, but with each of these omissions, your capacity to make milk decreases. If you have given birth and lactated before, you may not need the full protocol to regain lactation, but this depends on whether you had a full supply the first time around, and how long it's been since you last lactated.

CO-NURSING AND BONDING

If you are partnered and both planning to lactate and feed, keep in mind that you may have varying levels of success in how much milk you are each able to produce. At certain times, your baby might prefer to feed from one parent more than the other, but that doesn't mean they love that parent more; it just means they are going for the food that is most copious and available, or maybe they prefer one type of nipple over the other. Some parents find that the reality of life with a newborn makes all the extra work involved with pumping simply not worth it—however, you might worry that if you don't continue with lactation, your baby won't bond with you as much. If you find yourself in this situation, make sure you take time to hold, rock, dress, change, sing, and talk to your baby a lot. Don't allow your fears to lead you to withdraw. Instead, use the extra time and energy you would have spent pumping in direct connection with your baby. And keep in mind that while the nursing relationship can be quite special, as your baby grows, they will eventually be interested in much more than milk. And no matter how your infant is fed, it is normal for babies, toddlers, and kids to prefer one parent over another at any given point. While it can be heartbreaking the first time it happens, it tends to come and go in phases. At some point in time, you will be the favorite, and the pendulum will swing back again.

FEEDING AFTER CHEST MASCULINIZATION SURGERY

Even if you completed top surgery prior to considering pregnancy, or as a prerequisite to carrying a pregnancy, don't discount the idea that you may potentially consider chestfeeding. Once you experience the awe of what your body can do after gestating a child, the possibility of feeding a child with your body may take on new meaning. The first time your baby starts rooting around to find your nipple and feed, you may open your mind to the possibility of making it happen. And if your chest starts to leak some milk after giving birth, you may feel moved to take advantage of what your body is offering to your baby.

It is possible for any (or all) of these things to happen to you and still feel overwhelming dysphoria while nursing your baby. Each and every one of us is a complex human being, and nursing a baby is certainly wrought with complexity. If you find that you do want to feed your baby with your body, you can do that by using a feeding tube that provides supplemental milk or formula in addition to any milk your body makes, or even if you don't make any milk at all. If your body does make some milk but chestfeeding is not feasible for you, you can hand express and give the milk to your baby with a syringe, a feeding tube and syringe attached to your finger, or in a small cup. If you find that you appreciate the value of skin-to-skin contact to support relaxation and bonding, you can make that happen without doing *any* feeding with your body. Ultimately, the goal is to feel comfortable and embodied in your parenting. For you, that may be accomplished by not using your body to feed at all, by making milk but not feeding with your body, by chestfeeding with a supplemental feeding tube, or by making milk and chestfeeding. Take your time and see what happens. Follow your own body's reactions as you experiment to find the option that is going to work best for you.

Keep in mind that any milk-making cells that remain in your chest after surgery will respond to the hormones that initiate lactation. Your chest might start to appear lumpy during pregnancy, and after birth, any milk-making framework that is no longer connected to a nipple will swell up and become painful, especially under the arms. This is a self-correcting process due to the role of feedback inhibitor of lactation (FIL), which turns off milk production when milk is not removed from the ducts, and turns milk production up when the ducts are emptied. It is important to be on the lookout for signs of mastitis, which is an infection of the milk-producing anatomy. Mastitis results in fever accompanied by pain and redness in the chest tissue, and it can easily be treated with an expeditious use of antibiotics.

If you do have some milk and you decide to remove it, you will relieve the pressure in the ducts that do have an exit, but you may also be stimulating the ducts that don't have an exit. This can extend the engorgement period; however, the ducts that are not emptied will eventually stop filling with milk. If you are chestfeeding, you may need to soften your chest tissue so that baby can latch, which can be done with a warm shower or warm washcloth compress and hand expression before feeding, followed by a flexible ice pack or cold, cleaned cabbage leaves applied to the chest afterward.

If you are not chestfeeding after giving birth, you can speed up the cessation of milk production with a twenty-four-hour regimen of over-the-counter (or behind-the-counter) antihistamines, along with ibuprofen, ice, and cabbage leaves for as long as you need them. While some people find lymphatic massage to be helpful for pain relief, others say to avoid stimulating the chest tissue until milk production stops. The best herbal support is sage tea or tincture, although some people find peppermint tea to be helpful and more readily available.

With these measures, the engorgement will be much improved within twenty-four hours, and milk production will stop all together within a few days. There is also a medication called cabergoline (brand name Dostinex) that decreases prolactin levels; however, it can cause nausea, vomiting, constipation, and dizziness, which are not very compatible with caring for a newborn and recovering from birth.

If you are reading this chapter prior to having top surgery, there are a few things to know. One is that binding quickly becomes unbearably painful once you are pregnant because the hormones of pregnancy cause the milk-making anatomy to start expanding almost immediately. It also may be a while before you can start binding after birth, because chest compression can lead to blocked ducts and mastitis. If you are planning to get top surgery after giving birth (or if you opt for an additional surgery to correct changes in the chest after pregnancy), you may need to allow time for lactation to stop completely before the surgery is performed. This is because any milk-making framework that remains in the chest after surgery will become engorged and complicate the healing process if it is still producing milk. Once lactation is established, it can take up to six months (or longer if you lactate for more than a year) for lactation to stop. You can speed up the process by drinking a cup or two of sage tea daily and avoiding any stimulation of the chest. Starting testosterone may also help reduce your milk supply, although many transmasculine people take testosterone while chestfeeding. (Testosterone is not secreted in large amounts in human milk, and no risks have been shown to the babies whose nursing parent is receiving gender-affirming testosterone.)

If you are planning top surgery prior to giving birth, be sure to discuss your plans for pregnancy with your surgeon. Regardless of whether or not you end up feeding your baby with your body, a surgical technique that protects the connection between any remaining milk ducts and the nipple will allow you to remove milk and/or ease engorgement after birth. This is called a periareolar technique, which involves making incisions around the outer edge of the areola, protecting the connective framework that leads to the nipple.

USING A SUPPLEMENTAL NURSING SYSTEM

You can feed your baby with your body and also use supplemental milk or formula at the same time by using a supplemental nursing system (SNS). This involves putting baby's liquid food into a container, inserting a feeding tube into the liquid, and allowing baby to siphon the liquid out by putting the other end of the tube into the corner of baby's mouth as they suck at the chest. There are special SNS products that have everything ready-made in one kit. These kits have a string attached to the liquid reservoir so that you can hang it around your neck, although you may do better by hanging it over your shoulder so that it doesn't get in the way when baby is trying to latch. You can also create a makeshift SNS by simply running a feeding tube from a container of milk or formula to baby's mouth, although for long-term use, it's easier to use a ready-made SNS.

In the beginning, using an SNS requires two people. In fact, latching a newborn often requires two people even without an SNS! Once you get baby latched, your helper can gently work the feeding tube into the corner of baby's mouth. You may need to prime the tube first in order for baby to get the liquid to flow, which can be done by placing the end of the tube lower than the reservoir and letting gravity do its thing.

Some people prefer to tape the feeding tube to the chest so that the end of the tube rests at the tip of the nipple; however, if you and your baby are still in the learning process of getting a deep latch, the tube may complicate things and cause a lot of frustration. Until you get used to latching, you may want to latch baby first, and then apply the tube. You may find that the taping method is a pain and instead opt to hold the tube in place with your finger as you latch baby on, but this is most definitely an advanced latching technique.

GETTING THE LATCH RIGHT

Feeding your baby with your body may be the most natural thing in the world, but like so many human skills, we have to learn. Many a new parent has wept while trying to feed their baby through seething pain, believing that if they are not able to muscle through it, then they are failing as a parent already, in the first week of life. Well-meaning words of advice that "some pain is normal in the beginning" and "your nipples will toughen up" are just plain wrong. You probably wouldn't let anyone else bite your nipples enough to cause cracks, blisters, bleeding, and infection, so why wouldn't you intervene immediately if your baby is doing it—especially if that is supposed to be the way they get their food?

The culmination of the lactation process relies on adequate emptying of the milk ducts in order for lactation to continue. If milk accumulates and is not removed, the feedback inhibitor of lactation (FIL) will cause milk production to stop. If milk keeps flowing, not only will FIL be suppressed, causing more milk to be produced, it will also allow your prolactin receptors to multiply and flourish, ensuring your body's ability to make a full milk supply for as long as your baby will need it. The first two weeks after birth is a sensitive period for the expansion of prolactin receptors, which means that if the milk ducts are not adequately emptied during this time, your long-term ability to produce enough milk for your baby will be diminished.

If you are removing your milk by allowing your baby to latch and suck, your job is to position them in a way that allows them to drain the milk efficiently. Getting the position right is imperative for the baby to get a deep latch, which is the only way to help them get ample calories without damaging the part of your body that feeds them. Positioning for a deep latch is not something you can learn in the twenty-four hours you are in the hospital recovering from birth, nor is a quick visit or two with your midwife always sufficient. If this is all the support you get and it isn't working, it doesn't mean there is something wrong with you. You and your baby simply need guidance from a provider who specializes in lactation and feeding so that you can learn how to position your baby effectively. Do not wait to get the support you need during this crucial time!

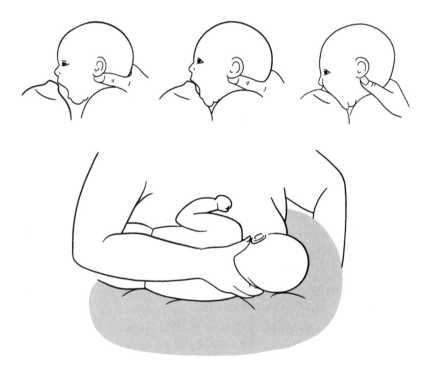

ANATOMY AND PHYSIOLOGY OF INFANT LATCH

Infants don't nipple feed—they chest- or breastfeed. The anatomy inside the baby's mouth is the same as an adult's—the top part of our mouths has a hard palate in front and a soft palate in back. A strong jaw and tongue that compresses the nipple against the hard palate will do damage, but a deep latch that places the nipple at the back of the baby's throat, against the soft palate, will protect the nipple. This also provides much more leverage for the lower jaw and tongue to remove milk from deep within the ducts.

STEPS TO GETTING A GOOD LATCH

- Sit in a comfortable chair and put your feet up on a small stool (a nursing stool has the perfect tilt and height) to raise your lap slightly and support your back. Do not skip this step—make sure you have this vital equipment on hand before your baby arrives.

- Use pillows to bring baby up to nipple level. A special nursing pillow can be helpful eventually, but if you've recently been pregnant, simple bed pillows will fit better around your postpartum belly.

- Position baby so that they don't have to turn their head to reach your chest. You can do this by placing them tummy to tummy with you. Check yourself by noting that baby's ear, shoulder, and hip are in a straight line.

- Bring baby in close so that your nipple rests just above baby's upper lip. This may seem counterintuitive, but it's actually a very important step because the baby will tilt their head back as they open their mouth wide. Starting high means that lots of chest tissue will end up over the baby's lower jaw, ensuring a deep latch.

- Make sure nothing is pressing against the back of the baby's head, which would inhibit them from achieving the head tilt that is necessary for a deep latch. The traditional cradle-type hold is actually notorious for causing a shallow latch with newborns. Instead, use a crossover hold, lying the baby in front of you, tummy to tummy, and placing the palm of your hand across the baby's shoulder blades, creating a cradle for baby's head with your thumb and forefinger behind baby's ears. This supports baby's upper body while allowing them to tilt their head back while latching. You can do the same in a football hold, placing baby alongside you and turning their hips in toward you, then putting your hand on their upper back and cradling the base of baby's head with your thumb and forefinger.

- In the beginning, you will want to make a "nipple sandwich" to support getting lots of chest tissue into the baby's mouth. This is similar to how you would squish a big sandwich in order to take a bite. Make sure that you match up your tissue compression with the baby's nose and chin (if baby is lying across your front, your hand will make a U shape; if baby is lying alongside you, your hand will make a C shape).

- Wait for your baby to open their mouth super wide, like a hungry baby bird. You will soon learn the difference between a wide-open mouth versus one that is only halfway open. Insist on a wide-open mouth before bringing baby onto the chest, or else baby will clamp down right on your nipple! You will note how baby tilts their head back as they open wide, sometimes even rapidly moving their head slightly back and forth with enthusiasm.

- Once baby opens their mouth super wide, bring them onto the chest very quickly. You are literally placing the nipple at the back of the baby's throat faster than they are able to close their mouth again. There is really no such thing as doing this too quickly.

- As soon as baby latches, take a deep breath and relax your body as you breathe out again. If the pain is less than a three or four on a scale of one to ten, and you are not on any pain medication, you have a deep latch. If the pain is more than a three or four, the latch is shallow and will damage your nipple while preventing baby from getting enough milk. Use your finger to press against the chest and break the suction so that you can take baby off and latch them again.

- If you are on pain medication, even ibuprofen, you will need to use visual cues to ensure that baby is latched properly, because you won't be able to use your pain level for feedback. Baby's upper and lower lip should be open at almost 180 degrees (a shallow latch produces a 90-degree angle). The upper and lower lip should both be flared out, not sucked in. Baby should be taking long, drawing sucks, not short, choppy ones. Note how your own facial muscles move all the way up to your temples when your mouth is wide open—this is what you should observe when baby is latched deeply.

- Listen closely. You will begin to hear baby swallowing every two to three sucks, which may sound like a high-pitched gulp or simply a pause in their exhale. If you hear a clicking sound, such as you might make with your own tongue pressed against the roof of your mouth, the latch is too shallow.

- After feeding, your nipple should be round and normal in color—not pinched, compressed, blanched, or creased, which happens when the latch is shallow, causing baby to press the tip of the nipple against the hard palate combined with enough suction to rid the tip of the nipple of blood flow.

- When in doubt, ask. That's what lactation professionals are for!

BONDING WITH YOUR BABY

Chest- or breastfeeding is not necessary to bond with your baby, nor is it required for your baby to develop a secure attachment to you. What is required is your presence and consistency in responding to your baby's needs. How your baby gets fed is secondary. If you are unable to feed your baby with your body, you can still bond with your baby. If you choose not to feed your baby with your body, no matter what the reason, you can still bond with your baby. Your newborn needs to be fed, held, kept warm, have their bum cleaned, and be rocked, walked, or bounced to sleep. Feeding is but one of the ways an infant needs to be cared for, but the others are equally important. Your emotional presence and your dedication to providing care for your baby are all that is required for bonding.

Many people emphasize the importance of the first hour after birth for "bonding time"; however, this is a true misnomer. Bonding takes place over weeks, months, and years. It doesn't happen immediately for everyone, so if you don't instantly feel overwhelming, endless love for your newborn, you're not doing it wrong, and you are actually in good company with many a loving parent. The only reason we emphasize the bonding potential of the first hour after birth is that hospital routines used to require newborns to be whisked away to the nursery before parents even had a chance to meet them! Now that this is no longer the routine practice for a well baby, many prefer the term "the golden hour" to reflect the sense of magic and awe as a newborn, in full awareness, investigates the world around them. Your baby will turn toward the sound of your voice. They will open their eyes and look around. They will snuggle, smell, taste, and root against your skin. They will grasp your finger with their little hand. The golden hour is simply a time to get acquainted with this little human who has come into your life. In time, your heart will swell with the greatest love you have ever known.

GUIDANCE FOR CARE PROVIDERS

Information about the benefits of human milk and the value of chest- or breastfeeding is abundant, but the lived experience of new parents is more nuanced than lactation promotion campaigns suggest. The desire to provide our babies with the best possible start in life is universal; however, offering a single superior way to do that is not only shortsighted but also counter-productive. If the approach contributes to parental shame and stress rather than building confidence and calm, it inhibits attachment and can render trauma during the postpartum transition. I invite all providers who support lactation and feeding to do a thorough accounting of the words you say, the handouts you provide, and the way you go about ensuring feeding success to make sure that it is appropriate for all parents, regardless of the choices made around infant feeding.

As providers who care for queer and trans families during pregnancy, we have a responsibility to ensure that our practices are not only welcoming to but specifically inclusive of queer and trans identities and experiences. This extends to the language used on your website, educational materials, and medical forms. It includes the way your support staff answers the phone and gathers information about new patients or clients. It includes the way you hold space for the existence of people of all genders in all parenting roles, not only when speaking to queer or trans people in your care, but in how you discuss pregnancy and parenting with everyone. It is not enough to merely incorporate gender-inclusive language. Creating an inclusive practice means providing services that address the unique and specific needs of gender-diverse clientele. If there are services needed by your clientele that you are not able to provide yourself, have a solid referral network that you have personally vetted for gender inclusivity and trans competency.

The leadership role we inherently possess as health care providers requires that we must not only serve our own queer and trans clients well, but we also need to uphold expectations of inclusivity in everything we do. We must advocate within our professions, our jurisdictions, and our communities. Know that every time you go to bat for an individual family, you are making space for every family that follows. Pave the way especially for the nonbinary and transgender people in your care—if you are a hospital provider, take extra steps to ensure a smooth and affirming experience in triage, among nursing staff, among the colleagues you share call with, and the surgical staff for cesarean delivery. Know the resources for queer and trans parents in your community, and if resources don't exist, do what you can to help create them.

Resources

MAIA Midwifery's Queer & Trans Pregnancy Program: www.maiamidwifery.com/services/midwifery-care

Queer and Transgender Midwives Association: www.elephantcircle.net/qtma

Postpartum Support International: Postpartum.net

Newman-Goldfarb protocols for induced lactation: www.canadianbreastfeedingfoundation.org/induced/induced.shtml

ACKNOWLEDGMENTS

To my queer community, specifically those of you who have entrusted me to midwife your journey to parenthood, I could not have written this book without each and every one of you. Your willingness to share your vulnerability and your truths have informed my practice in ways that reverberate throughout all I do. You have made me the midwife I am today, and I am honored to play this role in the community we all share.

To my editor at Sasquatch Books, Hannah Elnan: I am ever grateful that you reached out to offer your support and advocacy in publishing this book. I needed a literary midwife, and your sound advice, kind words, and patient reassurance have kept me pushing on.

To Yemisi "Yemi" Miller-Tonnet, Clare Heimer, Mac Brydum, Òscar Viñas Rodriguez, and Juan Jose Pedro Frasquet, your insights as inclusivity readers have been crucial, and your words of affirmation and praise have carried me through the final edits. You have my heartfelt appreciation for both. Thanks also to Adrienne Black for your heart-centered wisdom and well-honed insights about surrogacy, and for taking the time to share them with me; to Caroline Sausler, for testing *all* the OPKs; to Annie Moffat, for seeing me; to Tracy Cooper for making sure everyone got pregnant when I was away on writing retreats; and to Brad Farmer, for anchoring me in a sailboat on the Alaskan coast to conceive this book in the company of moon jellies, bald eagles, and the occasional grizzly bear.

Although writing a book during this first pandemic year has been a lonesome endeavor, I have felt the love, support, and encouragement of many. In return, I extend my gratitude to the Jacobs-Brown family, Geraldine Lee, Karma Augerot, Henry Brown, Tree Willard, Rick Deiss, and Jackie Bauer. And to Clementine, the best quarantine companion I ever could have asked for: thank you for naps on my chest, talking to me every day, and for being the most beautiful, stiletto-pawed, green-eyed calico kitten ever.

A lifetime of gratitude belongs to my baby, Finley Ataienne, for initiating me into parenthood and becoming my greatest teacher, and to Gi, Danny, and Prana for coming into my life and expanding my heart. I love you, always.

BIBLIOGRAPHY

Chapter 1: Making Decisions and Creating a Timeline

Bortoletto, P., et al. "Reproductive outcomes of women 40 and older undergoing IVF with donor sperm." *Fertility and Sterility* - International edition 114, no. 3 (September 2020): E102–E103.

Brandt, J., et al. "Transgender men, pregnancy, and the "new" advanced paternal age: A review of the literature." *Maturitas* 128 (October 2019): 17–21.

Cano, F., et al. "Effect of aging on the female reproductive system: Evidence for a role of uterine senescence in the decline in female fecundity." *Fertility and Sterility* 64, no. 3 (September 1995): 584–9.

Carpinello, O., et al. "Does ovarian stimulation benefit ovulatory women undergoing therapeutic donor insemination?" *Fertility and Sterility* 115, no. 3 (March 2021): 638–45.

Cohlen, B., et al. "IUI: Review and systematic assessment of the evidence that supports global recommendations." *Human Reproduction Update* 24, no. 3 (May 2018): 300–319.

Ferrara, I., et al. "Intrauterine insemination with frozen donor sperm. Pregnancy outcome in relation to age and ovarian stimulation regime." *Human Reproduction (Oxford, England)* 17, no. 9 (September 2002): 2320–4.

Ghuman, N., et al. "Does age of the sperm donor influence live birth outcome in assisted reproduction?" *Human Reproduction (Oxford, England)* 31, no. 3 (March 2016): 582–92.

Hawkins Bressler, L., et al. "Does empiric superovulation improve fecundity in healthy women undergoing therapeutic donor insemination without a male partner?" *Fertility and Sterility* 113, no. 1 (January 2020): 114–120.

Magnus, M., et al. "Role of maternal age and pregnancy history in risk of miscarriage: Prospective register based study." *BMJ* (2019): 364:l869.

Pirhonen, J., et al. "Effect of maternal age on uterine flow impedance." *Journal of Clinical Ultrasound* 33, no. 1 (January 2005): 14–7.

Ripley, M., et al. "Does ovarian reserve predict egg quality in unstimulated therapeutic donor insemination cycles?" *Fertility and Sterility* 103, no. 5 (May 2015): 1170–5.e2

Sheen, J., et al. "Maternal age and risk for adverse outcomes." *American Journal of Obstetrics and Gynecology* 219, no. 4 (October 2018): 390.e1–390.e15.

Ubaldi, F., et al. "Implantation in patients over 40 and raising FSH levels—a review." *Placenta* 24 Supplement B (October 2003): S34–8.

Chapter 2: Fertile Health for Every Body

Adeleye, A., et al. "Semen parameters among transgender women with a history of hormonal treatment." *Urology* 124, (February 2019): 136–141.

Allen, K., and M. Harris. "The role of n-3 fatty acids in gestation and parturition." *Experimental Biology and Medicine (Maywood, N.J.)* 226, no. 6 (June 2001): 498–506.

Alshahrani, S., et al. "Infertile men older than 40 years are at higher risk of sperm DNA damage." *Reproductive Biology and Endocrinology* 12, no. 1 (November 20, 2014): 103.

Augood, C., et al. "Smoking and female infertility: A systematic review and meta-analysis." *Human Reproduction (Oxford, England)* 13, no. 6 (June 1998): 1532–9.

Bacon, L. *Health at Every Size.* BenBella Books. Dallas, TX. 2008.

Baker F., and H. Driver. "Circadian rhythms, sleep, and the menstrual cycle." *Sleep Medicine* 8, no. 6 (September 2007): 613–22.

Banihani, S. "Vitamin B12 and semen quality." *Biomolecules* 7, no. 2 (June 9, 2017): 42.

Belloc, S., et al. "How to overcome male infertility after 40: Influence of paternal age on fertility." *Maturitas* 78, no. 1 (May 2014): 22–9.

Bisanti, L., et al. "Shift work and subfecundity: A European multicenter study." *Journal of Occupational and Environmental Medicine* 38, no. 4 (April 1996): 352–8.

Blumenthal, J., et al. "Is exercise a viable treatment for depression?" *ACSM's Health & Fitness Journal* 16, no. 4 (July 2012): 14–21.

Bracci, M., et al. "Influence of night-shift and napping at work on urinary melatonin, 17-beta-estradiol and clock gene expression in pre-menopausal nurses." *Journal of Biological Regulators and Homeostatic Agents* 27, no. 1 (January–March 2013): 267–74.

Brandt, J., et al. "Advanced paternal age, infertility, and reproductive risks: A review of the literature." *Prenatal Diagnosis* 39, no. 2 (January 2019): 81–87.

Brandt, J., et al. "Transgender men, pregnancy, and the 'new' advanced paternal age: A review of the literature." *Maturitas* 128 (October 2019): 17–21.

Brar, B. K., et al. "Effect of intrauterine marijuana exposure on fetal growth patterns and placental vascular resistance." *Journal of Maternal-Fetal and Neonatal Medicine* (November 1, 2019): 1–5.

Cardoso, J., et al. "Optimizing male fertility: Oxidative stress and the use of antioxidants." *World Journal of Urology* 37, no. 6 (June 2019): 1029–1034.

Chavarro, J., et al. "Diet and lifestyle in the prevention of ovulatory disorder infertility." *Obstetrics and Gynecology* 110, no. 5 (November 2007): 1050–8.

Chiu, Y., et al., "Association between pesticide residue intake from consumption of fruits and vegetables and pregnancy outcomes among women undergoing infertility treatment with assistance reproductive technology." *JAMA Internal Medicine* 178, no. 1 (January 1, 2018): 17–26.

Chiu, Y., et al. "Comparison of questionnaire-based estimation of pesticide residue intake from fruits and vegetables with urinary concentrations of pesticide biomarkers." *Journal of Exposure Science & Environmental Epidemiology* 28, no. 1 (January 2018): 31–9.

Chrousos, G., et al. "Interactions between the hypothalamic-pituitary-adrenal axis and the female reproductive system: Clinical implications." *Annals of Internal Medicine* 129, no. 3 (August 1, 1998): 229–40.

Cito, G., et al. "Vitamin D and male fertility: An updated review." *World Journal of Men's Health* 38, no. 2 (April 2020): 164–77.

Collodel, G., et al. "Fatty acid profile and metabolism are related to human sperm parameters and are relevant in idiopathic infertility and varicocele." *Mediators of Inflammation* 2020, no. 2020 (August 31, 2020): 1–13.

Conner, S., et al. "Maternal marijuana use and adverse neonatal outcomes: A systematic review and meta-analysis." *Obstetrics and Gynecology* 128, no. 4 (October 2016): 713–723.

Cooper, A., et al. "To eat soy or to not eat soy: The ongoing look at phytoestrogens and fertility." *Fertility and Sterility* 112, no. 5 (November 2019): 825–826.

Corsi, D., et al. "Association between self-reported prenatal cannabis use and maternal, perinatal, and neonatal outcomes." *JAMA* 322, no. 2 (2019): 145–152.

de Angelis, C., et al. "The role of vitamin D in male fertility: A focus on the testis." *Reviews in Endocrine & Metabolic Disorders* 18, no. 3 (September 2017): 285–305.

den Biggelaar, L., et al. "Prospective associations of dietary carbohydrate, fat, and protein intake with ß-cell function in the CODAM study." *European Journal of Nutrition* 58, no. 2 (March 2019): 597–608.

Djulus, J., et al. "Marijuana use and breastfeeding." *Canadian Family Physician Medecin de Famille Canadien* 51, no. 3 (March 2005): 349–50.

Doepker, C., et al. "Key findings and implications of a recent systematic review of the potential adverse effects of caffeine consumption in healthy adults, pregnant women, adolescents, and children." *Nutrients* 10, no. 10 (October 18, 2018): 1536.

Dordević, M., et al. "Morbidity in newborns exposed to organophosphorus pesticides." *Medicinski Pregled* 63, no. 5–6 (May–June 2010): 414–7.

Eisenberg, M., et al. "Relationship between physical occupational exposures and health on semen quality: Data from the Longitudinal Investigation of Fertility and the Environment (LIFE) Study." *Fertility and Sterility* 103, no. 5 (May 2015): 1271–7.

Environmental Working Group. "Dirty dozen endocrine disruptors" October 28, 2013. https://www.ewg.org/research/dirty-dozen-list-endocrine-disruptors.

Eskiocak, S., et al. "Effect of psychological stress on the L-arginine-nitric oxide pathway and semen quality." *Brazilian Journal of Medical and Biological Research* 39, no. 5 (May 2006): 581–8.

Eslamian, G., et al. "Effects of coadministration of DHA and vitamin E on spermatogram, seminal oxidative stress, and sperm phospholipids in asthenozoospermic men: a randomized controlled trial." *American Journal of Clinical Nutrition* 112, no. 3 (September 1, 2020): 707–19.

Esmaeili, V., et al. "Dietary fatty acids affect semen quality: A review." *Andrology* 3, no. 3 (May 2015): 450–61.

Ferin, M. "Clinical review 105: Stress and the reproductive cycle." *Journal of Clinical Endocrinology and Metabolism* 84, no. 6 (June 1999): 1768–74.

Fontana, R., and S. Della Torre. "The deep correlation between energy metabolism and reproduction: A view on the effects of nutrition for women fertility." *Nutrients* 8, no. 2 (February 11, 2016): 87.

Foran, J., et al. "Risk-based consumption advice for farmed Atlantic and wild Pacific salmon contaminated with dioxins and dioxin-like compounds." *Environmental Health Perspectives* 113, no. 5 (May 2005): 552–6.

Garolla, A., et al. "Dietary supplements for male infertility: A critical evaluation of their composition." *Nutrients* 12, no. 5 (May 19, 2020): E1472.

Gaskins, A., et al. "Paternal physical and sedentary activities in relation to semen quality and reproductive outcomes among couples from a fertility center." *Human Reproduction (Oxford, England)* 29, no. 11 (November 2014): 2575–82.

Gaskins, A., et al. "Dietary patterns and outcomes of assisted reproduction." *American Journal of Obstetrics and Gynecology* 220, no. 6 (June 2019): 567.e1–18.

Grant, K., et al. "Cannabis use during pregnancy: Pharmacokinetics and effects on child development." *Pharmacology & Therapeutics* 182 (February 2018): 133–151.

Haight, S., et al. "Frequency of cannabis use during pregnancy and adverse infant outcomes, by cigarette smoking status - 8 PRAMS states, 2017." *Drug and Alcohol Dependence* 220 (2021): 108507.

Halis, G., and A. Arici. "Endometriosis and inflammation in infertility." *Annals of the New York Academy of Sciences* 1034, no. 1 (December 2004): 300–15.

Hayden, R., et al. "The role of lifestyle in male infertility: Diet, physical activity, and body habitus." *Current Urology Reports* 19, no. 7 (May 17, 2018): 56.

Hearing, C., et al. "Physical exercise for treatment of mood disorders: A critical review." *Current Behavioral Neuroscience Reports* 3, no. 4 (December 2016): 350–9.

Hollis, B. W., and C. L. Wagner. "Vitamin D requirements during lactation: High-dose maternal supplementation as therapy to prevent hypovitaminosis D for both the mother and the nursing infant." *American Journal of Clinical Nutrition,* edited by D. J. Raiten, 80, no. 6(S) (2004): 1752S–1758S.

Homayouni, A., et al. "Effects of probiotics on the recurrence of bacterial vaginosis: A review." *Journal of Lower Genital Tract Disease* 18, no. 1 (January 2014): 79–86.

Huizink, A. "Prenatal cannabis exposure and infant outcomes: Overview of studies." *Progress in Neuro-Psychopharmacology & Biological Psychiatry* 52 (July 3, 2014): 45–52.

Hull, M., et al. "Delayed conception and active and passive smoking." *Fertility and Sterility* 74, no. 4 (October 2000): 725–33.

Isoyama, R., et al. "Clinical experience with methylcobalamin (CH3-B12) for male infertility." *Hinyokika Kiyo. Acta Urologica Japonica* 30, no. 4 (April 1984): 581–6.

Iszatt, N., et al. "Environmental toxicants in breast milk of Norwegian mothers and gut bacteria composition and metabolites in their infants at 1 month." *Microbiome* 7, no. 1 (February 27, 2019): 34.

Jansson, L., et al. "Perinatal marijuana use and the developing child." *JAMA* 320, no. 6 (2018): 545–6.

Kennedy, D., and G. Koren. "Identifying women who might benefit from higher doses of folic acid in pregnancy." *Canadian Family Physician Medecin de Famille Canadien* 58, no. 4 (April 2012): 394–7.

Kharbanda, E., et al. "Birth and early developmental screening outcomes associated with cannabis exposure during pregnancy." Journal of Perinatology: Official Journal of the California Perinatal Association 40, no. 3 (March 2020): 473–480.

Kim, T., et al. "Associations of mental health and sleep duration with menstrual cycle irregularity: A population-based study." *Archives of Women's Mental Health* 21, no. 6 (December 2018): 619–26.

Kloss, J., et al. "Sleep, sleep disturbance, and fertility in women." *Sleep Medicine Reviews* 22 (August 2015): 78–87.

Leproult, R., et al. "Circadian misalignment augments markers of insulin resistance and inflammation, independently of sleep loss." *Diabetes* 63, no. 6 (June 2014): 1860–9.

Light, A., et al. "Transgender men who experienced pregnancy after female-to-male gender transitioning." *Obstetrics and Gynecology* 124, no. 6 (December 2014): 1120–7.

Li, Q., et al. "Assessment of antihistamine use in early pregnancy and birth defects." *Journal of Allergy and Clinical Immunology. In Practice* 1, no. 6 (November–December 2013): 666–74.e1.

Liu, M., et al. "Sleep deprivation and late bedtime impair sperm health through increasing antisperm antibody production: A prospective study of 981 healthy men." *Medical Science Monitor* 23 (April 16, 2017): 1842–8.

Lopez-Garcia, E., et al. "Consumption of trans fatty acids is related to plasma biomarkers of inflammation and endothelial dysfunction." *Journal of Nutrition* 135, no. 3 (March 2005): 562–6.

Lynch, C., et al. "Preconception stress increases the risk of infertility: Results from a couple-based prospective cohort study—the LIFE study." *Human Reproduction (Oxford, England)* 29, no. 5 (May 2014): 1067–75.

Mahmoud, B., et al. "The impact of nutrition and lifestyle on male fertility." *Archivio Italiano di Urologia, Andrologia* 92, no. 2 (June 24, 2020).

Marschalek, J., et al. "Influence of orally administered probiotic lactobacillus strains on vaginal microbiota in women with breast cancer during chemotherapy: A randomized placebo-controlled double-blinded pilot study." *Breast Care (Basel, Switzerland)* 12, no. 5 (October 2017): 335–9.

Martin-Hidalgo, D., et al. "Antioxidants and male fertility: From molecular studies to clinical evidence." *Antioxidants* 8, no. 4 (April 5, 2019): 89.

McKinnon, C., et al. "Body mass index, physical activity and fecundability in a North American preconception cohort study." *Fertility and Sterility* 106, no. 2 (August 2016): 451–9.

Metz, T., and E. Stickrath. "Marijuana use in pregnancy and lactation: A review of the evidence." *American Journal of Obstetrics and Gynecology* 213, no. 6 (December 2015): 761–78.

Mingian, S., and S. Haifei. "Sex hormones and their receptors regulate liver energy homeostasis." *International Journal of Endocrinology* 2015, Article ID 294278, 12 pages.

Moreno, I., et al. "Evidence that the endometrial microbiota has an effect on implantation success or failure." *American Journal of Obstetrics and Gynecology* 215, no. 6 (December 2016): 684–703.

Moslemi, M., and S. Tavanbakhsh. "Selenium-vitamin E supplementation in infertile men: Effects on semen parameters and pregnancy rate." *International Journal of General Medicine* 4 (January 23, 2011): 99–104.

Nehra, D., et al. "Prolonging the female reproductive lifespan and improving egg quality with dietary omega-3 fatty acids." *Aging Cell* 11, no. 6 (December 2012): 1046–54.

Ness, R. "Cocaine and tobacco use and the risk of spontaneous abortion." *New England Journal of Medicine* 340, no. 5 (February 4, 1999): 333–9.

Nguyen-Powanda, P., and B. Robaire. "Oxidative stress and reproductive function in the aging male." *Biology (Basel)* 9, no. 282 (2020): 282.

"Organic foods: Health and environmental advantages and disadvantages." American Academy of Pediatrics Committee on Nutrition and Council on Environmental Health, 2012.

Palacios, C., et al. "Regimens of vitamin D supplementation for women during pregnancy." *Cochrane Database of Systematic Reviews* 10 (October 3, 2019): CD013446.

Palma, E., et al. "Long-term lactobacillus rhamnosus BMX 54 application to restore a balanced vaginal ecosystem: A promising solution against HPV-infection." *BMC Infectious Diseases* 18, no. 1 (January 5, 2018): 13.

Papadopoulou, E., et al. "Diet as a source of exposure to environmental contaminants for pregnant women and children from six European countries." *Environmental Health Perspectives* 127, no. 10 (October 2019): 107005.

Park, J., et al. "Daily perceived stress and time to pregnancy: A prospective cohort study of women trying to conceive." *Psychoneuroendocrinology* 110 (December 2019): 104446.

Paul, S., et al. "Associations between prenatal cannabis exposure and childhood outcomes: Results from the ABCD study." *JAMA Psychiatry* 78, no. 1 (2021): 64–76.

Pauli, J., et al. "Current perspectives of insulin resistance and polycystic ovary syndrome." *Diabetic Medicine* 28, no. 12 (December 2011): 1445–54.

Penzias, A., et al. "Smoking and infertility: A committee opinion." *Fertility and Sterility* 110, no. 4 (September 2018): 611–8.

Perez-Reyes, M., and M. Wall. "Presence of delta9-tetrahydrocannabinol in human milk." *New England Journal of Medicine* 307, no. 13 (September 23, 1982): 819–20.

"Physical activity and exercise during pregnancy and the postpartum period: ACOG Committee opinion summary, Number 804." *Obstetrics and Gynecology* 135, no. 4 (April 2020): 991–3.

Qian, J., et al. "Impacts of caffeine during pregnancy." *Trends in Endocrinology and Metabolism* 31, no. 3 (March 2020): 218–27.

Radwanska, E., et al. "Nocturnal prolactin levels in infertile women with endometriosis." *Journal of Reproductive Medicine* 32, no. 8 (August 1987): 605–8.

Raichlen, D., et al. "Wired to run: Exercise-induced endocannabinoid signaling in humans and cursorial mammals with implications for the 'runner's high'." *Journal of Experimental Biology* 215, no. 8 (April 15, 2012): 1331–6.

Recine, N., et al. "Restoring vaginal microbiota: Biological control of bacterial vaginosis. A prospective case-control study using lactobacillus rhamnosus BMX 54 as adjuvant treatment against bacterial vaginosis." *Archives of Gynecology and Obstetrics* 293, no. 1 (January 2016): 101–7.

Rembiakowska, E. "The impact of organic agriculture on food quality." *Agricultura (Slovenia)* 3, no. 1 (2004): 19–26.

Ricci, E., et al. "Semen quality and alcohol intake: A systematic review and meta-analysis." *Reproductive Biomedicine Online* 34, no. 1 (January 2017): 38–47.

Richardson, M., et al. "Environmental and developmental origins of ovarian reserve." *Human Reproduction Update* 20, no. 3 (May–June 2014): 353–69.

Russo, R., et al. "Randomised clinical trial in women with recurrent vulvovaginal candidiasis: Efficacy of probiotics and lactoferrin as maintenance treatment." *Mycoses* 62, no. 4 (April 2019): 328–35.

Safarinejad, M., et al. "Relationship of omega-3 and omega-6 fatty acids with semen characteristics, and anti-oxidant status of seminal plasma: A comparison between fertile and infertile men." *Clinical Nutrition (Edinburgh, Lothian)* 29, no. 1 (February 2010): 100–5.

Semet, M., et al. "The impact of drugs on male fertility: A review." *Andrology* 5, no. 4 (07 2017): 640–63.

Shechter, A., et al. "Circadian rhythms and shift working women." *Sleep Medicine Clinics* 3, no. 1 (2008): 13–24.

Showell, M., et al. "Antioxidants for female subfertility." *Cochrane Database of Systematic Reviews* 8 (August 27, 2020): CD007807.

Skoracka, K., et al. "Diet and nutritional factors in male (in)fertility—Underestimated factors." *Journal of Clinical Medicine* 9, no. 5 (May 9, 2020): 1400.

Speroff, L., and M. Fritz. *Clinical Gynecologic Endocrinology and Infertility*. 8th ed. Philadelphia: Lippincott Williams & Wilkins, 2005.

Storgaard, L., et al. "Does smoking during pregnancy affect sons' sperm counts?" *Epidemiology (Cambridge, Mass.)* 14, no. 3 (May 2003): 278–86.

Tennes, K., et al. "Marijuana: Prenatal and postnatal exposure in the human." *NIDA Research Monograph* 59 (1985): 48–60.

Tirabassi, G., et al. "Association between vitamin D and sperm parameters: Clinical evidence." *Endocrine* 58, no. 1 (October 2017): 194–8.

Touzet, S., et al. "Relationship between sleep and secretion of gonadotropin and ovarian hormones in women with normal cycles." *Fertility and Sterility* 77, no. 4 (April 2002): 738–44.

U.S. Department of Agriculture, Agricultural Research Service. FoodData Central, 2019. fdc.nal.usda .gov.

Vigar, V., et al. "A systematic review of organic versus conventional food consumption: Is there a measurable benefit on human health?" *Nutrients* 12, no. 1 (December 18, 2019): 7.

Wald, N., et al. "Quantifying the effect of folic acid." *Lancet* 358, no. 9298 (December 15, 2001): 2069–73.

Wesselink, A., et al. "Dietary phytoestrogen intakes of adult women are not strongly related to fecundability in 2 preconception cohort studies." *Journal of Nutrition* 150, no. 5 (May 1, 2020): 1240–51.

Willis, S., et al. "Female sleep patterns, shift work, and fecundability in a North American preconception cohort study." *Fertility and Sterility* 111, no. 6 (June 2019): 1201–1210.e1.

Wilson, R., et al. "Pre-conception folic acid and multivitamin supplementation for the primary and secondary prevention of neural tube defects and other folic acid-sensitive congenital anomalies." *Journal of Obstetrics and Gynaecology Canada* 37, no. 6 (June 2015): 534–52.

Wise, L., et al. "A prospective cohort study of physical activity and time to pregnancy." *Fertility and Sterility* 97, no. 5 (May 2012): 1136–42.e1: 4.

Woods, M., ed. "Maternal caffeine intake may be associated with low birth weight." Health Library: Evidence-Based Information. October 2014.

Wymore, E., et al. "Persistence of Δ-9-tetrahydrocannabinol in human breast milk." *JAMA Pediatrics* 175, no. 6 (June 2021): 632–634.

Young, K., et al. "The cascade of positive events: Does exercise on a given day increase the frequency of additional positive events?" *Personality and Individual Differences* 120 (2018): 299–303.

Yu, Y., et al. "Maternal exposure to the mixture of organophosphorus pesticides induces reproductive dysfunction in the offspring." *Environmental Toxicology* 28, no. 9 (September 2013): 507–15.

Zhang, L., et al. "Optimizing fertility part 2: Environmental toxins." *BC Medical Journal* 62, no. 9 (November 2020): 323–7.

Chapter 3: Lab Tests and Fertility Evaluations

Adeleye, A., et al. "Semen parameters among transgender women with a history of hormonal treatment." *Urology* 124 (February 2019): 136–41.

Alexander, E., et al. "Guidelines of the American thyroid association for the diagnosis and management of thyroid disease during pregnancy and the postpartum." *Thyroid* 27, no. 3 (March 2017): 315–89.

Alshahrani, S., et al. "Infertile men older than 40 years are at higher risk of sperm DNA damage." *Reproductive Biology and Endocrinology* 12, no. 1 (November 20, 2014): 103.

American College of Obstetricians and Gynecologists (ACOG). "ACOG Practice Bulletin No. 192: Management of Alloimmunization During Pregnancy." *Obstetrics and Gynecology* 131, no. 3 (March 2018): e82–90.

Banihani, S. "Vitamin B12 and semen quality." *Biomolecules* 7, no. 2 (June 9, 2017): 42.

Barber, V., et al. "Prevention of acquisition of cytomegalovirus infection in pregnancy through hygiene-based behavioral interventions: A systematic review and gap analysis." *Pediatric Infectious Disease Journal* 39, no. 10 (October 2020): 949–54.

Belloc, S., et al. "How to overcome male infertility after 40: Influence of paternal age on fertility." *Maturitas* 78, no. 1 (May 2014): 22–9.

Benatta, M., et al. "The impact of nutrition and lifestyle on male fertility." *Archivio Italiano di Urologia, Andrologia* 92, no. 2 (June 24, 2020): 121–131.

Brandt, J., et al. "Advanced paternal age, infertility, and reproductive risks: A review of the literature." *Prenatal Diagnosis* 39, no. 2 (January 2019): 81–7.

Cardoso, J., et al. "Optimizing male fertility: Oxidative stress and the use of antioxidants." *World Journal of Urology* 37, no. 6 (June 2019): 1029–34.

Catalano, P., et al. HAPO Study Cooperative Research Group. "The hyperglycemia and adverse pregnancy outcome study: Associations of GDM and obesity with pregnancy outcomes." *Diabetes Care* 35, no. 4 (April 2012): 780–6.

Cito, G., et al. "Vitamin D and male fertility: An updated review. *World Journal of Men's Health* 38, no. 2 (April 2020): 164–77.

Collodel, G., et al. "Fatty acid profile and metabolism are related to human sperm parameters and are relevant in idiopathic infertility and varicocele." *Mediators of Inflammation* 2020 (August 31, 2020): 1–13.

Crispin, P., et al. "First trimester ferritin screening for pre-delivery anaemia as a patient blood management strategy." *Transfusion and Apheresis Science* 58, no. 1 (February 2019): 50–7.

Crowther, C., et al. "Interventions to prevent women from developing gestational diabetes mellitus: An overview of cochrane reviews." *Cochrane Database of Systematic Reviews* 2020, no. 6. (September 3, 2020): CD012394.

de Angelis, C., et al. "The role of vitamin D in male fertility: A focus on the testis." *Reviews in Endocrine & Metabolic Disorders* 18, no. 3 (September 2017): 285–305.

Dolitsky, S., et al. "Beyond the 'Jewish panel': The importance of offering expanded carrier screening to the Ashkenazi Jewish population." *F&S Reports* 1, no. 3 (December 2020): 294–8.

Eisenberg, M., et al. "Relationship between physical occupational exposures and health on semen quality: Data from the Longitudinal Investigation of Fertility and the Environment (LIFE) Study." *Fertility and Sterility* 103, no. 5 (May 2015): 1271–7.

Eskiocak, S., et al. "Effect of psychological stress on the L-arginine-nitric oxide pathway and semen quality." *Brazilian Journal of Medical and Biological Research* 39, no. 5 (May 2006): 581–8.

Eslamian, G., et al. "Effects of coadministration of DHA and vitamin E on spermatogram, seminal oxidative stress, and sperm phospholipids in asthenozoospermic men: a randomized controlled trial." *American Journal of Clinical Nutrition* 112, no. 3 (September 1, 2020): 707–19.

Esmaeili, V., et al. "Dietary fatty acids affect semen quality: A review." *Andrology* 3, no. 3 (May 2015): 450–61.

Ethics Committee of the American Society for Reproductive Medicine. "Access to fertility services by transgender and nonbinary persons: An ethics committee opinion." *Fertility and Sterility* 115, no. 4 (April 2021): 874–8.

Fung, J., et al. "Association of vitamin D intake and serum levels with fertility: Results from the Lifestyle and Fertility Study." *Fertility and Sterility* 108, no. 2 (August 2017): 302–11.

Garolla, A., et al. "Dietary supplements for male infertility: A critical evaluation of their composition." *Nutrients* 12, no. 5 (May 19, 2020): E1472.

Gaskins, A., et al. "Paternal physical and sedentary activities in relation to semen quality and reproductive outcomes among couples from a fertility center." *Human Reproduction (Oxford, England)* 29, no. 11 (November 2014): 2575–82.

Georgieff, M. "Iron deficiency in pregnancy." *American Journal of Obstetrics and Gynecology* 223, no. 4 (October 2020): 516–24.

Gregg, A., and J. Edwards. "Prenatal genetic carrier screening in the genomic age." *Seminars in Perinatology* 42, no. 5 (August 2018): 303–6.

Hayden, R., et al. "The role of lifestyle in male infertility: Diet, physical activity, and body habitus." *Current Urology Reports* 19, no. 7 (May 17, 2018): 56.

Hyde, T., et al. "Cytomegalovirus seroconversion rates and risk factors: Implications for congenital CMV." *Reviews in Medical Virology* 20, no. 5 (September 2010): 311–26.

Johnson, K., et al. "Recommendations to improve preconception health and health care—United States: A report of the CDC/ATSDR preconception care work group and the select panel on preconception care." *MMWR. Recommendations and Reports* 55, RR-6 (April 21, 2006): 1–23.

Kronemyer, B. "Prepregnancy hemoglobin A1c and risk of maternal complications." *Contemporary Ob/Gyn* 65, no. 7 (2020): 24.

Martin-Hidalgo, D., et al. "Antioxidants and male fertility: From molecular studies to clinical evidence." *Antioxidants* 8, no. 4 (April 5, 2019): 89.

Moslemi, M., and S. Tavanbakhsh. "Selenium-vitamin E supplementation in infertile men: Effects on semen parameters and pregnancy rate." *International Journal of General Medicine* 4 (January 23, 2011): 99–104.

Muscogiuri, G., et al. "Shedding new light on female fertility: The role of vitamin D." *Reviews in Endocrine & Metabolic Disorders* 18, no. 3 (September 2017): 273–83.

Nguyen-Powanda, P., and B. Robaire. "Oxidative stress and reproductive function in the aging male." *Biology (Basel)* 9, no. 282 (2020): 282.

Penzias, A., et al., and the Practice Committee of the American Society for Reproductive Medicine. "Testing and interpreting measures of ovarian reserve: A committee opinion." *Fertility and Sterility* 114, no. 6 (December 2020): 1151–7.

Penzias, A., et al., and the Practice Committee of the American Society for Reproductive Medicine. "Recommendations for reducing the risk of viral transmission during fertility treatment with the use of autologous gametes: A committee opinion." *Fertility and Sterility* 114, no. 6 (December 2020): 1158–1164.

Reichman, O., et al. "Preconception screening for cytomegalovirus: An effective preventive approach." *BioMed Research International* 2014, no. 10 (2014): 135416.

Ricci, E., et al. "Semen quality and alcohol intake: A systematic review and meta-analysis." *Reproductive Biomedicine Online* 34, no. 1 (January 2017): 38–47.

Rodger, A., et al. "Sexual activity without condoms and risk of HIV transmission in serodifferent couples when the HIV-positive partner is using suppressive antiretroviral therapy." *Journal of the American Medical Association* 316, no. 2 (July 12, 2016): 171–181.

Safarinejad, M., et al. "Relationship of omega-3 and omega-6 fatty acids with semen characteristics, and anti-oxidant status of seminal plasma: A comparison between fertile and infertile men." *Clinical Nutrition (Edinburgh, Lothian)* 29, no. 1 (February 2010): 100–5.

Skoracka, K., et al. "Diet and nutritional factors in male (in)fertility—Underestimated factors." *Journal of Clinical Medicine* 9, no. 5 (May 9, 2020): 1400.

Thomas, L., et al. "Which types of conditions should be included in reproductive genetic carrier screening? Views of parents of children with a genetic condition." *European Journal of Medical Genetics* 63, no. 12 (December 2020): 104075.

Tirabassi, G., et al. "Association between vitamin D and sperm parameters: Clinical evidence." *Endocrine* 58, no. 1 (October 2017): 194–8.

Tourtelot, E., et al. "Women who received varicella vaccine versus natural infection have different long-term T cell immunity but similar antibody levels." *Vaccine* 38, no. 7 (February 11, 2020): 1581–5. Accessed January 25, 2021.

Unuane, D., and B. Velkeniers. "Impact of thyroid disease on fertility and assisted conception." *Best Practice & Research. Clinical Endocrinology & Metabolism* 34, no. 4 (July 2020): 101378.

Zolton, J., et al. "Preconception A1c and time to pregnancy, pregnancy loss, and live birth." *Fertility and sterility* - International edition 112, no. 3 Supplement (September 1, 2019): e82–83.

Chapter 4: Gamete Donors

Crawshaw, M. "Direct-to-consumer DNA testing: The fallout for individuals and their families unexpectedly learning of their donor conception origins." *Human Fertility (Cambridge, England)* 21, no. 4 (December 2018): 225–8.

Grilli, S. "Making bodies, making relatives. Family resemblances and relatedness in the age of assisted reproductive technologies." *Antropologia* 6, no. 2 (2019): 27–44.

Hadizadeh-Talasaz, F., et al. "Exploring infertile couples' decisions to disclose donor conception to the future child." *International Journal of Fertility & Sterility* 14, no. 3 (October 2020): 240–6.

Hudson, N. *Gamete Donation and 'Race'. In eLS.* Chichester: John Wiley & Sons, 2015.

Newman, A. "Mixing and matching: Sperm donor selection for interracial lesbian couples." *Medical Anthropology* 38, no. 8 (November–December 2019): 710–24.

Raes, I., et al. "Parental (in)equality and the genetic link in lesbian families." *Journal of Reproductive and Infant Psychology* 32, no. 5 (2014): 457–68.

Schrijvers, A., et al. "Being a donor-child: Wishes for parental support, peer support and counseling." *Journal of Psychosomatic Obstetrics and Gynaecology* 40, no. 1 (March 2019): 29–37.

Chapter 5: Surrogacy

Bergman, K. *Your Future Family*. Newburyport, MA: Canari Press, 2019.

Black, Adrienne, interview. Conducted by Kristin L. Kali, February 9, 2021.

"Men Having Babies." https://www.menhavingbabies.org/

Chapter 6: Insemination Methods and Timing

Arab-Zozani, M., and C. Nastri. "Single versus double intrauterine insemination (IUI) for pregnancy: A systematic review and meta-analysis." *European Journal of Obstetrics and Gynecology* 215 (August 2017): 75–84.

Behre, H., et al. "Prediction of ovulation by urinary hormone measurements with the home use Clear-Plan Fertility Monitor: Comparison with transvaginal ultrasound scans and serum hormone measurements." *Human Reproduction (Oxford, England)* 15, no. 12 (December 2000): 2478–82.

Bigelow, J., et al. "Mucus observations in the fertile window: A better predictor of conception than timing of intercourse." *Human Reproduction (Oxford, England)* 19, no. 4 (April 2004): 889–892.

Blasco, V., et al. "Influence of follicle rupture and uterine contractions on intrauterine insemination outcome: A new predictive model." *Fertility and Sterility* 102, no. 4 (October 2014): 1034–40.

Blockeel, J., et al. "Should an intrauterine insemination with donor semen be performed 1 or 2 days after the spontaneous LH rise? A prospective RCT." *Human Reproduction (Oxford, England)* 29, no. 4 (April 2014): 697–703.

Brezina, P., et al. "At home testing: Optimizing management for the infertility physician." *Fertility and Sterility* 95, no. 6 (May 2011): 1867–78.

Byrd, W., et al. "A prospective randomized study of pregnancy rates following intrauterine and intra-cervical insemination using frozen donor sperm." *Fertility and Sterility* 53, no. 3 (March 1990): 521–7.

Cantineau, A., et al. "Synchronised approach for intrauterine insemination in subfertile couples." *Cochrane Database of Systematic Reviews* no. 12 (December 21, 2014): CD006942.

Carpinello, O., et al. "Does ovarian stimulation benefit ovulatory women undergoing therapeutic donor insemination?" *Fertility and Sterility* 115, no. 3 (March 2021): 638–45.

Carroll, N., and J. Palmer. "Comparison of intrauterine versus intracervical insemination in fertile single women." *Fertility and Sterility* 75, no. 4 (April 2001): 656–60.

Cohlen, B. *Intra-Uterine Insemination: Evidence Based Guidelines for Daily Practice*. Boca Raton, FL: CRC Press, 2011. Kindle.

Custers, I., et al. "Immobilisation versus immediate mobilization after intrauterine insemination: Randomised controlled trial." *BMJ (Clinical Research Ed.)* 339 (October 29, 2009): b4080.

Ecochard, R., et al. "Chronological aspects of ultrasonic, hormonal, and other indirect indices of ovulation." *BJOG* 108, no. 8 (August 2001): 822–9.

Ecochard, R., et al. "Self-identification of the clinical fertile window and the ovulation period." *Fertility and Sterility* 103, no. 5 (May 2015): 1319–1325.e3.

El Hachem, H., et al. "Timing therapeutic donor inseminations in natural cycles: Human chorionic gonadotrophin administration versus urinary LH monitoring." *Reproductive Biomedicine Online* 35, no. 2 (August 2017): 174–179.

Fauser, B., et al. "Multiple birth resulting from ovarian stimulation for subfertility treatment." *Lancet* 365, no. 9473 (May 21–27, 2005): 1807–16.

Ferrara, I., et al. "Intrauterine insemination with frozen donor sperm. Pregnancy outcome in relation to age and ovarian stimulation regime." *Human Reproduction (Oxford, England)* 17, no. 9 (September 2002): 2320–4.

Hawkins Bressler, L., et al. "Does empiric superovulation improve fecundity in healthy women undergoing therapeutic donor insemination without a male partner?" *Fertility and Sterility* 113, no. 1 (01 2020): 114–20.

Kissler, S., et al. "Uterine contractility and directed sperm transport assessed by hysterosalpingoscintigraphy (HSSG) and intrauterine pressure (IUP) measurement." *Acta Obstetricia et Gynecologica Scandinavica* 83, no. 4 (April 2004): 369–374.

Kop, P., et al. "Intracervical insemination and intrautrerine insemination for donor sperm treatment in the natural cycle: A randomized controlled trial." *Fertility and Sterility* 114, no. 3 (2020): e101–2.

Kunz, G., et al. "The dynamics of rapid sperm transport through the female genital tract: Evidence from vaginal sonography of uterine persitalsis and hysterosalpingoscintigraphy." *Human Reproduction (Oxford, England)* 11, no. 3 (March 1996): 627–632.

Kyrou, D., et al. "Spontaneous triggering of ovulation versus HCG administration in patients undergoing IUI: A prospective randomized study." *Reproductive Biomedicine Online* 25, no. 3 (September 2012): 278–83.

Lloyd, R., and C. Coulam. "The accuracy of urinary luteinizing hormone testing in predicting ovulation." *American Journal of Obstetrics and Gynecology* 160, no. 6 (June 1989): 1370–2, discussion: 1373–5.

Oruç, A., et al. "Influence of ultrasound-guided artificial insemination on pregnancy rates: A randomized study." *Archives of Gynecology and Obstetrics* 289, no. 1 (January 2014): 207–12.

Peters, A., et al. "Comparison of the methods of artificial insemination on the incidence of conception in single unmarried women." *Fertility and Sterility* 59, no. 1 (January 1993): 121–4.

Pistorius, L., et al. "A comparative study using prepared and unprepared frozen semen for donor insemination." *Archives of Andrology* 36, no. 1 (January–February 1996): 81–6.

Practice Committee of American Society for Reproductive Medicine in collaboration with Society for Reproductive Endocrinology and Infertility. "Optimizing natural fertility." *Fertility and Sterility* 90, no. 5, Suppl (November 2008): S1–6.

Roos, J., et al. "Monitoring the menstrual cycle: Comparison of urinary and serum reproductive hormones referenced to true ovulation." *European Journal of Contraception & Reproductive Health Care* 20, no. 6 (2015): 438–50.

Saleh, A., et al. "A randomized study of the effect of 10 minutes of bedrest after intrauterine insemination." *Fertility and Sterility* 74, no. 3 (September 2000): 509–11.

Saleh, A., et al. "A randomized study of the effect of 10 minutes of bedrest after intrauterine insemination." *Fertility and Sterility* 74, no. 3 (September 2000): 509–11.

Subak, L., et al. "Therapeutic donor insemination: A prospective randomized trial of fresh versus frozen sperm." *American Journal of Obstetrics and Gynecology* 166, no. 6 Pt. 1 (June 1992): 1597–604, discussion: 1604–6.

Thijssen, A., et al. "Predictive factors influencing pregnancy rates after intrauterine insemination with frozen donor semen: A prospective cohort study." *Reproductive Biomedicine Online* 34, no. 6 (June 2017): 590–7.

Wilcox, A., et al. "Timing of sexual intercourse in relation to ovulation. Effects on the probability of conception, survival of the pregnancy, and sex of the baby." *New England Journal of Medicine* 333, no. 23 (December 7, 1995): 1517–21.

Wilcox, A., et al. "Likelihood of conception with a single act of intercourse: Providing benchmark rates for assessment of post-coital contraceptives." *Contraception* 63, no. 4 (April 2001): 211–5.

Williams, D., et al. "Does intrauterine insemination offer an advantage to cervical cap insemination in a donor insemination program?" *Fertility and Sterility* 63, no. 2 (February 1995): 295–8.

Chapter 7: Troubleshooting and Complicated Conceptions

PCOS

Alur-Gupta, S., et al. "Postpartum complications increased in women with polycystic ovary syndrome." *American Journal of Obstetrics and Gynecology* 224, no. 3 (March 1, 2021): 280.e1–280.e13.

Arentz, S., et al. "Combined lifestyle and herbal medicine in overweight women with polycystic ovary syndrome (PCOS): A randomized controlled trial." *Phytotherapy Research* 31, no. 9 (September 2017): 1330–40.

Bashir, M., et al. "Vitamin D deficiency and PCOS: Association between vitamin D deficiency and PCOS in females presenting in a tertiary care hospital." *Professional Medical Journal* 26, no. 1 (2019): 40–3.

Borzoei, A., et al. "Effects of cinnamon supplementation on antioxidant status and serum lipids in women with polycystic ovary syndrome." *Journal of Traditional and Complementary Medicine* 8, no. 1 (January 2018): 128–133.

Butts, S., et al. "Vitamin D deficiency is associated with poor ovarian stimulation outcome in PCOS but not unexplained infertility." *Journal of Clinical Endocrinology and Metabolism* 104, no. 2 (February 1, 2019): 369–78.

Crawford, T., et al. "Antenatal dietary supplementation with myo-inositol in women during pregnancy for preventing gestational diabetes." *Cochrane Database of Systematic Reviews* no. 12 (December 17, 2015): CD011507.

Daneshbodi, H., et al. "Effect of omega-3 supplementation on gonadotropins and prolactin levels in women with polycystic ovary syndrome: A double blinded randomized controlled trial." *Iranian Journal of Reproductive Medicine* (April 2013): 58–9.

Dokras, A., et al. "Androgen excess- polycystic ovary syndrome society: Position statement on depression, anxiety, quality of life, and eating disorders in polycystic ovary syndrome." *Fertility and Sterility* 109, no. 5 (May 2018): 888–99.

El Refaeey, A., et al. "Combined coenzyme Q10 and clomiphene citrate for ovulation induction in clomiphene-citrate-resistant polycystic ovary syndrome." *Reproductive Biomedicine Online* 29, no. 1 (July 2014): 119–124.

Guo, S., et al. "Vitamin D supplementation ameliorates metabolic dysfunction in patients with PCOS: A systematic review of RCTs and insight into the underlying mechanism." *International Journal of Endocrinology* 2020. (December 2020): 1–18.

Izadi, A., et al. "Independent and additive effects of coenzyme Q10 and vitamin E on cardiometabolic outcomes and visceral adiposity in women with polycystic ovary syndrome." *Archives of Medical Research* 50, no. 2 (February 2019): 1–10.

Jamilian, M., et al. "A trial on the effects of magnesium-zinc-calcium-vitamin D co-supplementation on glycemic control and markers of cardio-metabolic risk in women with polycystic ovary syndrome." *Archives of Iranian Medicine* 20, no. 10 (October 2017): 640–5.

Jamilian, M., et al. "The influences of vitamin D and omega-3 co-supplementation on clinical, metabolic and genetic parameters in women with polycystic ovary syndrome." *Journal of Affective Disorders* 238 (October 1, 2018): 32–8.

Jedel, E., et al. "Impact of electro-acupuncture and physical exercise on hyperandrogenism and oligo/amenorrhea in women with polycystic ovary syndrome: A randomized controlled trial." *American Journal of Physiology. Endocrinology and Metabolism* 300, no. 1 (January 2011): E37–45.

Martelli, A., et al. "Coenzyme Q10: Clinical applications in cardiovascular diseases." *Antioxidants* 9, no. 4 (April 22, 2020): 341.

Moazami Goudarzi, Z., et al. "Laparoscopic ovarian electrocautery versus gonadotropin therapy in infertile women with clomiphene citrate-resistant polycystic ovary syndrome: A systematic review and meta-analysis." *Iranian Journal of Reproductive Medicine* 12, no. 8 (August 2014): 531–8.

Mohammadi, E., and M. Rafraf. "Benefits of omega-3 fatty acids supplementation on serum paraoxonase 1 activity and lipids ratios in polycystic ovary syndrome." *Health Promotion Perspectives* 2, no. 2 (December 28, 2012): 197–204.

Moini Jazani, A., et al. "A comprehensive review of clinical studies with herbal medicine on polycystic ovary syndrome (PCOS)." *Daru: Journal of Faculty of Pharmacy, Tehran University of Medical Sciences* 27, no. 2 (December 2019): 863–77.

Nas, K., and L. Tűű. "A comparative study between myo-inositol and metformin in the treatment of insulin-resistant women." *European Review for Medical and Pharmacological Sciences* 21, no. 2, Suppl (June 2017): 77–82.

Omran, E., et al. "Relation of serum vitamin D level in polycystic ovarian syndrome (PCOS) patients to ICSI outcome." *Middle East Fertility Society Journal* 25, no. 1 (2020): 1–8.

Pourghasem, S., et al. "The effectiveness of inositol and metformin on infertile polycystic ovary syndrome women with resistant to letrozole." *Archives of Gynecology and Obstetrics* 299, no. 4 (April 2019): 1193–9.

Shahin, A., and S. Mohammed. "Adding the phytoestrogen cimicifugae racemosae to clomiphene induction cycles with timed intercourse in polycystic ovary syndrome improves cycle outcomes and pregnancy rates—A randomized trial." *Gynecological Endocrinology* 30, no. 7 (July 2014): 505–510.

Shokrpour, M., et al. "Comparison of myo-inositol and metformin on glycemic control, lipid profiles, and gene expression related to insulin and lipid metabolism in women with polycystic ovary syndrome: a randomized controlled clinical trial." *Gynecological Endocrinology* 35, no. 5 (May 2019): 406–11.

Stener-Victorin, E., et al. "Acupuncture and physical exercise for affective symptoms and health-related quality of life in polycystic ovary syndrome: Secondary analysis from a randomized controlled trial." *BMC Complementary and Alternative Medicine* 13, no. 1 (June 13, 2013): 131.

Teede, H., et al. "Recommendations from the international evidence-based guideline for the assessment and management of polycystic ovary syndrome." *Fertility and Sterility* 110, no. 3 (August 2018): 364–379.

Trummer, C., et al. "Effects of vitamin D supplementation on metabolic and endocrine parameters in PCOS: A randomized-controlled trial." *European Journal of Nutrition* 58, no. 5 (August 2019): 2019–28.

"UBIQUINONE vs. UBIQUINOL: What's the difference?" *Better Nutrition* 80, no. 8 (2018): 12.

ENDOMETRIOSIS

Arablou, T., et al. "Resveratrol reduces the expression of insulin-like growth factor-1 and hepatocyte growth factor in stromal cells of women with endometriosis compared with nonendometriotic women." *Phytotherapy Research* 33, no. 4 (April 2019): 1044–54.

Arablou, T., and R. Kolahdouz-Mohammadi. "Curcumin and endometriosis: Review on potential roles and molecular mechanisms." *Biomedicine and Pharmacotherapy* 97 (January 2018): 91–7.

Attaman, J., et al. "The anti-inflammatory impact of omega-3 polyunsaturated fatty acids during the establishment of endometriosis-like lesions." *American Journal of Reproductive Immunology (New York, N.Y.)* 72, no. 4 (October 2014): 392–402.

Ballard, K., et al. "Can specific pain symptoms help in the diagnosis of endometriosis? A cohort study of women with chronic pelvic pain." *Fertility and Sterility* 94, no. 1 (June 2010): 20–7.

Ballard, K., et al. "Can symptomatology help in the diagnosis of endometriosis? Findings from a national case-control study—Part 1." *BJOG* 115, no. 11 (October 2008): 1382–91.

Brown, V., et al. "Repeat dose study of the cancer chemopreventive agent resveratrol in healthy volunteers: Safety, pharmacokinetics, and effect on the insulin-like growth factor axis." *Cancer Research* 70, no. 22 (November 15, 2010): 9003–11.

Dull, A., et al. "Therapeutic approaches of Resveratrol on endometriosis via anti-inflammatory and anti-angiogenic pathways." *Molecules (Basel, Switzerland)* 24, no. 4 (February 13, 2019): 667.

Fauconnier, A., et al. "Relation between pain symptoms and the anatomic location of deep infiltrating endometriosis." *Fertility and Sterility* 78, no. 4 (October 2002): 719–26.

Fjerbaek, A., and U. Knudsen. "Endometriosis, dysmenorrhea and diet—What is the evidence?" *European Journal of Obstetrics, Gynecology, and Reproductive Biology* 132, no. 2 (June 2007): 140–7

Giudice, L. "Clinical practice. Endometriosis." *New England Journal of Medicine* 362, no. 25 (June 24, 2010): 2389–98.

Grandi, G., et al. "The association between endometriomas and ovarian cancer: Preventive effect of inhibiting ovulation and menstruation during reproductive life." *BioMed Research International* 2015 (2015): 751571.

Grassi, P., et al. "Polychlorobiphenyls (PCBs), polychlorinated dibenzo-p-dioxins (PCDDs) and dibenzofurans (PCDFs) in fruit and vegetables from an industrial area in northern Italy." *Chemosphere* 79, no. 3 (April 2010): 292–8.

Halpern, G., et al. "Nutritional aspects related to endometriosis." *Revista da Associação Médica Brasileira* 61, no. 6 (November–December 2015): 519–23.

Ham, J., et al. "Silibinin-induced endoplasmic reticulum stress and mitochondrial dysfunction suppress growth of endometriotic lesions." *Journal of Cellular Physiology* 234, no. 4 (April 2019): 4327–41.

Harris, H., et al. "Dairy-food, calcium, magnesium, and vitamin D intake and endometriosis: A prospective cohort study." *American Journal of Epidemiology* 177, no. 5 (March 1, 2013): 420–30.

Harris, H., et al. "Early life abuse and risk of endometriosis." *Human Reproduction (Oxford, England)* 33, no. 9 (September 1, 2018): 1657–68.

Heard, M., et al. "High-fat diet promotion of endometriosis in an immunocompetent mouse model is associated with altered peripheral and ectopic lesion redox and inflammatory status." *Endocrinology* 157, no. 7 (July 2016): 2870–82.

Heilier, J., et al. "Environmental and host-associated risk factors in endometriosis and deep endometriotic nodules: A matched case-control study." *Environmental Research* 103, no. 1 (January 2007): 121–9.

Howells, L., et al. "Curcumin combined with FOLFOX chemotherapy is safe and tolerable in patients with metastatic colorectal cancer in a randomized phase IIa trial." *Journal of Nutrition* 149, no. 7 (July 1, 2019): 1133–9.

Itoh, H., et al. "Lactobacillus gasseri OLL2809 inhibits development of ectopic endometrial cell in peritoneal cavity via activation of NK cells in a murine endometriosis model." *Cytotechnology* 63, no. 2 (March 2011): 205–10.

Khanaki, K., et al. "Evaluation of the relationship between endometriosis and omega-3 and omega-6 polyunsaturated fatty acids." *Iranian Biomedical Journal* 16, no. 1 (2012): 38–43.

Khodaverdi, S., et al. "Beneficial effects of oral lactobacillus on pain severity in women suffering from endometriosis: A pilot placebo-controlled randomized clinical trial." *International Journal of Fertility & Sterility* 13, no. 3 (October 2019): 178–183.

Kocher, A., et al. "Highly bioavailable micellar curcuminoids accumulate in blood, are safe and do not reduce blood lipids and inflammation markers in moderately hyperlipidemic individuals." *Molecular Nutrition & Food Research* 60, no. 7 (July 2016): 1555–63.

Lalani, S., et al. "Endometriosis and adverse maternal, fetal and neonatal outcomes, a systematic review and meta-analysis." *Human Reproduction (Oxford, England)* 33, no. 10 (October 1, 2018): 1854–65.

La Rocca, C., and A. Mantovani. "From environment to food: The case of PCB." *Annali dell'Istituto Superiore di Sanita* 42, no. 4 (2006): 410–6.

Laschke, M., and M. Menger. "The gut microbiota: A puppet master in the pathogenesis of endometriosis?" *American Journal of Obstetrics and Gynecology* 215, no. 1 (July 2016): 68.e1–4.

Leone, R., et al. "A systematic review on endometriosis during pregnancy: Diagnosis, misdiagnosis, complications and outcomes." *Human Reproduction Update* 22, no. 1 (January–February 2016): 70–103.

Lete, I., et al. "Effectiveness of an antioxidant preparation with N-acetyl cysteine, alpha lipoic acid and bromelain in the treatment of endometriosis-associated pelvic pain: LEAP study." *European Journal of Obstetrics, Gynecology, and Reproductive Biology* 228 (September 2018): 221–4.

Lucero, J., et al. "Early follicular phase hormone levels in relation to patterns of alcohol, tobacco, and coffee use." *Fertility and Sterility* 76, no. 4 (October 2001): 723–9.

Marziali, M., et al. "Gluten-free diet: A new strategy for management of painful endometriosis related symptoms?" *Minerva Chirurgica* 67, no. 6 (December 2012): 499–504.

Matalliotakis, I., et al. "Epidemiological characteristics in women with and without endometriosis in the Yale series." *Archives of Gynecology and Obstetrics* 277, no. 5 (May 2008): 389–93.

Mier-Cabrera, J., et al. "Women with endometriosis improved their peripheral antioxidant markers after the application of a high antioxidant diet." *Reproductive Biology and Endocrinology* 7, no. 1 (May 28, 2009): 54.

Milić, N., et al. "New therapeutic potentials of milk thistle (silybum marianum)." *Natural Product Communications* 8, no. 12 (December 2013): 1801–10.

"Milk Thistle." Susan G. Komen Breast Cancer Foundation. https://ww5.komen.org/BreastCancer/Milk-Thistle.html.

Missmer, S., et al. "A prospective study of dietary fat consumption and endometriosis risk." *Human Reproduction (Oxford, England)* 25, no. 6 (June 2010): 1528–35.

Missmer, S., et al. "Reproductive history and endometriosis among premenopausal women." *Obstetrics and Gynecology* 104, no. 5 Pt. 1 (November 2004): 965–74.

Moore, J., et al. "Low FODMAP diet—Efficacy in managing abdominal symptoms in patients with endometriosis." *Journal of Nutrition & Intermediary Metabolism* 1, no. C (2014): 14.

Nnoaham, K., et al. "Is early age at menarche a risk factor for endometriosis? A systematic review and meta-analysis of case-control studies." *Fertility and Sterility* 98, no. 3 (September 2012): 702–712.e6.

Onalan, G., et al. "Effects of amifostine on endometriosis, comparison with N-acetyl cysteine, and leuprolide as a new treatment alternative: A randomized controlled trial." *Archives of Gynecology and Obstetrics* 289, no. 1 (January 2014): 193–200.

Parazzini, F., et al. "Diet and endometriosis risk: A literature review." *Reproductive Biomedicine Online* 26, no. 4 (April 2013): 323–36.

Parazzini, F., et al. "Selected food intake and risk of endometriosis." *Human Reproduction (Oxford, England)* 19, no. 8 (August 2004): 1755–9.

Pittaluga, E., et al. "More than antioxidant: N-acetyl-L-cysteine in a murine model of endometriosis." *Fertility and Sterility* 94, no. 7 (December 2010): 2905–8.

Porpora, M., et al. "A promise in the treatment of endometriosis: An observational cohort study on ovarian endometrioma reduction by N-acetylcysteine." *Evidence-Based Complementary and Alternative Medicine* 2013 (2013): 1–7.

Practice Committee of the American Society for Reproductive Medicine. "Endometriosis and infertility: A committee opinion." *Fertility and Sterility* 98, no. 3 (September 2012): 591–8.

Sesti, F., et al. "Hormonal suppression treatment or dietary therapy versus placebo in the control of painful symptoms after conservative surgery for endometriosis stage III-IV. A randomized comparative trial." *Fertility and Sterility* 88, no. 6 (December 2007): 1541–7.

Sesti, F., et al. "Recurrence rate of endometrioma after laparoscopic cystectomy: A comparative randomized trial between post-operative hormonal suppression treatment or dietary therapy vs. placebo." *European Journal of Obstetrics, Gynecology, and Reproductive Biology* 147, no. 1 (November 2009): 72–7.

Simoens, S., et al. "The burden of endometriosis: Costs and quality of life of women with endometriosis and treated in referral centres." *Human Reproduction (Oxford, England)* 27, no. 5 (May 2012): 1292–9.

Tomio, K., et al. "Omega-3 polyunsaturated fatty acids suppress the cystic lesion formation of peritoneal endometriosis in transgenic mouse models." *PLoS One* 8, no. 9 (September 10, 2013): e73085.

Trabert, B., et al. "Diet and risk of endometriosis in a population-based case-control study." *British Journal of Nutrition* 105, no. 3 (February 2011): 459–67.

Treloar, S., et al. "Early menstrual characteristics associated with subsequent diagnosis of endometriosis." *American Journal of Obstetrics and Gynecology* 202, no. 6 (June 2010): 534.e1–6.

Tsuchiya, M., et al. "Effect of soy isoflavones on endometriosis: Interaction with estrogen receptor 2 gene polymorphism." *Epidemiology (Cambridge, Mass.)* 18, no. 3 (May 2007): 402–8.

"Turmeric." National Institutes of Health: National Center for Complementary and Integrative Health. https://nccih.nih.gov/health/turmeric/ataglance.htm. Published September 2016.

Upson, K., et al. "Early-life factors and endometriosis risk." *Fertility and Sterility* 104, no. 4 (October 2015): 964–971.e5.

Vassilopoulou, L., et al. "Endometriosis and *in vitro* fertilisation." *Experimental and Therapeutic Medicine* 16, no. 2 (August 2018): 1043–51.

"Vitamin B6." National Institutes of Health: Office of Dietary Supplements. https://ods.od.nih.gov /factsheets/VitaminB6-HealthProfessional/. Published March 2, 2018.

Woroń, J., and M. Siwek. "Unwanted effects of psychotropic drug interactions with medicinal products and diet supplements containing plant extracts." *Psychiatria Polska* 52, no. 6 (December 29, 2018): 983–96.

Yang, K., et al. "Effectiveness of omega-3 fatty acid for polycystic ovary syndrome: A systematic review and meta-analysis." *Reproductive Biology and Endocrinology* 16, no. 1 (March 27, 2018): 27.

Youseflu, S., et al. "Dietary phytoestrogen intake and the risk of endometriosis in Iranian women: A case-control study." *International Journal of Fertility & Sterility* 13, no. 4 (January 2020): 296–300.

Zhang, Y., et al. "Curcumin inhibits endometriosis endometrial cells by reducing estradiol production." *Iranian Journal of Reproductive Medicine* 11, no. 5 (May 2013): 415–22.

FIBROIDS

Arjeh, S., et al. "Effect of oral consumption of vitamin D on uterine fibroids: A randomized clinical trial." *Complementary Therapies in Clinical Practice* 39 (May 2020): 101159.

Ciebiera, M., et al. "The evolving role of natural compounds in the medical treatment of uterine fibroids." *Journal of Clinical Medicine* 9, no. 5 (May 14, 2020): E1479.

Ciebiera, M., et al. "Vitamins and uterine fibroids: Current data on pathophysiology and possible clinical relevance." *International Journal of Molecular Sciences* 21, no. 15 (August 1, 2020): 5528.

"Common questions about contaminants in seafood." Environmental Defense Fund. http://seafood .edf.org/common-questions-about-contaminants-seafood.

Dalton-Brewer, N. "The role of complementary and alternative medicine for the management of fibroids and associated symptomatology." *Current Obstetrics and Gynecology Reports* 5, no. 2 (2016): 110–8.

"Eating fish: What pregnant women and parents should know." U.S. Food and Drug Administration. https://www.fda.gov/food/foodborneillnesscontaminants/metals/ucm393070.htm.

Gao, M., and H. Wang. "Frequent milk and soybean consumption are high risks for uterine leiomyoma: A prospective cohort study." *Medicine* 97, no. 41 (October 2018): e12009.

Guo, X., and J. Segars. "The impact and management of fibroids for fertility: An evidence-based approach." *Obstetrics and Gynecology Clinics of North America* 39, no. 4 (December 2012): 521–33.

Harris, H., et al. "Dietary fat intake, erythrocyte fatty acids, and risk of uterine fibroids." *Fertility and Sterility* 114, no. 4 (October 2020): 837–47.

"Healthy fish, healthy families." Physicians for Social Responsibility. http://action.psr.org/site /DocServer/HFHF_English.pdf?docID=703.

He, Y., et al. "Associations between uterine fibroids and lifestyles including diet, physical activity and stress: A case-control study in China." *Asia Pacific Journal of Clinical Nutrition* 22, no. 1 (2013): 109–17.

Islam, M., et al. "Molecular targets of dietary phytochemicals for possible prevention and therapy of uterine fibroids: Focus on fibrosis." *Critical Reviews in Food Science and Nutrition* 57, no. 17 (November 22, 2017): 3583–600.

Islam, M., et al. "Dietary phytochemicals for possible preventive and therapeutic option of uterine fibroids: Signaling pathways as target." *Pharmacological Reports* 69, no. 1 (February 2017): 57–70.

Khan, J., and M. Islam. "Effect of green tea epigallocatechin gallate on fibroid uterus." *International Medical Journal* 22, no. 6 (2015): 489–91.

Kondo, A., et al. "Epigallocatechin-3-gallate potentiates curcumin's ability to suppress uterine leiomyosarcoma cell growth and induce apoptosis." *International Journal of Clinical Oncology* 18, no. 3 (June 2013): 380–8.

Parazzini, F., et al. "Dietary components and uterine leiomyomas: A review of published data." *Nutrition and Cancer* 67, no. 4 (2015): 569–79.

"Polychlorinated byphenyls (PCBs): Basic information." Environmental Protection Agency. https://www.epa.gov/pcbs/learn-about-polychlorinated-biphenyls-pcbs.

"Polychlorinated biphenyls (PCBs)." Centers for Disease Control and Prevention. http://www.atsdr.cdc.gov/phs/phs.

Roshdy, E., et al. "Treatment of symptomatic uterine fibroids with green tea extract: A pilot randomized controlled clinical study." *International Journal of Women's Health* 5, no. 1 (2013): 477–486.

Sabry, M., et al. "Serum vitamin D3 level inversely correlates with uterine fibroid volume in different ethnic groups: A cross-sectional observational study." *International Journal of Women's Health* 5, no. 1 (2013): 93–100.

Shen, Y., et al. "Vegetarian diet and reduced uterine fibroids risk: A case-control study in Nanjing China." *Journal of Obstetrics and Gynaecology Research* 42, no. 1 (January 2016): 87–94.

"Should I eat the fish I catch?" Environmental Protection Agency. https://www.epa.gov/choose-fish-and-shellfish-wisely/should-i-eat-fish-i-catch-brochure.

Sparic, R., et al. "Epidemiology of uterine myomas: A review." *International Journal of Fertility & Sterility* 9, no. 4 (January–March 2016): 424–35.

Tempest, M. "Uterine fibroids and nutrition." *Today's Dietitian* 14, no. 5 (2012): 40–3.

Wise, L., et al. "Prospective study of dietary fat and risk of uterine leiomyomata." *American Journal of Clinical Nutrition* 99, no. 5 (May 2014): 1105–16.

POLYPS

Izhar, R., et al. "Fertility outcome after saline sonography guided removal of intrauterine polyps in women with unexplained infertility." *Journal of Ultrasonography* 19, no. 77 (2019): 113–9.

Chapter 8: In Vitro Fertilization and Embryo Transfer

Anderson, A., et al. "Simplified culture conditions: Comparing invocell culture device to in vitro culture." *Fertility and Sterility* 108, no. 3 (2017): e110.

Arredondo, F., et al. "Increase access to care with invocell." *Fertility and Sterility* 108, no. 3 (2017): e7.

Bortoletto, P., et al. "Reproductive outcomes of women 40 and older undergoing IVF with donor sperm." *Fertility and Sterility* - International edition 114, no. 3 (September 1, 2020): e102–e103.

García-Ferreyra, J., et al. "In vivo culture system using the INVOcell device shows similar pregnancy and implantation rates to those obtained from in vivo culture system in ICSI procedures." *Clinical Medicine Insights. Reproductive Health* 9, no. 9 (June 10, 2015): 7–11.

Ghuman, N., et al. "Does age of the sperm donor influence live birth outcome in assisted reproduction?" *Human Reproduction (Oxford, England)* 31, no. 3 (March 2016): 582–90.

Knopman, J., et al. "What makes them split? Identifying risk factors that lead to monozygotic twins after in vitro fertilization." *Fertility and Sterility* 102, no. 1 (July 2014): 82–9.

Lasiuk, G., et al. "Unexpected: An interpretive description of parental traumas associated with preterm birth." *BMC Pregnancy and Childbirth* 13, no. Suppl 1 (2013): S13.

Peipert, B., et al. "Analysis of state mandated insurance coverage for infertility treatment and fertility preservation in the United States." *Fertility and Sterility* - International edition 114, no. 3 (September 1, 2020): e4–e5.

Penzias, A., et al., and the Practice Committees of the American Society for Reproductive Medicine and the Society for Assisted Reproductive Technology. "The use of preimplantation genetic testing for aneuploidy (PGT-A): A committee opinion." *Fertility and Sterility* 109, no. 3 (March 2018): 429–36.

Roeca, C., et al. "Preimplantation genetic testing and chances of a healthy live birth amongst recipients of fresh donor oocytes in the United States." *Journal of Assisted Reproduction and Genetics* 37, no. 9 (September 2020): 2283–92.

Sunkara, S., et al. "Perinatal outcomes following assisted reproductive technology." *Journal of Human Reproductive Sciences* 12, no. 3 (July–September 2019): 177–81.

Chapter 9: Coping with Cycle Attempts

Brown, B. *Daring Greatly: How the Courage to Be Vulnerable Transforms the Way We Live, Love, Parent, and Lead.* Penguin Random House, 2012.

Gottman, J., and N. Silver. *What Makes Love Last? How to Build Trust and Avoid Betrayal.* Simon & Schuster, 2011.

Grewen, K., et al. "Warm partner contact is related to lower cardiovascular reactivity." *Behavioral Medicine (Washington, D. C.)* 29, no. 3 (Fall 2003): 123–30.

Johnson, S. *Hold Me Tight: Your Guide to the Most Successful Approach to Building Loving Relationships.* Little, Brown, 2008.

Nagoski, E., and A. Nagoski. *Burnout: The Secret to Unlocking the Stress Cycle.* Ballantine Books, 2020.

Patel, A., et al. "Application of Mindfulness-Based Psychological Interventions in Infertility." *Journal of Human Reproductive Sciences* 13, no. 1 (January–March 2020): 3–21.

Tatkin, S. *Wired for Love: How Understanding Your Partner's Brain and Attachment Style Can Help You Defuse Conflict and Build a Secure Relationship.* New Harbinger, 2012.

Taylor, S. *The Body Is Not an Apology: The Power of Radical Self-Love.* Berrett-Koehler Publishers, 2018.

Chapter 10: Miscarriage

"ACOG Practice Bulletin No. 200: Early Pregnancy Loss." *Obstetrics and Gynecology* 132, no. 5 (November 2018): e197–207.

Black, B., and W. Fields. "Contexts Reproductive Loss in Lesbian Couples." *MCN. The American Journal of Maternal Child Nursing* 39, no. 3 (May–June 2014): 157–62, quiz: 163–4.

Magnus, M., et al. "Role of maternal age and pregnancy history in risk of miscarriage: Prospective register based study." *BMJ (Clinical Research Ed.)* 364 (March 20, 2019): l869.

Peel, E. "Pregnancy loss in lesbian and bisexual women: An online survey of experiences." *Human Reproduction (Oxford, England)* 25, no. 3 (March 2010): 721–7.

Riggs, D., et al. "Men, trans/masculine, and non-binary people's experiences of pregnancy loss: An international qualitative study." *BMC Pregnancy and Childbirth* 20, no. 1 (August 24, 2020): 482.

Wojnar, D., et al. "Confronting the inevitable: A conceptual model of miscarriage for use in clinical practice and research." *Death Studies* 35, no. 6 (July 2011): 536–58.

Chapter 11: Early Pregnancy and Lactation Induction

"ACOG committee opinion number 804: Physical activity and exercise during pregnancy and the postpartum period." April 2020.

Bazzano, A., et al. "A review of herbal and pharmaceutical galactagogues for breast-feeding." *Ochsner Journal* 16, no. 4 (Winter 2016): 511–24.

Brouwers, J., et al. "Plasma prolactin levels after acute and subchronic oral administration of domperidone and of metoclopramide: A cross-over study in healthy volunteers." *Clinical Endocrinology* 12, no. 5 (May 1980): 435–40.

Cheyney, M., et al. "Outcomes of care for 16,924 planned home births in the United States: The Midwives Alliance of North America statistics project, 2004 to 2009." *Journal of Midwifery & Women's Health* 59, no. 1 (January–February 2014): 17–27.

Coad, J., and M. Dunstall. *Anatomy and physiology for midwives.* Harcort Publishers, 2001.

da Silva, O., et al. "Effect of domperidone on milk production in mothers of premature newborns: A randomized, double-blind, placebo-controlled trial." *Canadian Medical Association Journal* 164, no. 1 (January 9, 2001): 17–21.

Denton, Y. "Induced lactation in the nulliparous adoptive mother." *British Journal of Midwifery* 18, no. 2 (2010): 84–7.

"Domperidone." In *Drugs and Lactation Database (LactMed) Bethesda (MD).* US: National Library of Medicine, 2006.

Ely, D., and A. Driscoll. "Infant mortality in the United States, 2017: Data from the period linked birth/infant death file." *National Vital Statistics Reports* 68, no. 10 (August 1, 2019): 1–20. Hyattsville, MD: National Center for Health Statistics.

García-Acosta, J., et al. "Trans* pregnancy and lactation: A literature review from a nursing perspective." *International Journal of Environmental Research and Public Health* 17, no. 1 (December 19, 2019): 44.

Handout #19a. *Domperidone.* January 2005. Written by Jack Newman, MD: FRCPC 2005.

Hofmeyr, G., et al. "Domperidone: Secretion in breast milk and effect on puerperal prolactin levels." *British Journal of Obstetrics and Gynaecology* 92, no. 2 (February 1985): 141–4.

Hutton, E., et al. "Outcomes associated with planned home and planned hospital births in low-risk women attended by midwives in Ontario, Canada, 2003–2006: A retrospective cohort study." *Birth (Berkeley, Calif.)* 36, no. 3 (September 2009): 180–9.

Hutton, E., et al. "Outcomes associated with planned place of birth among women with low-risk pregnancies." *Canadian Medical Association Journal* 188, no. 5 (March 15, 2016): E80–90.

Janssen, P., et al. "Outcomes of planned home birth with registered midwife versus planned hospital birth with midwife or physician." *Canadian Medical Association Journal* 181, no. 6–7 (September 15, 2009): 377–83.

Johnson, K., and B. Daviss. "Outcomes of planned home births with certified professional midwives: Large prospective study in North America." *BMJ (Clinical Research Ed.)* 330, no. 7505 (June 18, 2005): 1416.

Luo, L., et al. "Interventions for leg cramps in pregnancy." *Cochrane Database of Systematic Reviews* 12, no. 12 (December 4, 2020): CD010655.

Marasco, L. "Increasing your milk supply with galactogogues." *Journal of Human Lactation* 24, no. 4 (November 2008): 455–6.

McCarthy, F., et al. "Hyperemesis gravidarum: Current perspectives." *International Journal of Women's Health* 6 (August 5, 2014): 719–25.

McGuire, E. "Induced lactation and mothers sharing breastfeeding: A case report." *Breastfeeding Review* 27, no. 2 (2019): 37–41.

"Milk Production." https://kellymom.com/hot-topics/milkproduction.

"Newman-Goldfarb Protocols." Jack Newman, MD FRCPC, and Lenore Goldfarb, PhD., IBCLC. November 2002.

Olsen, O., and J. Clausen. "Planned hospital birth versus planned home birth." *Cochrane Database of Systematic Reviews* (September 12, 2012).

Petersen, E., et al. Racial/ethnic disparities in pregnancy-related deaths—United States, 2007–2016. *MMWR. Morbidity and Mortality Weekly Report* 68, no. 35 (September 6, 2019): 762–5.

Reisman, T., and Z. Goldstein. "Case report: Induced lactation in a transgender woman." *Transgender Health* 3, no. 1 (January 1, 2018): 24–6.

Silver, R., et al. "Nulliparous pregnancy outcomes study: Monitoring mothers-to-be (NuMoM2b) study. Prospective evaluation of maternal sleep position through 30 weeks of gestation and adverse pregnancy outcomes." *Obstetrics and Gynecology* 134, no. 4 (October 2019): 667–76.

Souter, V., et al. "Comparison of midwifery and obstetric care in low-risk hospital births." *Obstetrics and Gynecology* 134, no. 5 (November 2019): 1056–65.

Spencer, R., and D. Fraser. "You're kinda passing a test: A phenomenological study of women's experiences of breastfeeding." *British Journal of Midwifery* 26, no. 11 (2018): 724–30.

Trautner, E., et al. "Knowledge and practice of lactation in trans women among professionals working in trans health." *International Breastfeeding Journal* 15, no. 1 (July 16, 2020): 63.

Ureño, T., et al. "Dysphoric milk ejection reflex: A case series." *Breastfeeding Medicine* 13, no. 1 (January/February 2018): 85–8.

INDEX

D

E

F

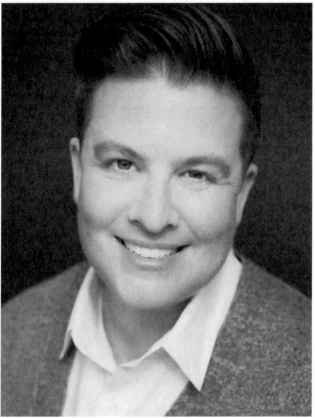

Timeca Briggs

ABOUT THE AUTHOR

KRISTIN L. KALI, Licensed Midwife, (they/them) is the owner of MAIA Midwifery & Fertility Services, PLLC, currently based in Seattle, Washington, with a long-standing history in the San Francisco Bay Area. They have supported thousands of LGBTQ+ parents through fertility and preconception care; in-home insemination; prenatal care; childbirth education; delivery in hospitals, homes, and birth centers; postpartum care; lactation management; and parenting groups. As a public speaker, educator, and consultant, they have trained hundreds of midwives and childbirth professionals to serve the queer and trans community with humility, respect, and the widespread use of gender-inclusive language.

QUEER CONCEPTION

The **COMPLETE
FERTILITY GUIDE**
for **QUEER** and **TRANS
PARENTS**-to-**BE**

KRISTIN L. KALI
LICENSED MIDWIFE

SASQUATCH BOOKS
SEATTLE

Printed in the United States of America

SASQUATCH BOOKS with colophon is a registered trademark of Penguin Random House LLC

26 25 24 23 22   9 8 7 6 5 4 3 2 1

Editor: Hannah Elnan
Production editor: Bridget Sweet
Designer: Alicia Terry

Library of Congress Cataloging-in-Publication Data
Names: Kali, Kristin L., author.
Title: Queer conception : the complete fertility guide for queer and trans
    parents-to-be / Kristin L. Kali, Licensed Midwife.
Description: Seattle : Sasquatch Books, [2022] | Includes index.
Identifiers: LCCN 2021024227 | ISBN 9781632173980 (paperback) | ISBN
    9781632173997 (ebook)
Subjects: LCSH: Human reproductive technology. | Gay parents. | Lesbians. |
    Bisexual women.
Classification: LCC RG133.5 .K35 2022 | DDC 618.1/78008664—dc23
LC record available at https://lccn.loc.gov/2021024227

ISBN: 978-1-63217-398-0

Sasquatch Books
1325 Fourth Avenue, Suite 1025
Seattle, WA 98101
SasquatchBooks.com

This book was created on stolen lands that have been tended for generations by the Coast Salish, Duwamish, Lummi, and Lingít people.

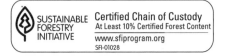

SUSTAINABLE FORESTRY INITIATIVE

Certified Chain of Custody
At Least 10% Certified Forest Content
www.sfiprogram.org
SFI-01028